# SUPERFOODS

## The Healthiest Foods on the Planet

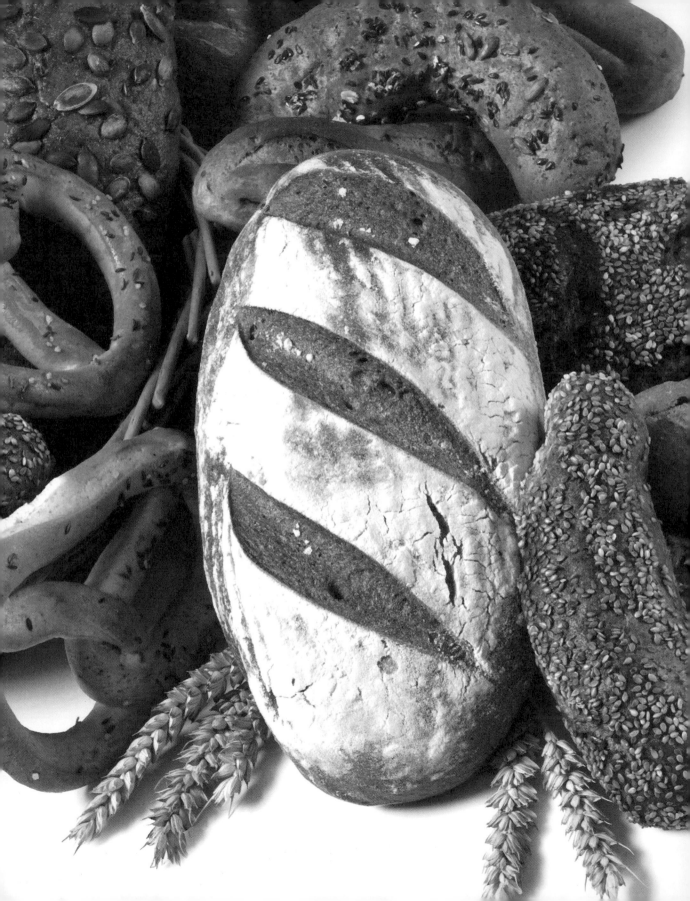

# SUPERFOODS
## The Healthiest Foods on the Planet

FIREFLY BOOKS

# A FIREFLY BOOK

Published by Firefly Books Ltd. 2010

**Publisher Cataloging-in-Publication Data (U.S.)**
Reinhard, Tonia.
   Superfoods : the healthiest foods on the planet /
Tonia Reinhard.
[256] p. :  col. photos. ;  cm.
Includes index.
Summary: A comprehensive reference to the world's
superfoods, including fruits, vegetables, nuts, grains,
cereals, and meat and dairy products.
ISBN-13: 978-1-55407-684-0
ISBN-10: 1-55407-684-6
   1. Nutrition. 2. Natural foods – Health aspects.
   3. Health.  I. Title.
641.5/63 dc22      RA784.R456 2010

**Library and Archives Canada Cataloguing in
Publication**
Reinhard, Tonia
Superfoods : the healthiest foods on the planet /
Tonia Reinhard.
Includes index.
ISBN-13: 978-1-55407-684-0
ISBN-10: 1-55407-684-6
   1. Nutrition.  2. Health--Nutritional aspects.  I. Title.
RA784.R454 2010          613.2          C2009-907514-8

Published in the United States by
Firefly Books (U.S.) Inc.
P.O. Box 1338, Ellicott Station
Buffalo, New York 14205

Published in Canada by
Firefly Books Ltd.
66 Leek Crescent
Richmond Hill, Ontario L4B 1H1

The moral rights of the author have been asserted.

Printed in China by 1010 Printing International Ltd
Color separation Pica Digital Pte Ltd, Singapore

Developed by Global Book Publishing
Level 8, 15 Orion Road, Lane Cove,
NSW 2066, Australia
Ph: (612) 9425 5800   Fax: (612) 9425 5804
Email: rightsmanager@globalpub.com.au

**MANAGING DIRECTOR** Chryl Campbell
**PUBLISHER** Roz Hopkins
**EDITORIAL DIRECTOR** Sarah Anderson
**MANAGING EDITOR** John Mapps
**PROJECT EDITOR** Scott Forbes
**AUTHOR** Tonia Reinhard
**COVER DESIGN** Cathy Campbell and Kylie Mulquin
**DESIGNER** Cathy Campbell
**DESIGN CONCEPT** Lena Lowe
**PICTURE RESEARCH** Scott Forbes and Kylie Mulquin
**INDEXER** Jo Rudd
**PROOFREADER** Kevin Diletti
**PUBLISHING COORDINATOR** Jessica Luca
**ADMINISTRATIVE ASSISTANT** Kristen Donath

Photographs from the Global Book Publishing Photo Library
(except where credited otherwise on page 256)
Front cover image: Fresh Berries with Meringue
(Getty Images/Gentl & Hyers)
Back cover images: Walnuts (t), Cherry tomatoes (c),
Plums (b) (Shutterstock)

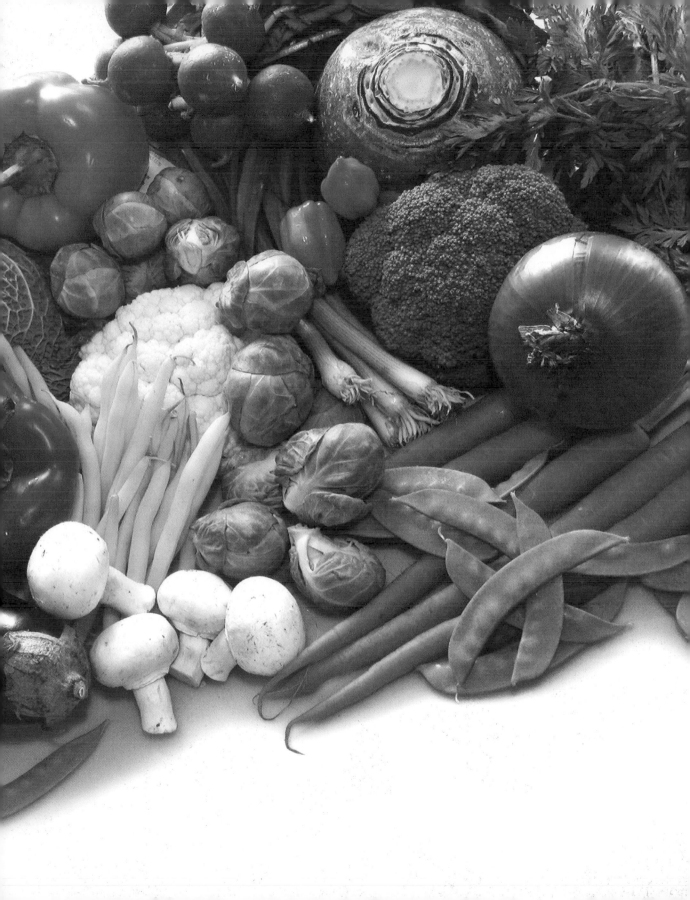

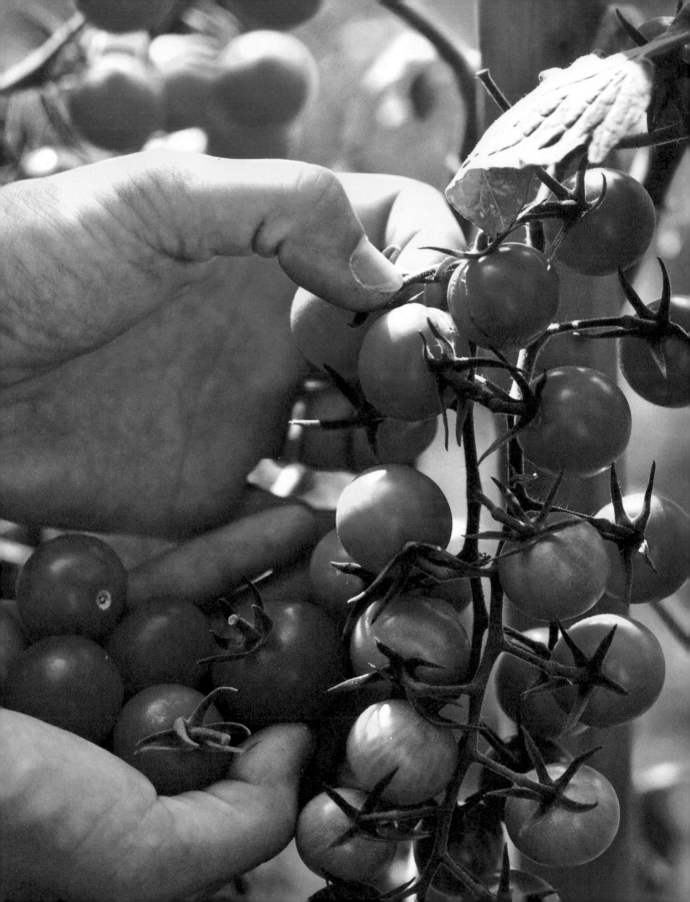

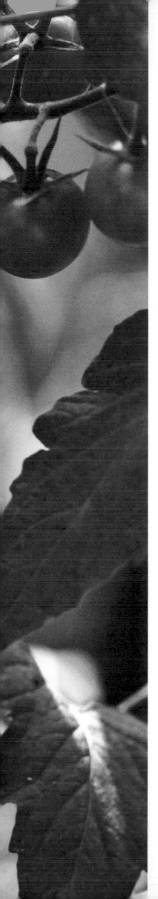

# Contents

# Foreword

If you're like most people, you probably first heard the word "superfood" fairly recently. It may have sounded more like a clever marketing term than a reasonable way to describe a specific food, and, indeed, few government health authorities have yet come up with a precise meaning for the term. A simple definition, however, is that a superfood is a food that contains a high level of essential nutrients and other compounds that may benefit your health. And, with both scientific and public interest in health and nutrition at an all-time high, it's a term that's here to stay—and with good reason.

Barely a day goes by without the announcement of another scientific study on a specific food and its link to disease prevention. An example is a recent study published in the *European Heart Journal* on the benefits of chocolate. The largest observational study conducted thus far on chocolate and cardio-vascular-disease risk, it found that people who ate the most chocolate had a 39 percent lower risk of heart attack and stroke than those who ate almost no chocolate. Good news indeed, if you like chocolate!

What such studies underline is the effectiveness of individual foods in warding off chronic diseases. Of course, researchers have not only known this for some time, but have also shown how certain foods can be used to combat particular conditions. Dr. David Jenkins, a preeminent researcher and professor at the University of Toronto, first showed in 2002 that a dietary plan incorporating specific foods lowered blood cholesterol levels as effectively as statins (powerful medications), with no side effects. Rather than focus on one or two foods, Dr. Jenkins's approach involved using what he called "a dietary portfolio of cholesterol-lowering foods"; in other words, a range of recommended foods from which the user could select according to taste preferences and availability, while still achieving the desired outcome.

The wisdom of this approach had already been proved to me in my own practice, several years before I read about Dr. Jenkins's study. I was counseling a 30-something man on hypercholesterolemia, or a high level of cholesterol in the blood, whose physician was ready to prescribe drugs. His father had died at the age of 51 of a heart attack, but he was reluctant to use the drugs. I started out our second session in typical "small steps" mode, suggesting we make gradual changes to his eating pattern. But the patient's sense of urgency soon made me take a different tack. He was aiming for dramatic change, so we put together a plan that focused on a range of foods, many of which would later be in Dr. Jenkins's portfolio. The patient came back less than two months later with significant improvements in his test results and a bonus: modest weight loss.

All this goes to show that by eating a range of foods with proven benefits you can achieve major improvements in your health and lifestyle. And that's where this book comes in. Whether you want to make dramatic changes to your diet or take small steps toward better health, this comprehensive guide will help you design your own portfolio of powerful foods. I'm confident you will find it an indispensable companion on your journey toward healthier eating and a greater sense of wellbeing.

*Tonia Reinhard*

RIGHT A diet based on superfoods can be varied and enjoyable as well as healthful, as the term covers a huge range of foods, from fresh fruit and vegetables to meats, fish, herbs, and even chocoloate.

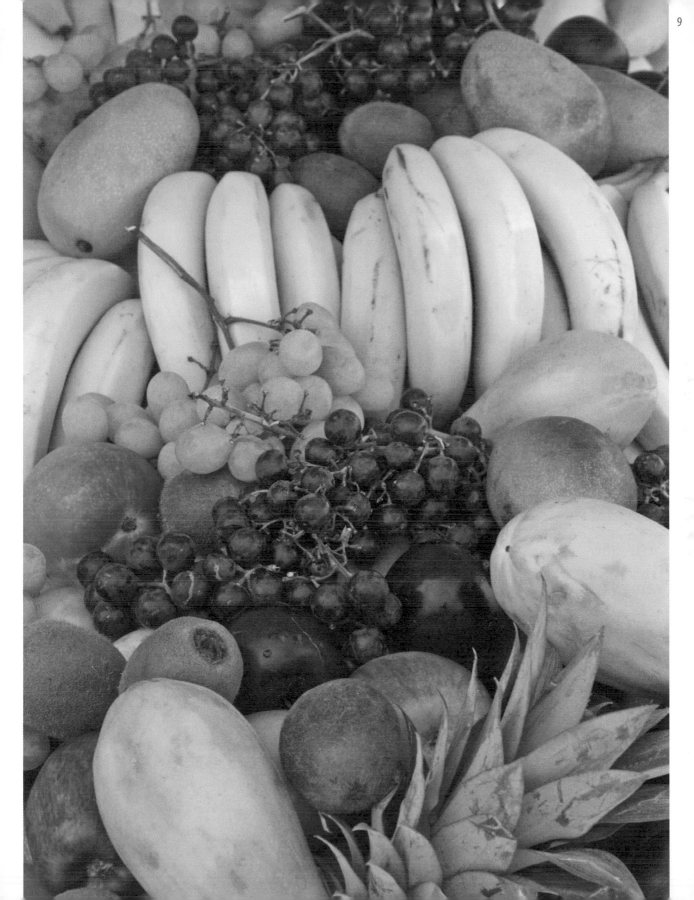

# Introduction

The meaning of the word "superfood" has evolved over time and taken on specific connotations in different parts of the world. According to the *Oxford English Dictionary (OED)*, the term dates back to two early usages in print media in 1915 and 1949. The *OED* entry provides an adequate general definition: "food considered especially nutritious or otherwise beneficial to health and well-being." In recent years, however, some more specific definitions have had to be created, partly to protect consumers against unscrupulous marketing practices.

A concept that has been widely employed to help better define the meaning of "superfood" is that of the "nutrient density" of foods, whereby foods are described as either "nutrient-dense" (or "nutrient-rich") or "nutrient-poor." The so-called essential nutrients are compounds that we need to grow and maintain our bodies and can only obtain from food; they include protein, carbohydrates, fat, minerals, and vitamins. A nutrient-dense or nutrient-rich food is one that provides significant levels of these nutrients *in a reasonable number of calories*. A useful way to get to grips with this concept is to think of your optimal daily calorie level, a level that does not promote weight gain, as money. When we buy things, we all want to get the best product for our dollars; likewise, we have a limited number of calories that we can use each day, so we want to obtain the highest possible levels of essential nutrients for those limited calories.

And it's certainly true that many superfoods are nutrient-rich foods—dark, leafy vegetables, for example, are high in vitamin A and other essential nutrients, and low in calories. But superfoods also include foods that are high in other compounds that are not essential nutrients but may still offer health benefits—most notably, the compounds collectively known as phytochemicals.

According to current scientific understanding, the potential benefits of eating foods that are high in either nutrients or phytochemicals, or both, include the fact that they may help lower our risk of developing certain chronic diseases, including cancer, cardiovascular disease, and type 2 diabetes. In the majority of Western countries, these are the leading causes of death. So, by incorporating the foods in this book into your eating plan, you might well increase your likelihood of living longer.

BELOW Superfoods are loaded with compounds beneficial to your health. Chili peppers, for example, contain capsaicin, a substance that has been shown to inhibit the growth of cancer cells.

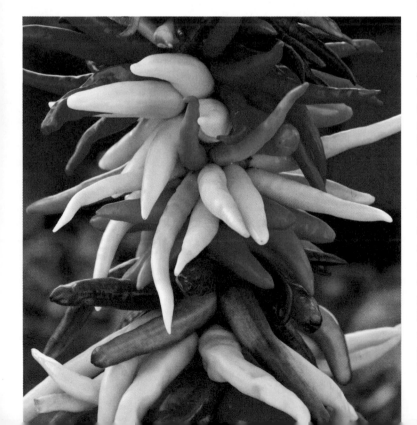

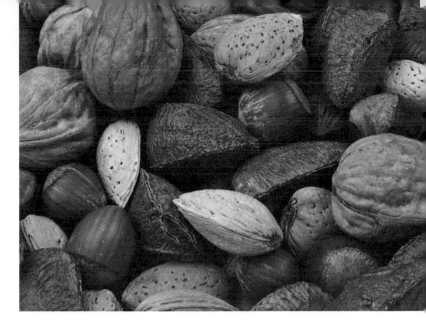

## BENEFICIAL COMPOUNDS

The best yardstick for evaluating the level of a particular nutrient in a food is the Daily Value (DV), known in some places as the Daily Intake (DI). This usually appears on food labels and indicates the percentage of the desired daily intake of a particular nutrient that the food in question provides. So, for example, a packet of Brazil nuts may indicate that a serving of the nuts will supply 25 percent of the copper we need for the day.

The individual essential nutrients for which a DV has been established include:

- Vitamins: A, C, D, E, K, thiamine (B1), riboflavin (B2), niacin (B3), pantothenic acid (B5), B6 (pyridoxine), biotin (B7), B12 (cobalamin), folate, and choline.
- Minerals: calcium, chloride, copper, chromium, fluoride, iodine, iron, magnesium, manganese, molybdenum, phosphorus, potassium, selenium, sodium, and zinc.

Phytochemicals are naturally occurring compounds in plant foods, which are biologically active in the body; some animal foods also contain other non-nutrient compounds that scientists have found to be beneficial. A comprehensive database of all the unique compounds in foods has yet to be compiled, but, for each superfood in this book, we have highlighted those that have been shown, in scientific studies, to enhance health in one way or another. The biological activities of these compounds include but are not limited to antioxidant effects, immune-system enhancement, estrogen-metabolism alteration, apoptosis (inducing the suicide of cancer cells), DNA damage repair, and detoxification of carcinogens (cancer-causing agents).

## THE ROLE OF ANTIOXIDANTS

Much recent scientific research has focused on antioxidants because of the key role they seem to play in disease prevention. Scientists believe that compounds known as reactive oxygen species, which are produced in the body in response to environmental pollutants, cigarette smoke, sunlight, oxidized compounds in foods, and certain normal metabolic processes, cause oxidative damage in cells of the body. This can in turn trigger chronic diseases and conditions, including cardiovascular disease, cancer, and diabetes. Antioxidants appear to combat this oxidative damage.

Vitamins C and E and the mineral selenium function as antioxidants, but of particular interest are the phytochemical antioxidants, of which more than 4,000 are currently known. The following are major classes of some of these compounds:

- Carotenoids: These include beta-carotene, which can be converted to active vitamin A (retinol) in the body, and lycopene, lutein, and zeaxanthin.
- Polyphenols: Subgroups include flavonoids, phenolic acids, lignans, and stilbenes; subgroups of the flavonoids include flavanols (which include catechins), flavones, flavonols, flavanones, isoflavones, and anthocyanins.

ABOVE You can select superfoods according to taste and nutritional requirements. Nuts are a good choice if you want to increase your intake of fiber and minerals such as copper and magnesium.

## GOING ORGANIC

Many people have concerns about the use of pesticides on food plants. Government agencies routinely test foods for pesticide residue and have reassured consumers that the benefits of eating healthy foods outweigh any potential dangers. If you are still concerned, however, you can opt for organic foods, which are becoming more widely available; make sure, however, that you choose those that are certified by a national body, such as the US Department of Agriculture (USDA).

## HOW TO USE THIS BOOK

The foods in this book are divided into chapters covering broad categories, such as fruits. Within these chapters, the entries are arranged in subcategories, such as citrus and vine fruits within fruits. Foods derived from plants are listed in alphabetical order of the plant's scientific name. Some foods are covered by entries relating to different products: wheat, for example, is discussed under Whole Wheat Berries, Wheat Germ, Whole-wheat Pasta, and Whole-wheat Bread. Each entry includes background information on the food, details of the nutrients and other compounds it contains, and tips on how to obtain the greatest benefit from the food.

It's a good idea to follow the portfolio approach described in the Foreword (p. 8). As you read the book, jot down the foods you want to try. To start slowly, put one new superfood on your grocery list each week; to quickly overhaul your eating plan, add three to your diet every day, one at each meal. If the foods are as super as we think they are, you'll soon find yourself with an expanding porfolio, and a great investment in your health.

Chapter name ●

# Pears

☺ *Pyrus communis* Pear, European Pear, Wild Pear
☺ *Pyrus pyrifolia* Asian Pear, Nashi Pear

Pears originated in the coastal and temperate regions of Europe and western Asia. The Asian or nashi pear has been cultivated in Asia for over 4,000 years; it is more round in shape and has a grainier texture than the more familiar European pear.

### In a Nutshell

**Origin:** Europe and western Asia
**Season:** Autumn
**Why they're super:** High in fiber; good source of vitamins C and K, potassium, and copper; contain antioxidant phenols
**Growing at home:** Easily grown at home

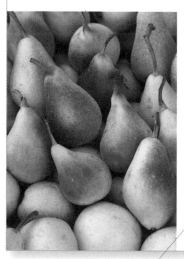

Pears are cultivated and propagated in much the same way as apples, and the two fruits are related and can even be similar in appearance—some pears resemble apples and the only difference is in the texture of the flesh. The flesh of pears contains stone cells, often called "grit."

Pears are an excellent source of fiber as well as a good source of vitamins C and K, potassium, and copper. They also contain antioxidant phenols.

### THE HEALTHY EVIDENCE

A 2009 study published in the *European Journal of Nutrition* reported on the health benefits of chlorogenic acid, a phenol found in pears (and some other fruits) at a high level. They tested the compound on human endothelial cells and found that it exhibited potent anti-inflammatory effects and countered some of the other processes involved in atherosclerosis, an underlying cause of cardiovascular disease. The chlorogenic acid also functioned as a powerful antioxidant. The authors concluded that these effects "suggest that chlorogenic acid could be useful in the prevention of atherosclerosis."

LEFT 'Forelle' is a popular European pear cultivar. The *Pyrus* genus includes 20 or so species, but *P. communis* and *P. pyrifolia* are the most common.

| What's in a Serving? |
|---|
| **FRESH PEAR** |
| **1 medium** |
| **(6.3 ounces/178 g)** |
| **Calories:** 103 (431 kJ) |
| **Protein:** 0.7 g |
| **Total fat:** 0.2 g |
| **Saturated fat:** 0 g |
| **Carbohydrates:** 27.5 g |
| **Fiber:** 5.5 g |

### Making the Most of Pears

The important antioxidants in pears and the high level of fiber will be retained in cooking. This makes pears versatile from a nutritional standpoint, in that their health benefits can be incorporated into flavorful entrées and desserts. A pear treat that also includes other health-promoting ingredients is roasted pears drizzled with a mixture of honey, fresh lemon juice, and cinnamon.

● **MAKING THE MOST OF ...**
Describes ways to add the superfood to your eating plan, or provides tips on how to optimize its nutrients and phytochemicals. Some nutrients are sensitive to heat and may therefore be lost in cooking; those most sensitive to heat are vitamin C, folate, and riboflavin. In addition, some vitamins and all minerals are water-soluble and will therefore be lost in cooking water, while other vitamins—notably A, D, E, and K—dissolve in fat but are not lost in cooking water. Some phytochemicals, notably the carotenoids, are also fat-soluble. In general, the best cooking methods for retaining nutrients are steaming, microwaving with little or no water, and quick stir-frying.

ROPICAL FRUITS ●

# Pineapple

● *Ananas comosus* ●

● **Section name**
● **Scientific name**

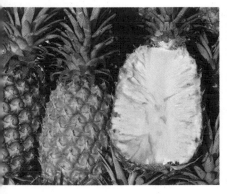

### Making the Most of Pineapples

Pineapple is best eaten fresh to capitalize on all the nutrients, but many important minerals and antioxidants will be present in canned pineapple, too. Choose products packed in 100 percent juice, and be sure to use the liquid to obtain all the water-soluble nutrients.

LEFT When Columbus first saw the pineapple, he described it as "in the shape of a pine cone, twice as big, which fruit is excellent and it can be cut with a knife, like a turnip, and it seems to be wholesome."

spread it throughout South America and the Caribbean. Spanish explorers took the pineapple back to Europe, where it became wildly popular and, notably in painting and sculpture, a symbol of all things exotic.

Pineapple is an excellent source of vitamin C, with one serving providing 131 percent of the Daily Value, and manganese. It is also a good source of vitamin B6, folate, thiamine, magnesium, potassium, and copper. In addition, pineapple contains several antioxidant flavonoids that may help combat chronic diseases.

## What's in a Serving?

**FRESH PINEAPPLE**
**(1 cup/165 g)**
**Calories:** 82 (345 kJ)
**Protein:** 0.1 g
**Total fat:** 0.2 g
**Saturated fat:** 0 g
**Carbohydrates:** 21.7 g
**Fiber:** 2.3 g

Pineapple is a multiple fruit, in that it forms as the fruits (drupelets) of individual flowers on the plant merge and grow together. Pineapple is most often associated with Hawaii, but was not introduced there until 1813. It is in fact native to Paraguay and southern Brazil, and the indigenous peoples of those regions

### In a Nutshell

**Origin:** Brazil and Paraguay
**Season:** Year-round
**Why it's super:** High in vitamin C and manganese; good source of vitamin B6, folate, thiamine, magnesium, potassium, and copper; contains antioxidant flavonoids
**Growing at home:** Can be grown at home; pineapples do well in containers in warm climates

### THE HEALTHY EVIDENCE ●

A 2009 study published in the journal *Food and Chemical Toxicology* reported on the analysis of the antioxidant compounds in pineapple. The results showed that the antioxidant potency of pineapple extract was high, and either similar to or higher than that of other fruits and vegetables. In addition to the abundant vitamin C, an antioxidant nutrient, they found important flavonoids such as quercetin.

● **THE HEALTHY EVIDENCE**
Provides a brief survey of the key scientific studies that indicate a potential benefit of the food. The principal source for this information was the online PubMed utility (www.ncbi.nlm.nih.gov/pubmed), a US National Library of Medicine and National Institutes of Health database. It is important to keep in mind that research is ongoing, and that we cannot rely on any one study for proof of a particular health benefit. The gold standard for scientific evidence is the human clinical trial, and even with that kind of study you need to consider the number of subjects and whether the results may have been duplicated by another study.

● **WHAT'S IN A SERVING?**
Shows the size of a typical serving of the food, the calories the serving supplies, and the content (in grams) of the energy-yielding nutrients, carbohydrate, fat, and protein, as well as fiber. This information is derived from the Nutrient Database (www.nal.usda.gov/fnic/foodcomp/search) maintained by the US Department of Agriculture (USDA), except for specialized foods, for which manufacturer data were used. Due to the fact that the USDA uses direct measurement and analysis of foods and also rounds off figures, the typical conversion factor of 4.184 for calories to kilojoules may not apply; however, these are the most accurate measurements available.

● **IN A NUTSHELL**
Summarizes information on the food's origin, the season in which it is harvested or is most widely available, why it can be considered a superfood, and whether it can be grown at home. If a serving of a superfood contains 10 percent or more of the Daily Value (DV) for an essential nutrient, it is described as "high in" or "an excellent source of" that nutrient, and if it contains 5–9 percent of the DV it is termed "a good source." The levels of nutrients contained in each food are also shown in the nutritional tables on pages 232–45.

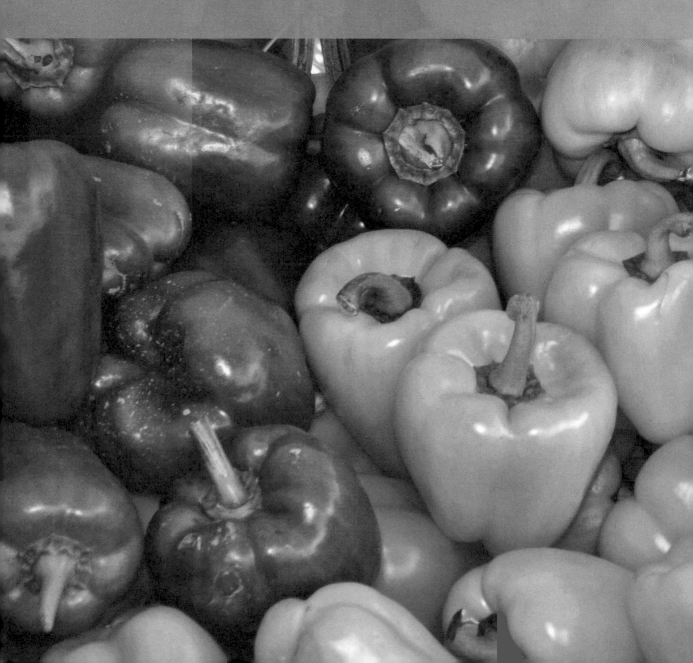

# 1 Vegetables

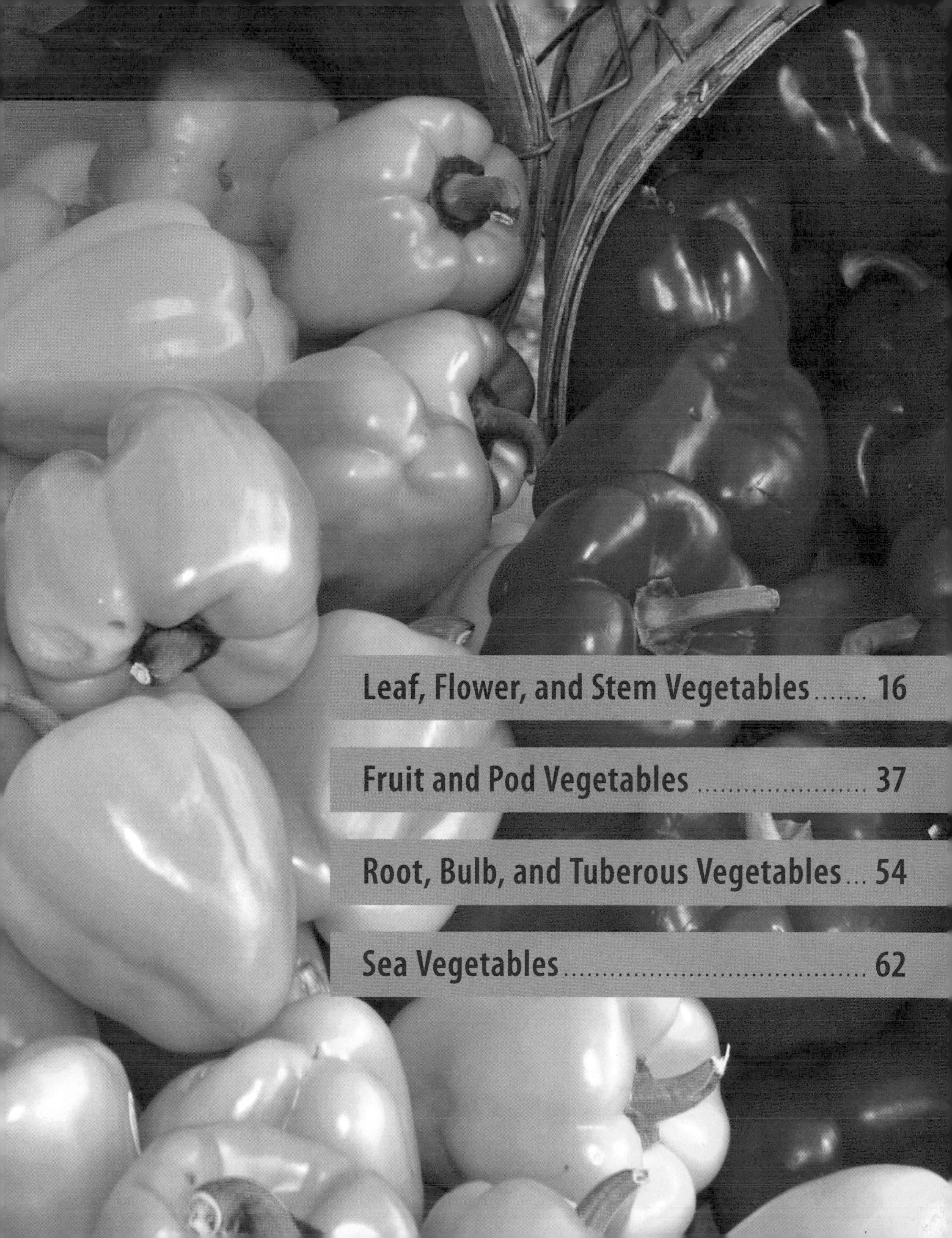

## LEAF, FLOWER, AND STEM VEGETABLES

# Asparagus

✪ *Asparagus officinalis*

Even in the health-promoting food group of vegetables, asparagus is a standout. An excellent source of vitamins A, C, and K, as well as folate, riboflavin, and thiamine, it is also high in fiber and the minerals manganese, copper, and potassium. A serving of asparagus packs an antioxidant punch, containing both beta-carotene and lutein. This bevy of nutrients is accompanied by only 20 calories per serving. Last but by no means

least, asparagus is high in compounds known as fructooligosaccharides (FOS), a type of soluble fiber.

Although asparagus was a relatively rare delicacy until quite recently, it is now available year-round in many countries. White asparagus, which has a lower beta-carotene and lutein content than the green variety, can also be found in most grocery stores.

### THE HEALTHY EVIDENCE

Folate is important for pregnant women in the prevention of neural tube defects, such as spina bifida, in the fetus. In addition, it lowers blood levels of homocysteine, a compound linked to heart disease, strokes, and dementia. Antioxidants may protect against cardiovascular disease and cancer; furthermore, a recent study in the *American Journal of Ophthalmology* reported lower risk for macular degeneration at the highest dietary lutein intake.

Research also suggests that FOS are highly beneficial. Not only do they help lower blood lipids, such as cholesterol and triglycerides, but they also act as a prebiotic, a substance that promotes the growth of healthy bacteria in the intestine.

---

### What's in a Serving?

**COOKED ASPARAGUS
(1 cup/180 g)**
**Calories:** 20 (85 kJ)
**Protein:** 2.2 g
**Total fat:** 0.2 g
**Saturated fat:** 0 g
**Carbohydrates:** 1.8 g
**Fiber:** 1.8 g

---

### In a Nutshell

**Origin:** Native to most of Europe, northern Africa, and western Asia
**Season:** Spring
**Why it's super:** High in vitamins A, C, and K, folate, fiber, riboflavin, thiamine, potassium, manganese, copper, and antioxidants
**Growing at home:** Can be grown at home

---

BELOW Asparagus was highly popular with the ancient Romans, who valued it as a food and for its medicinal properties.

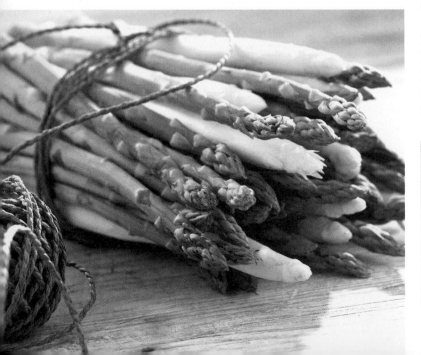

---

### Making the Most of Asparagus

To preserve nutrients, refrigerate asparagus after purchase and use as soon as possible. The best cooking method for nutrient retention is steaming; however, roasting asparagus also preserves nutrients and brings out excellent flavor. Whether the asparagus is steamed or roasted, sprinkling it with fresh lemon juice adds vitamin C and tart flavor.

# Chard and Leaf Beets

✪ *Beta vulgaris* var. *flavescens* Chard
✪ *Beta vulgaris* var. *flavescens* subsp. *cicla* Spinach Beet

Particularly popular among Mediterranean cultures, chard, also called Swiss chard, silver beet, and seakale beet, has large puckered leaves and broad white or colored stems. (The name Swiss chard was coined to distinguish this vegetable from French spinach.) Its close relative, spinach beet or perpetual spinach, has smaller leaves and a more slender stem. Both come from the same family as beetroot (see p. 57), but only the leaves and stem are eaten. They generally have a bitter taste.

A serving of chard or leaf beets provides seven times the Daily Value of vitamin K, 100 percent of the Daily Value for vitamin A, half of the daily need for vitamin C, and about a fifth of the Daily Value for vitamin E. Chard and leaf beets are high in antioxidants and are an excellent source of fiber, potassium, manganese, magnesium, and iron, and a good source of calcium and copper.

### THE HEALTHY EVIDENCE

High levels of antioxidants, as found in these vegetables, have been shown to help prevent cardiovascular diseases and cancer. A 2008 study in the *American Journal of Clinical Nutrition* reported that higher dietary intakes of potassium lowered risk for heart attack and stroke. Other studies showed that consuming chard reduced precancerous colon lesions.

| What's in a Serving? |
| --- |
| **COOKED CHARD AND LEAF BEETS** |
| **(1 cup/175 g)** |
| **Calories:** 35 (147 kJ) |
| **Protein:** 3.3 g |
| **Total fat:** 0.1 g |
| **Saturated fat:** 0 g |
| **Carbohydrates:** 7.2 g |
| **Fiber:** 3.7 g |

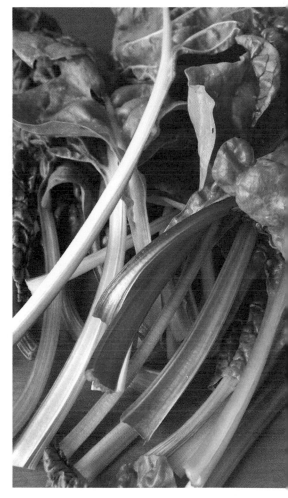

RIGHT The white or colored stems of Swiss chard are an excellent vegetable in their own right. They are often prepared separately, in the manner of asparagus or celery.

## Making the Most of Chard and Leaf Beets

To retain nutrients, avoid boiling and sauté instead. The stems take longer to cook, so put them in the skillet first with a few tablespoons of olive oil and chopped onion. When the stems are tender, toss in the leaves, cover, and sauté until the leaves are also tender. To enhance iron absorption, add some acidic juice, such as orange or lemon.

### In a Nutshell

**Origin:** Sicily
**Season:** Late spring through late autumn
**Why they're super:** High in vitamins A, C, E, and K, fiber, magnesium, manganese, potassium, iron, and antioxidants; also a good source of calcium and copper
**Growing at home:** Easily grown at home

# Chinese Mustard

✪ *Brassica juncea* var. *rugosa*

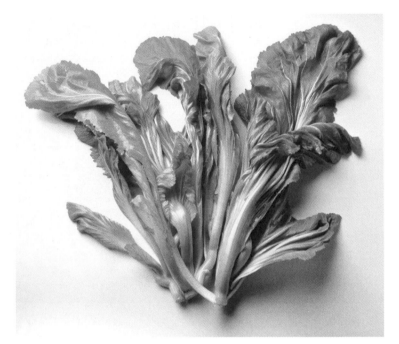

LEFT Chinese mustard greens add a pungent flavor to a salad when mixed with milder greens, such as kale, cabbage, or collard greens.

## Making the Most of Chinese Mustard

Chinese mustard has a pungent flavor, so it does not require additional flavoring. Add 6 cups (336 g) of the stems to hot olive oil and sauté in garlic, for added nutrients. Pour in 1 cup (235 ml) of chicken broth and simmer for ten minutes. Add leaves to the mixture and continue simmering until the broth has reduced.

## What's in a Serving?

**COOKED CHINESE MUSTARD**

**(1 cup/140 g)**

**Calories:** 21 (88 kJ)

**Protein:** 3.2 g

**Total fat:** 0.3 g

**Saturated fat:** 0 g

**Carbohydrates:** 2.9 g

**Fiber:** 2.8 g

Chinese mustard, also known as gai choy, is a species of mustard plant that has long been cultivated for its leaves and seeds. A subvariety is southern giant curled mustard, which resembles kale, but has a horseradish flavor. The leaves are widely used in Asian cooking, and can be cooked like spinach. The seeds of Chinese mustard are among the smallest of seeds, about ⅛ inch (3 mm) in diameter, and vary in color from yellowish to white to brown or black; they are important in many regional Indian and Bangladeshi cuisines, as is the oil extract from the seeds.

One serving of Chinese mustard provides five times the Daily Value of vitamin K and is high in vitamins A and C and folate. Chinese mustard is also an excellent source of the minerals manganese, potassium, copper, and calcium. Furthermore, it is a good source of fiber and provides a high level of antioxidants, including beta-carotene, lutein, and zeaxanthin.

## THE HEALTHY EVIDENCE

The high antioxidant content of Chinese mustard may help prevent diseases in which oxidative damage plays a role, such as cardiovascular disease and cancer. A large epidemiological study in 2007 showed modest support for the hypothesis that higher intakes of brassicas, including Chinese mustard, is linked to lower risk of prostate cancer. The researchers believe that the cancer protection arises from sulforaphane compounds, which protect DNA from damage.

## In a Nutshell

**Origin:** Foothills of the Himalayas

**Season:** Harvested early summer through late autumn

**Why it's super:** High in vitamins A, C, and K, folate, fiber, potassium, copper, manganese, calcium, sulforaphane, and antioxidants

**Growing at home:** Easily grown in the home garden

# Kale

*✿ Brassica oleracea, Acephala Group*

## What's in a Serving?

**COOKED KALE**
**(1 cup/130 g)**
**Calories:** 36 (152 kJ)
**Protein:** 2.5 g
**Total fat:** 0.5 g
**Saturated fat:** 0.1 g
**Carbohydrates:** 7.3 g
**Fiber:** 2.6 g

Kale, also called borecole, is a type of cabbage in which the central leaves do not form a head. For this reason, it is more similar to wild cabbage than to domesticated forms. Kale is one of many nutritious cultivars of *Brassica oleracea*; others include broccoli, cauliflower, collard, and Brussels sprouts.

Kale contains more than twice the level of antioxidants contained in other leafy greens, which are themselves excellent sources. Kale's antioxidants include beta-carotene, lutein, and zeaxanthin. One serving contains nearly eight times the Daily Value of vitamin K and twice the Daily Value of vitamin A. Kale is also low in calories and a good source of folate, fiber, vitamin C, and the minerals manganese, potassium, copper, and calcium.

### THE HEALTHY EVIDENCE

Kale's high levels of antioxidants make it effective in the prevention of cardiovascular disease and cancer. The high concentration of lutein and zeaxanthin in particular may help prevent degenerative eye diseases such as cataract, macular degeneration, and glaucoma. In addition, kale contains a high level of sulforaphane, a compound that studies have shown to be a potent anticancer agent. An article in the journal *Cancer Prevention Research* also reported that sulforaphane inhibits the bacteria that cause stomach and duodenal ulcers, and other studies have shown that it fights blood-vessel inflammation that contributes to heart disease.

### Making the Most of Kale

Sauté chopped onion in 2 tablespoons of olive oil, then add 1 tablespoon of vinegar and 1 cup (235 ml) of chicken broth. Add 4 cups (268 g) of kale, cover, and simmer for five minutes. Throw in ¼ cup (30 g) of dried cranberries, to boost the antioxidant content and add tart flavor, and simmer for ten minutes.

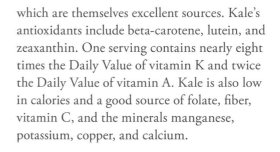

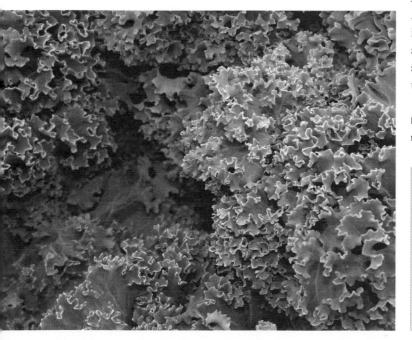

LEFT Kale tastes sweeter and more full of flavor after exposure to a frost. Once picked it will keep well in the freezer.

### In a Nutshell

**Origin:** Asia Minor
**Season:** Early spring to mid-summer
**Why it's super:** High in vitamins A and K, folate, sulforaphane, and antioxidants; good source of fiber, vitamin C, manganese, potassium, copper, and calcium
**Growing at home:** Suitable for home garden cultivation

# Collard

✿ *Brassica oleracea*, Acephala Group

## What's in a Serving?

**COOKED COLLARD
(1 cup/190 g)**
**Calories:** 49 (203 kJ)
**Protein:** 4 g
**Total fat:** 0.7 g
**Saturated fat:** 0.1 g
**Carbohydrates:** 9.3 g
**Fiber:** 5.3 g

Collard is a staple food in the southern United States. Although collard is related to kale and mustard greens, its greens have a milder taste. While generally available year-round, collard reaches its peak during late winter and early spring.

One cup of collard provides more than the Daily Value of vitamins K and A, and more than half of the recommended amount of vitamin C and manganese. Collard is also rich in folate, calcium, and potassium, in addition to being an excellent source of fiber, and is an outstanding source of antioxidants, particularly the antioxidants beta-carotene, lutein, and zeaxanthin.

RIGHT In the southern United States, eating collards and black peas on New Year's Day is said to bring good luck and prosperity.

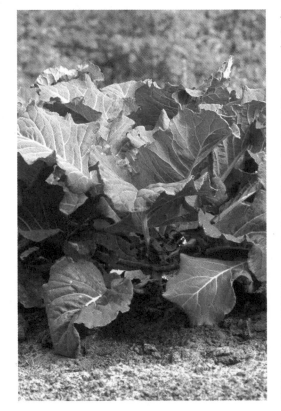

### In a Nutshell

**Origin:** Uncertain
**Season:** Mid-summer through autumn
**Why it's super:** High in vitamins A, C, and K, folate, fiber, manganese, potassium, calcium, sulforaphane, and antioxidants
**Growing at home:** Can be grown relatively easily in the home garden

## THE HEALTHY EVIDENCE

The high antioxidant levels of collard may help prevent diseases in which oxidative damage plays a major role, such as cardiovascular disease, dementia, and cancer. The *2008 Dallas Heart Study* showed that low dietary intake of potassium was associated with a higher risk of hypertension, a risk factor for stroke, so eating collard may counter this. The calcium in collard provides protection against bone loss; recent studies have also shown that calcium helps prevent migraine headaches and reduce symptoms associated with premenstrual syndrome (PMS). The anitoxidants lutein and zeaxanthin also help prevent eye diseases associated with ageing. Like other brassicas, collard contains sulforaphane, which may protect against cancer.

## Making the Most of Collard

The traditional method for cooking collard is to boil with salt pork. For a healthier approach, sauté in canola oil and add a tasty vegetable, such as red pepper (capsicum), to replace the flavor of the pork. This will also increase the nutrient level of the dish.

# Chinese Broccoli

✿ *Brassica oleracea*, Alboglabra Group

Also known as kai-lan, gai-lan, or Chinese kale, this leaf vegetable has a thick stem like broccoli, cauliflower, and Brussels sprouts, and flat, glossy, blue-green leaves. Overall, it looks similar to broccoli but with a longer stem and a small number of tiny flower heads. The flavor is very much like that of broccoli, but perhaps just a little sweeter. Although the plant's origin is uncertain, it may have been taken to the Orient by Portuguese explorers before developing to its present form through many generations of selection.

Widely used in Cantonese, Vietnamese, and Thai cuisine, Chinese broccoli is an excellent source of vitamins A, C, and K (just one serving provides almost the entire Daily Value for vitamin K), and folate, as well as a significant source of fiber, thiamine, riboflavin, calcium, potassium, and manganese. Like other brassicas, it also contains antioxidants and sulforaphane, as well as diindolylmethane (DIM).

## THE HEALTHY EVIDENCE

Folate is the main nutrient that protects against neural tube defects—the cause of

### Making the Most of Chinese Broccoli

Blanch 4 cups (360 g) of Chinese broccoli in boiling water for a few minutes. Stir-fry in 1 tablespoon of sesame oil and season with 2 tablespoons of oyster sauce, 3 tablespoons of chicken broth, 1 tablespoon of rice wine, and 1 teaspoon of sugar. Adding slices of ginger boosts the antioxidant content and flavor.

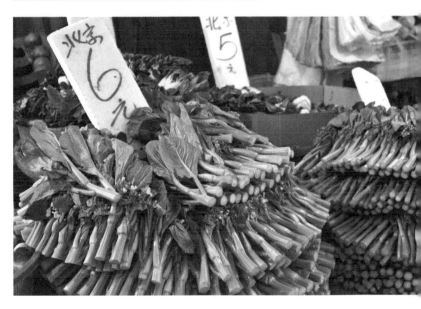

ABOVE When buying Chinese broccoli, look for crisp stalks with no sign of wilting. Check, too, that the leaves are free of soft spots and blemishes.

many common birth defects including spina bifida—and an adequate intake of folate is particularly important before and during pregnancy. Sulforaphane and DIM have been shown to protect against cancer: a 2010 study in *Cancer Research* reported that DIM is "an anticancer agent" that targets compounds involved in tumor promotion in human colon cancer cells.

### In a Nutshell

**Origin:** Uncertain

**Season:** Late spring through autumn, with mid-summer providing the best yields

**Why it's super:** High in vitamins A, C, and K and folate; good source of fiber, thiamine, riboflavin, calcium, potassium, manganese, sulforaphane, diindolyl-methane, and antioxidants

**Growing at home:** Can be cultivated in the home garden

### What's in a Serving?

**COOKED CHINESE BROCCOLI**

**(1 cup/88 g)**

**Calories:** 19 (83 kJ)

**Protein:** 1 g

**Total fat:** 0.6 g

**Saturated fat:** 0.1 g

**Carbohydrates:** 3.3 g

**Fiber:** 2.2 g

# Cauliflower

✿ *Brassica oleracea*, Botrytis Group

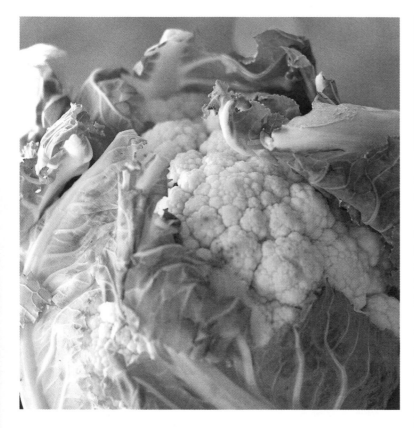

### Making the Most of Cauliflower

The best way to eat cauliflower is raw in fresh salads or with dips, as this will retain the vitamin C and other water-soluble nutrients. However, it can be boiled for a short time and puréed to make a lower-calorie replacement for mashed potatoes.

LEFT The part of the cauliflower that is most commonly eaten is known as the "curd." It consists of the undeveloped flowers of the plant.

L like its close relative broccoli, cauliflower is grown for its flowering parts. Its name comes from the Latin word *caulis*, which means "cabbage." The white color of cauliflower is caused by the leaves shielding the flowers from the sun during the early growth period. Although they are less common, other varieties of cauliflower are orange, green, or purple in color. The cauliflower head is the most commonly eaten part of the plant, but the leaves can be used in soups.

Cauliflower is an excellent source of vitamins C and K, and a significant source of vitamin B6, folate, fiber, manganese, and omega-3 fatty acids. The orange variety of cauliflower is 25 times higher in vitamin A than white cauliflower. Like other brassicas, cauliflower also contains sulforaphane. There is no substantial difference in nutrients between fresh and frozen cauliflower.

## THE HEALTHY EVIDENCE

Numerous studies have linked sulforaphane to a reduced cancer risk in humans. A study in the *Journal of Nutrition* reported that treating liver cells with compounds contained in cauliflower reduced the production of lipids that increase heart disease risk when present in high levels in the blood. Another study reported that a high intake of cauliflower was associated with a lower risk of an aggressive form of prostate cancer.

### What's in a Serving?

**COOKED CAULIFLOWER (1 cup/124 g)**

**Calories:** 29 (119 kJ)
**Protein:** 2.2 g
**Total fat:** 0.6 g
**Saturated fat:** 0.1 g
**Carbohydrates:** 5.1 g
**Fiber:** 2.9 g

### In a Nutshell

**Origin:** Northeastern Mediterranean
**Season:** Best in late summer, early autumn
**Why it's super:** High in vitamins C and K; good source of vitamin B6, folate, fiber, manganese, sulforaphane, and omega-3 fatty acids
**Growing at home:** Difficult to grow at home

# Cabbage

✪ *Brassica oleracea*, Capitata Group

Cabbage evolved along the Mediterranean coast from the wild mustard plant. The ancient Romans and Greeks believed it to have medicinal purposes. The most common cabbage plant is green, but other varieties may be red or purple in color. Savoy cabbage is a variety of green cabbage, but with a pale green, ruffled leaf.

Cabbage is an excellent source of vitamins C and K. It is also a good source of vitamin B6, folate, fiber, manganese, potassium, sulforaphane, and omega-3 fatty acids.

## THE HEALTHY EVIDENCE

The consumption of cabbage and other cruciferous vegetables has been consistently associated in both human and animal studies with a lower risk of many cancers such as those of the lung, colon, breast, stomach, and ovaries. A recent study in the *International Journal of Cancer* suggests that the inclusion of cabbage in the diet lowers the risk for bladder cancer. In another study of over 1,000 men at the Fred Hutchinson Cancer Research Center in Seattle, those men who consumed three or more servings of cruciferous vegetables, such as cabbage, each week had a 44 percent lower prostate-cancer risk. In the Netherlands, a study of over 100,000 people lasting more than six years showed a 49 percent lower risk of colorectal cancer with higher intakes of cruciferous vegetables.

### In a Nutshell

**Origin:** Mediterranean

**Season:** Early to late autumn

**Why it is super:** High in vitamins C and K; good source of vitamin B6, folate, fiber, manganese, potassium, sulforaphane, and omega 3 fatty acids

**Growing at home:** Cabbage is hardy and easy to grow

### What's in a Serving?

**COOKED CABBAGE (1 cup/150 g)**

**Calories:** 34 (142 kJ)

**Protein:** 1.9 g

**Total fat:** 0.1 g

**Saturated fat:** 0 g

**Carbohydrates:** 8.3 g

**Fiber:** 2.9 g

### Making the Most of Cabbage

Although boiling is the typical way to cook cabbage, shredding raw cabbage for use in various types of fresh salads will preserve its vitamin C and folate. Combine the raw cabbage with shredded carrots, dried cranberries, and walnuts, and toss with a honey vinaigrette dressing to increase antioxidant and omega-3 fatty acid intake.

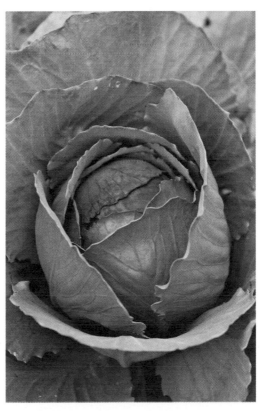

LEFT The color of red cabbage varies according to soil type, with acidic soils producing a redder vegetable and more alkaline soils yielding green or yellow leaves.

# Broccoli

✿ *Brassica oleracea*, Cymosa Group

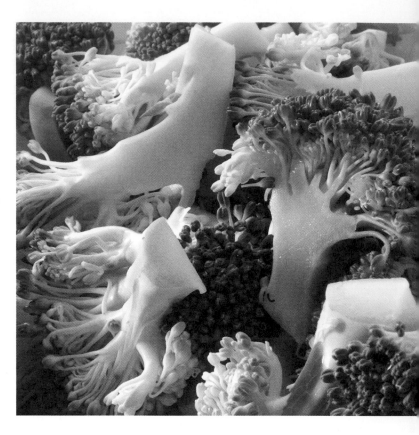

The name "broccoli" comes from the Latin *brachium*, meaning "branch" or "arm," and the vegetable is so named because of its similarity to a tree. Its common coloring is light to deep green, but certain varieties may also have a purplish cast. Broccolini, which has smaller buds and a stalk similar to that of asparagus or Chinese broccoli (gailan), is a cross between broccoli and kale.

One serving of broccoli provides twice the Daily Value of vitamins C and K, and half the daily requirement for vitamin A. Broccoli is also an excellent source of folate and fiber, and a good source of manganese, potassium, and magnesium. The nutrient profile for frozen broccoli is similar to that of fresh broccoli, although it contains 35 percent more beta-carotene by weight than fresh broccoli due to volume concentration.

## THE HEALTHY EVIDENCE

In addition to its abundant supply of vitamins and minerals, broccoli contains several important phytochemicals. It is high in the flavonoid quercetin and in sulforaphane, both of which protect against cancer. One study of 66,940 women showed that those with the highest flavonoid intake had a 25 percent

### What's in a Serving?

**COOKED BROCCOLI**
**(1 cup/156 g)**
**Calories:** 55 (231 kJ)
**Protein:** 3.7 g
**Total fat:** 0.6 g
**Saturated fat:** 0.1 g
**Carbohydrates:** 11.2 g
**Fiber:** 5.1 g

ABOVE Broccoli is a type of cabbage in which the flowers form a dense head. It was introduced to the United States and Britain in the eighteenth century.

reduced risk of ovarian cancer compared with those consuming the least, while a study from the *Journal of the National Cancer Institute* showed that a high intake of broccoli greatly reduced the risk of aggressive prostate cancer. The antioxidants, potassium, and folate in broccoli also help protect against cardiovascular disease.

### In a Nutshell

**Origin:** Italy
**Season:** Late summer through autumn
**Why it's super:** High in vitamins A, C, and K, folate, and fiber; good source of magnesium, manganese, potassium, sulforaphane, quercetin, and antioxidants
**Growing at home:** Grows best in cooler conditions, and is difficult to cultivate

### Making the Most of Broccoli

Broccoli's phytochemicals and heat-sensitive nutrients such as folate are best retained by either not cooking it at all or lightly sautéing. Steaming does not work well with cruciferous vegetables, as covering during cooking causes retention of sulfurous-smelling compounds. Raw broccoli florets can be added to salads or dipped in plain yogurt with various spices.

# Brussels Sprouts

✿ *Brassica oleracea,* Gemmifera Group

Brussels sprouts grow in bunches of from 20 to 40 on the stem of a plant measuring 2–3 feet (0.6–0.9 m) tall. They thrive best in cooler conditions, but may also be grown successfully in warmer climates. Their color ranges from sage green to red or purple. Descended from the cabbage, the Brussels sprout as we know it was first cultivated in Belgium in the 12th century, hence the name.

Brussels sprouts are rich in many nutrients. A 1-cup serving provides more than twice the Daily Value of vitamin K, 150 percent of vitamin C, and almost a quarter of the Daily Value for folate and vitamin A. Brussels sprouts are also a significant source of fiber, manganese, potassium, iron, antioxidants, and omega-3 fatty acids, in the form of alpha-linolenic acid (ALA).

## THE HEALTHY EVIDENCE

A study in the journal *Annals of the Rheumatic Diseases,* which involved more than 20,000 subjects, found that those who ate foods rich in vitamin C, such as Brussels sprouts, were protected against inflammatory polyarthritis, a form of rheumatoid arthritis. Studies in the *American Journal of Clinical Nutrition* have pointed to the cardio-protective effects of ALA. Like other brassicas, Brussels sprouts contain sulforaphane, which is linked to cancer prevention.

| What's in a Serving? |
| --- |
| **COOKED BRUSSELS SPROUTS** |
| **(1 cup/156 g)** |
| **Calories:** 56 (234 kJ) |
| **Protein:** 4 g |
| **Total fat:** 0.8 g |
| **Saturated fat:** 0.2 g |
| **Carbohydrates:** 11 g |
| **Fiber:** 14.1 g |

### In a Nutshell

**Origin:** Belgium
**Season:** Autumn
**Why they're super:** High in vitamins A, C, and K and folate; good source of fiber, manganese, potassium, iron, omega-3 fatty acids, sulforaphane, and antioxidants
**Growing at home:** Can be grown in the home garden

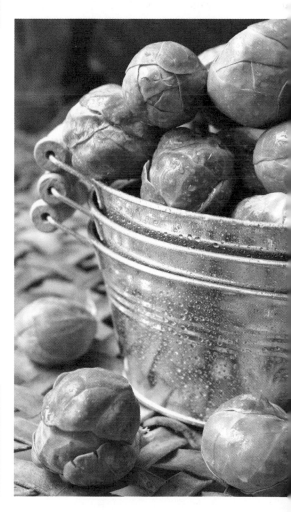

RIGHT Brussels sprouts are commonly eaten with poultry and game. In Belgium, their country of origin, they are traditionally served with peeled chestnuts.

## Making the Most of Brussels Sprouts

Cut the sprouts in half to reduce cooking time and thereby save nutrients. Add the sprouts to boiling water, and then lower the heat to simmer. Test with a fork, and cook just long enough that the sprouts are tender (six to seven minutes). To enhance iron absorption, season with a vinaigrette dressing.

# Asian Greens

✪ *Brassica rapa* var. *chinensis* Pak Choy
✪ *Brassica rapa* var. *nipposinica* Mizuna
✪ *Brassica rapa* var. *pekinensis* Chinese Cabbage
✪ *Brassica rapa* var. *rosularis* Chinese Flat Cabbage

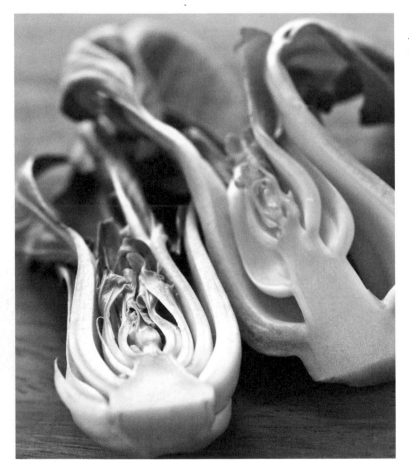

ABOVE Pak choy is a winter-hardy plant that is increasingly grown in Europe and other temperate climates. Sliced in half the plant has a rather elegant form that can enhance the appearance of some dishes.

*Life expectancy would grow by leaps and bounds if green vegetables smelled as good as bacon.*

Doug Larson, US journalist (1926– )

A wide range of Asian greens is available, both species and cultivars, but most are closely related and can be used interchangeably in cooking. Identifying Asian greens can be tricky, in that a number of names exist for each of the varieties, and the names in English do not always translate directly from those used in Chinese. To make matters worse, there is some disagreement over identification among botanists.

## CHINESE CABBAGES

In Chinese, there is no word for cabbage, so the various types of cabbage are named for their appearance. Pak choy, for example, means "white vegetable." In English, pak choy is also called bok choy or buk choy, among other names. A fast-growing plant that grows 16–20 inches (40–50 cm) tall, it is ready for harvest in just two months. It does not travel well, so it is seldom exported from Asian countries; however, it is now widely grown in the West. Pak choy has a white stalk with dark green leaves that grow loosely, like Swiss chard. It has higher nutritional content than cabbage and a slightly bitter flavor.

Mizuna has a mild peppery taste, similar to arugula (rocket) but not as strong. The plant produces stalks with deeply cut, serrated

## Making the Most of Asian Greens

With the exception of vitamin C and folate, the nutrients are not affected by cooking. The vitamin C and folate are best preserved by rapid stir-frying, which is typical in Asian cuisines. The iron available for absorption can be increased by adding an acidic ingredient, such as rice wine vinegar.

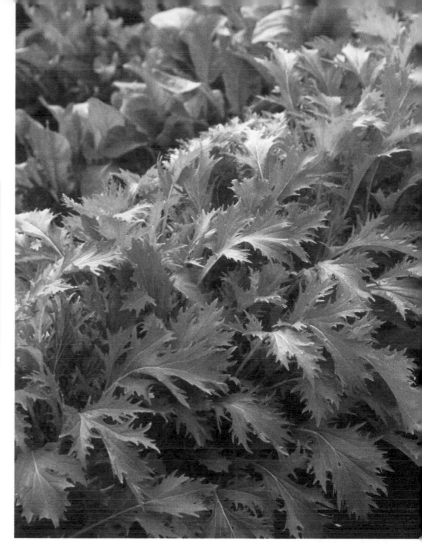

leaves. A single plant may have as many as 180 leaves clustered in a compact bunch, usually 12 inches (30 cm) or so in diameter. Mizuna is resistant to cold and may even grow during the winter months. It can be mixed with other greens in a salad to add variety and to boost the nutritional content of the salad.

So-called Chinese cabbage, or napa, is lighter in shade—pale yellow to light green—than the other cabbages. It grows in a barrel-like shape on a head about 12 inches (30 cm) long and 6 inches (15 cm) thick. Chinese flat cabbage, also called tatsoi, grows in a rosette that is the shape of a plate and may be 12 inches (30 cm) across. The individual leaves resemble those of its close relative, pak choy.

The nutrient profiles are similar for all Asian greens, though a paler color signals a slightly lower level of vitamin A. The greens are outstanding sources of vitamins A, C, and K, with one serving exceeding the Daily Value of vitamin A and meeting more than half the Daily Values for vitamins C and K. Moreover, Asian greens are an excellent source of vitamin B6, folate, pantothenic acid, calcium, iron, potassium, and manganese. They are also extremely high in beta-carotene and, like

other brassicas, they contain phytochemicals such as sulforaphane and isothiocyanates.

ABOVE An attractive plant, mizuna adapts well to most soils and is particularly easy to grow.

## THE HEALTHY EVIDENCE

The high levels of antioxidants make Asian greens powerhouses of protection against cardiovascular disease and cancer. In the case of cancer, there is an added benefit beyond the antioxidant content, from the phytochemicals sulforaphane and isothiocyanates. A review published in the journal *Nutrition and Cancer* reported that a diet high in brassicas, which included pak choy, was associated with a lower risk of prostate cancer. In addition, a 2009 study in the *Journal of Medicinal Food* reported that Chinese cabbage showed antidiabetic effects in rats.

## What's in a Serving?

**COOKED ASIAN GREENS**
**(1 cup/170 g)**

**Calories:** 20 (81 kJ)

**Protein:** 2.6 g

**Total fat:** 0.3 g

**Saturated fat:** 0 g

**Carbohydrates:** 3 g

**Fiber:** 1.7 g

# Endive

✪ *Cichorium endivia*

Endive is often used in salad mixtures. There are two varieties, curly endive, sometimes called chicory, which has narrow, green, curly outer leaves, and the broad-leafed variety, often called escarole. The endive plant grows as a head, and the outer leaves are a darker green and bitter, while the inner leaves are lighter in color and have a milder flavor. Both varieties of endive are available year-round, with the peak season being from June through October. Endive is rich in vitamins A and K, folate, fiber, and manganese, and it's a good source of vitamin C, potassium, pantothenic acid, and antioxidants.

## THE HEALTHY EVIDENCE

Endive contains several different nutrients and compounds that function as antioxidants, including beta-carotene, vitamin C, and manganese. These are important in protecting the body against diseases involving oxidative damage, such as cardiovascular disease, cancer, Alzheimer's, and even the ageing process. Studies in the *Journal of Nutrition* in the 1990s reported on the importance of manganese in maintaining normal blood

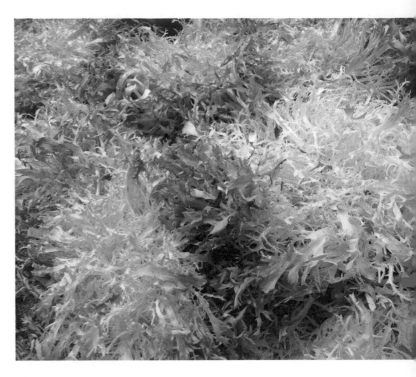

ABOVE Choose endive heads that are free of browning, crisp and bright green. Refrigerated in plastic bags, they will keep for about ten days.

glucose—animals fed manganese-deficient diets had fewer insulin receptors, key components that allow glucose to enter the cell for use as energy.

## Making the Most of Endive

Endive is highly perishable, so use it immediately or wrap it tightly and store it in the refrigerator for up to three days. The best way to eat endive is raw in a fresh salad, although it can be cooked. For a simple endive salad, select the lighter-colored leaves and tear them into small pieces; add cherry tomatoes, shredded carrots, dried cranberries, and almonds for added antioxidants, and toss with a vinaigrette or other dressing.

## In a Nutshell

**Origin:** Eastern Mediterranean

**Season:** Summer through autumn

**Why it's super:** High in vitamins A and K, folate, fiber, and manganese; good source of vitamin C, potassium, pantothenic acid, and antioxidants

**Growing at home:** Grows best in cooler conditions, but is easy to grow

## What's in a Serving?

**RAW ENDIVE**

**(2 cups/100 g)**

**Calories:** 17 (71 kJ)

**Protein:** 1.3 g

**Total fat:** 0.2 g

**Saturated fat:** 0 g

**Carbohydrates:** 3.4 g

**Fiber:** 3.1 g

# Globe Artichoke

✪ *Cynara scolymus*

The globe artichoke is a member of the thistle family. The plants grow to a height of 3–4 feet (0.9–1.2 m), producing large heads of violet or sometimes white flowers at the top of the stem. The edible part is the "heart" of the immature flower. Artichokes are available all year, with the peak season being in spring and autumn. France, Italy, and Spain are the main sources of artichokes, except in the United States, where nearly the entire crop comes from California.

Artichokes are an outstanding source of fiber, with one serving providing half of the Daily Value for most people. In addition, that one serving is an excellent source of vitamin K, folate, and potassium, and a good source of vitamin C, the antioxidant lutein, niacin, riboflavin, and iron. Artichokes also contain a phytochemical, cynarin, which researchers have studied in relation to several diseases.

## THE HEALTHY EVIDENCE

In the 1970s, European researchers documented cynarin's cholesterol-lowering effect in humans. A study published in 2000 reported that artichoke leaf containing a consistent amount of cynarin lowered cholesterol levels by up to 15 percent.

Scientists now believe that artichokes contain many other compounds that contribute to the cholesterol-lowering effect. A recent study published in the *Journal of Alternative and Complementary Medicine* reported that the extract also eased irritable bowel syndrome.

### In a Nutshell

**Origin:** Southern Europe through the Mediterranean
**Season:** All year, peaking in spring and autumn
**Why it's super:** High in vitamin K, folate, fiber, and potassium; good source of vitamin C, iron, niacin, riboflavin, lutein, and cynarin
**Growing at home:** Limited to warm areas

### What's in a Serving?

**COOKED ARTICHOKE (1 cup/168 g)**
**Calories:** 89 (370 kJ)
**Protein:** 4.9 g
**Total fat:** 0.6 g
**Saturated fat:** 0.1 g
**Carbohydrates:** 20 g
**Fiber:** 14 g

BELOW Artichokes are sometimes used to make herbal teas, and are the principal flavoring for the Italian apéritif liqueur Cynar.

### Making the Most of Globe Artichoke

Remove the outer leaves of the artichoke, until only the heart remains. Cut approximately 1 inch (2.5 cm) off the top. To retain heat-sensitive nutrients, place the heart in a shallow dish in less than 1 inch (2.5 cm) of water. Cover and microwave for five minutes, or until tender (test with a fork). Sprinkle with lemon juice to enhance iron absorption.

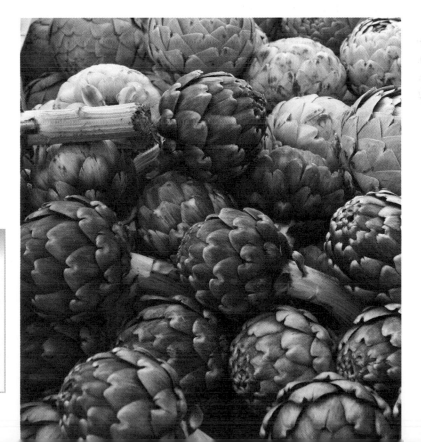

# Arugula or Rocket

✿ *Eruca sativa*

A member of the mustard family, arugula is also known as rocket, garden rocket, rughetta, and roquette. Its slightly pungent, peppery flavor makes an interesting addition to salads. The flavor is milder when the leaves are smaller and less mature, and it's best to pick them before they become too large, when the taste can be overwhelming. In some cultures the seeds are used for oil.

Arugula is low in calories and is an excellent source of vitamins A, C, and K and folate, as well as a good source of calcium and magnesium. The antioxidant content is high, in the

## What's in a Serving?

**RAW ARUGULA**
**(2 cups/40 g)**
**Calories:** 10 (42 kJ)
**Protein:** 1 g
**Total fat:** 0.3 g
**Saturated fat:** 0 g
**Carbohydrates:** 1.5 g
**Fiber:** 0.6 g

## In a Nutshell

**Origin:** Mediterranean
**Season:** Summer and autumn
**Why it's super:** High in vitamins A, C, and K, folate, and antioxidants; good source of calcium, magnesium, and ALA
**Growing at home:** Easily grown in the home garden. When the plants go to seed, the flowers can be picked for use in salads.

form of beta-carotene, lutein, and zeaxanthin. In addition, arugula is a good source of alpha-linolenic acid (ALA), an essential fatty acid—it contains 0.07 g in a 2-cup serving.

## THE HEALTHY EVIDENCE

In a recent review in the journal *Alternative Therapies in Health and Medicine*, a Harvard Medical School researcher reported that, "Presently, the weight of the evidence favors recommendations for modest dietary consumption of ALA (2–3 grams daily) for the primary and secondary prevention of heart disease." This protective effect may relate to ALA's ability to influence platelet function, inflammation, and blood-vessel function.

BELOW Rocket has been cultivated in the Mediterranean since the time of the Roman Empire, where it was considered an aphrodisiac.

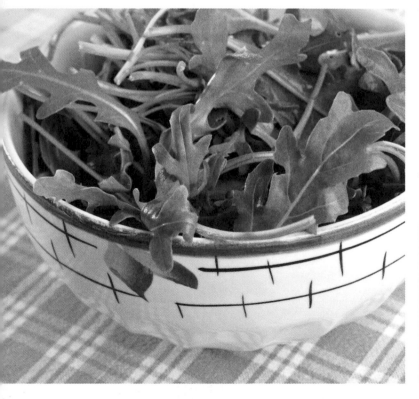

## Making the Most of Arugula

With the notable exception of vitamin C and folate, cooking does not reduce the levels of the key health-promoting nutrients; arugula can therefore be sautéed or made into pesto. However, people most often eat arugula in a fresh salad, where it blends well with other high-nutrient ingredients such as walnuts, raisins, and dried cranberries.

# Fennel

✿ *Foeniculum vulgare*

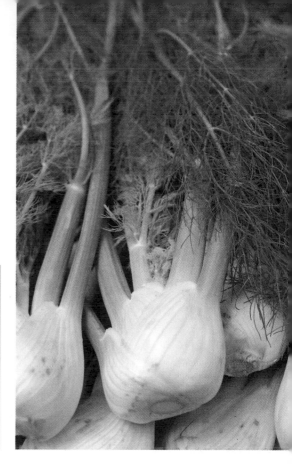

RIGHT In Greek mythology, Prometheus was said to have stolen fire from the gods and hidden it in a fennel stalk.

Fennel is widely valued for its leaves, edible seeds, bulb, and celery-like stalks. Its licorice flavor comes from the presence of anethole, an aromatic compound. It is also found in anise and star anise, though their flavors are not as strong as that of fennel. The fennel plant consists of stalks topped with feathery green leaves and flowers that produce "seeds" (actually a fruit); at their base the stalks form a broad bulb. It is sometimes used as a vegetable, often referred to as Florence fennel or finocchio.

Fennel is a highly aromatic herb with culinary and medicinal uses, and it is a main ingredient of the alcoholic spirit absinthe. The seeds are widely used to relieve flatulence in children; in India, they have long been used to calm the palate and rejuvenate digestion.

Of the edible parts of the plant, it is the fennel seeds that contain the highest levels of nutrients and phytochemicals. A single tablespoon of fennel seeds is low in calories yet high in fiber, protein, and essential fatty acids, and also a good source of calcium, iron, and manganese.

## What's in a Serving?

| RAW FENNEL SEEDS (1 tablespoon/5.8 g) | RAW FENNEL BULB (1 cup/87 g) |
|---|---|
| **Calories:** 20 (84 kJ) | **Calories:** 27 (113 kJ) |
| **Protein:** 0.9 g | **Protein:** 1.1 g |
| **Total fat:** 0.9 g | **Total fat:** 0.2 g |
| **Saturated fat:** 0 g | **Saturated fat:** 0 g |
| **Carbohydrates:** 3 g | **Carbohydrates:** 6.3 g |
| **Fiber:** 2.3 g | **Fiber:** 2.7 g |

## THE HEALTHY EVIDENCE

Fennel's unique combination of phytochemicals, including the flavonoids rutin, quercitin, and kacmpfcrol, rcsults in potent antioxidant activity. In several studies, anethole, the main component of fennel oil extract, was shown to reduce inflammation that contributes to heart disease, and it also exhibits anti-cancer effects. The University of Texas Anderson Cancer Center published an article on the biological mechanisms responsible for these effects.

## In a Nutshell

**Origin:** Mediterranean region

**Season:** Late summer through autumn

**Why it's super:** High in fiber, protein, essential fatty acids, antioxidants, and anethole; good source of calcium, iron, and manganese

**Growing at home:** Easy to grow in a home garden

## Making the Most of Fennel

The nutrients and antioxidants contained in fennel are not eliminated during cooking, therefore the bulb and seeds can be added to a wide variety of dishes, including soups, sauces, and vegetable dishes. In many cultures, people simply pick up a handful of fennel seeds and eat them raw. Bulbs are often eaten raw, but can also be braised.

# Romaine or Cos Lettuce

✪ *Lactuca sativa*

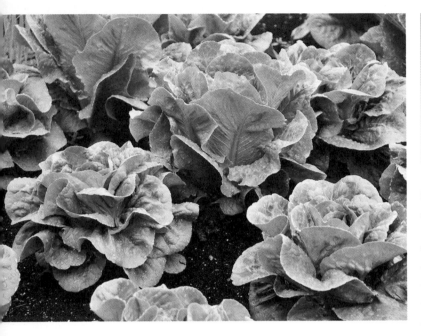

### Making the Most of Romaine Lettuce

Romaine makes an excellent fresh salad green, and in its raw state will retain all its water-soluble and heat-sensitive nutrients. Another way to include more of this health-promoting food in your diet is to wrap other ingredients, such as rice and meat mixtures, in the large leaves.

LEFT Romaine lettuce is often used as the maror, or bitter herb, in the Jewish Passover Seder, the ritual feast that marks the start of Passover.

Romaine lettuce, also known as cos, is a head-forming lettuce with deep green, long leaves and a crisp texture. The scientific name derives from the Latin word for milk—lettuces release a white, milk-like liquid when their leaves are broken, which provides the slightly bitter taste.

Most sources cite the eastern Mediterranean region as the plant's point of origin, and ancient Romans and Greeks valued it for medicinal purposes. Columbus introduced romaine and other lettuces to North America in 1493. In the 1700s, Spanish missionaries planted lettuce in California, which remains the lettuce capital of the United States.

Romaine is an excellent source of vitamins A, C, and K, folate, manganese and chromium, and is a good source of vitamins B1 and B2, fiber, potassium, molybdenum, iron, and phosphorus. A single serving contains 164 percent of the Daily Value for vitamin A in the form of the antioxidant carotenoids beta-carotene, lutein, and zeaxanthin. Romaine is also a significant source of alpha-linolenic acid (ALA).

### THE HEALTHY EVIDENCE

Romaine's mix of nutrients can help reduce the risk of cardiovascular disease. Folate, ALA, and carotenoids have all been shown to fight heart disease, as described in a recent article in *The American Journal of Clinical Nutrition*. In addition, potassium has been shown in numerous studies to protect against hypertension and stroke.

---

### What's in a Serving?

**RAW ROMAINE LETTUCE**
**(2 cups/94 g)**
**Calories:** 16 (68 kJ)
**Protein:** 1.2 g
**Total fat:** 0.3 g
**Saturated fat:** 0 g
**Carbohydrates:** 3 g
**Fiber:** 2 g

---

### In a Nutshell

**Origin:** Eastern Mediterranean region
**Season:** Summer
**Why it's super:** High in vitamins A, C, and K, folate, manganese, chromium, and antioxidants; good source of vitamins B1 and B2, fiber, potassium, molybdenum, iron, phosphorus, and ALA
**Growing at home:** Easy to grow in a home garden

# Alfalfa Sprouts

✪ *Medicago sativa*

Known also as lucerne, alfalfa is a perennial herb of the clover family. It was first grown in Persia, now Iran; in the late fifth century BCE, the Persians took the plant to Europe during their invasion of Greece. More than 400 years later, alfalfa was introduced to China. The mature plant is still widely used as feed for livestock. In the past, people have eaten the young leaves in times of famine, but it is the sprouted seeds that are used for human consumption these days.

Alfalfa grows best in warm temperate and cool subtropical regions. The seeds can be sprouted at home by rinsing, soaking overnight, draining, and then placing in a thin layer in a covered container. It takes a few days for the seeds to sprout in a warm environment, and they must be rinsed in the morning and evening during this time. The sprouts are a good source of vitamin C, folate, fiber, manganese, and copper.

## THE HEALTHY EVIDENCE

Alfalfa's complement of nutrients, notably vitamin C, fiber, and copper, helps protect against heart disease. A 2009 in-vitro study published in *Cardiovascular Research* reported that copper caused regression of cardiac hypertrophy, an adverse result of heart failure. The researchers stated that "regression of heart hypertrophy by copper supplementation would be a simple and less expensive therapy [than conventional treatments] for heart disease."

---

### In a Nutshell

**Origin:** Iran

**Season:** Summer

**Why they're super:** Good source of vitamin C, folate, fiber, manganese, and copper

**Growing at home:** Easy to grow in a container

---

### What's in a Serving?

**RAW ALFALFA SPROUTS**

**(2 cups/66 g)**

Calories: 15 (63 kJ)

Protein: 2.6 g

Total fat: 0.5 g

Saturated fat: 0 g

Carbohydrates: 1.4 g

Fiber: 1.3 g

---

RIGHT The nutty flavor and interesting texture of alfalfa sprouts make them an excellent addition to salads and sandwiches of all kinds.

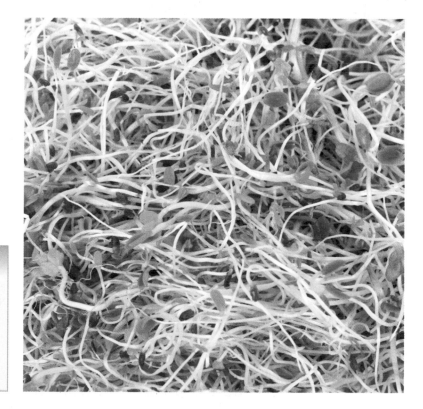

## Making the Most of Alfalfa Sprouts

For optimal retention of vitamin C and folate, use sprouts as a topper for fresh salads. Adding other fresh vegetables high in carotenoids, such as shredded carrots, diced tomatoes and red pepper (capsicum), will more than triple the antioxidant content, supplementing alfalfa's heart-protection effects.

# Watercress

✿ *Nasturtium officinale*

## What's in a Serving?

**RAW WATERCRESS**
**(2 cups/68 g)**
**Calories:** 7 (31 kJ)
**Protein:** 1.6 g
**Total fat:** 0.1 g
**Saturated fat:** 0 g
**Carbohydrates:** 0.9 g
**Fiber:** 0.3 g

Wild watercress has been a favorite food since ancient times, enjoyed notably by the Romans, Greeks, and Anglo-Saxons. Most likely, watercress was first cultivated by Germans in the 1500s.

The hairless perennial has white roots and small round leaves, and grows near streams. The leaves are a deep green color, which is a clue to the nutrients it contains. The flavor is somewhat pungent; for this reason watercress is often mixed with milder greens in salads.

A serving of watercress provides almost half the Daily Value of vitamins A and C, and more than double the Daily Value of vitamin K. It is also a significant source of potassium, manganese, and calcium, and an excellent source of the antioxidants beta-carotene, lutein, and zeaxanthin. Studies have shown that watercress is high in isothiocyanates, too.

### In a Nutshell

**Origin:** Europe
**Season:** Summer
**Why it's super:** High in vitamins A, C, and K, and antioxidants and isothiocyanates; good source of potassium, manganese, and calcium
**Growing at home:** Difficult to grow in a home garden

### Making the Most of Watercress

Many of the important nutrients, such as antioxidants and minerals, are not destroyed by cooking, so you can incorporate watercress in stir-fries and soups. However, eating watercress fresh in a salad will also preserve the vitamin C, which is in abundant supply.

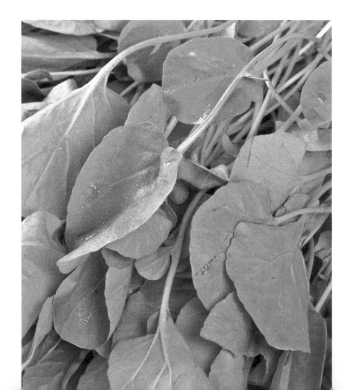

### THE HEALTHY EVIDENCE

Many recent studies have noted the significant anticancer and anti-inflammatory activity of isothiocyanates. A 2009 study in the journal *Free Radical Research Group* reported that consumption of watercress was associated with inhibition of compounds that cause inflammation and cancer. In addition, the high antioxidant content was shown to exert a potent and independent protective effect against both cancer and cardiovascular disease.

LEFT In late nineteenth-century England, watercress was sold in bunches by street vendors, to be eaten in the manner of an ice cream cone.

# Purslane

✿ *Portulaca oleracea*

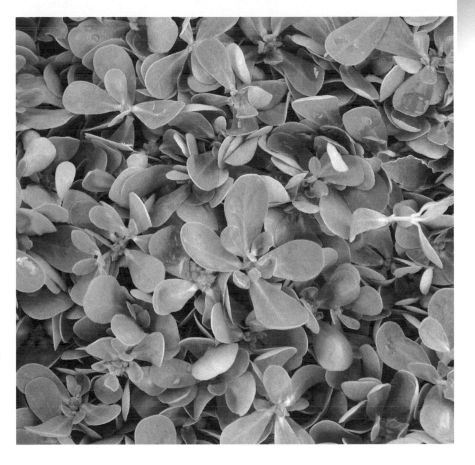

Other names for purslane include verdolaga, pigweed, little hogweed, and pusley. The plant spread from North Africa through the Middle East and the Indian subcontinent to Malaysia and Australia, and most likely arrived in North America during the pre-Columbian era; there it is considered an invasive weed in many regions.

All parts of the plant are edible, including the seeds. The leaves have a slight sour taste and are widely used in salads or cooked as other greens. Purslane holds a particularly important place in the traditional Japanese New Year ritual, being one of the seven special herbs used in a symbolic dish served on that occasion.

A serving of purslane provides 43 percent of the Daily Value for vitamin A and 20 percent of the Daily Value for vitamin C. The ample vitamin A level is present as the antioxidant carotenoids beta-carotene, lutein, and zeaxanthin. Purslane is also a significant source of calcium, magnesium, manganese, copper, and potassium, and other antioxidants.

ABOVE In ancient times, purslane's healing properties were said to be so great that Pliny advised wearing it as an amulet to ward off evil.

## Making the Most of Purslane

Since many of the important health benefits arise from the antioxidant and mineral content, cooking purslane will not result in significant nutrient losses. Try it in stir-fries or sauté it with a healthy vegetable oil. Purslane also makes an excellent salad green.

## In a Nutshell

**Origin:** North Africa

**Season:** Summer

**Why it's super:** High in vitamins A and C and antioxidants; good source of calcium, magnesium, manganese, copper, and potassium

**Growing at home:** Easy to grow in the home garden

## What's in a Serving?

**COOKED PURSLANE
(1 cup/115 g)**

**Calories:** 21 (86 kJ)

**Protein:** 1.7 g

**Total fat:** 0.2 g

**Saturated fat:** 0 g

**Carbohydrates:** 4 g

**Fiber:** 0 g

## THE HEALTHY EVIDENCE

Purslane has been the topic of numerous studies, including a recent study from the journal *Phytotherapy Research*. The authors discovered that three compounds contained in purslane—oleracein A, oleracein B, and oleracein E—had more antioxidant potency than vitamins C and E. Another study in 2009 reported that purslane was effective in treating post-menopausal women with abnormal uterine bleeding.

# Spinach

✿ *Spinacia oleracea*

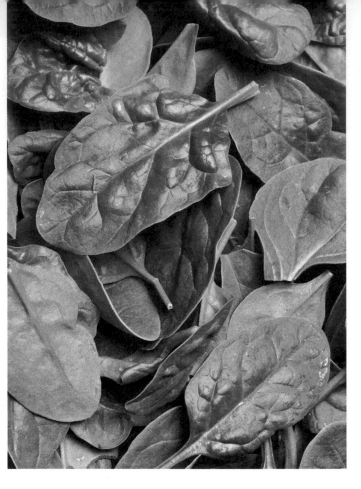

LEFT In medieval Europe and Asia, spinach was a common ingredient in sweet dishes. Sweet spinach tart is still a traditional Christmas dish in Provence, France.

Spinach originated in Nepal and spread from India to China by 647; in the eleventh century, it reached Europe via North Africa. Dishes prepared with spinach are often labeled "Florentine," a term that derives from its use in Florence in the 1500s: spinach was Catherine de' Medici's favorite food, and even when she moved to France to marry the future French king Henry II, she took cooks with her to prepare her spinach.

A serving of spinach provides an astonishing 1111 percent of the Daily Value for vitamin K and 377 percent of that for vitamin A. It is also high in vitamins B6, C, and E, folate, fiber, manganese, iron, magnesium, riboflavin, calcium, potassium, and copper, and a good source of thiamine, zinc and omega-3 fatty acids. Of particular note is the high level of antioxidants. Frozen and cooked spinach are actually higher in some nutrients because of the greater concentration in volume.

## THE HEALTHY EVIDENCE

The scientific literature is replete not only with studies of the benefits of these nutrients but of spinach itself. A 2010 study in the *International Journal of Molecular Medicine* reported improvement in the inflammation caused by asthma as a result of eating spinach extract. Another 2010 study reported that eating spinach reduced oxidation in the blood, which is associated with several diseases.

## What's in a Serving?

**COOKED SPINACH**
**(1 cup/180 g)**
**Calories:** 41 (173 kJ)
**Protein:** 5.4 g
**Total fat:** 0.5 g
**Saturated fat:** 0.1 g
**Carbohydrates:** 6.8 g
**Fiber:** 4.3 g

## Making the Most of Spinach

Cooking spinach for a short time causes minimal nutrient loss generally, and in fact increases nutrient levels in servings. An excellent cooking method for fresh or thawed frozen spinach is a light sauté in olive oil with other healthy ingredients such as onion or garlic. Using spinach in soups retains minerals and water-soluble vitamins.

## In a Nutshell

**Origin:** Nepal
**Season:** Summer
**Why it's super:** High in vitamins A, B6, C, K, and E, folate, fiber, manganese, magnesium, iron, riboflavin, calcium, potassium, copper, and antioxidants; good source of thiamine, zinc, and omega-3 fatty acids
**Growing at home:** Easy to grow in the home garden

# FRUIT AND POD VEGETABLES
# Okra

*Abelmoschus esculentus*

Okra is a perennial plant of the mallow family, cultivated for its green fruit, which grows up to 7 inches (18 cm) in length and has many seeds. It originated in Africa and spread to the Mediterranean region, only reaching the Americas in the 1600s, likely through the slave trade. Okra is both prized and maligned for its mucilaginous attributes, and is best known for being a key ingredient in the Creole spicy stew, gumbo.

A serving of okra provides 80 percent of the Daily Value for vitamin K and 44 percent of that for vitamin C, and is also high in fiber. In addition, okra is a significant source of vitamins A and B6, folate, niacin, riboflavin, manganese, calcium, magnesium, copper, and potassium. Antioxidants are present as beta-carotene, lutein, and zeaxanthin.

## THE HEALTHY EVIDENCE

Okra's ample supply of key nutrients makes it a beneficial food for disease prevention. A 2009 study in the journal *Food and Chemical Toxicology* also highlighted the antioxidant potential of okra seeds. As researchers add more diseases to the list of those involving oxidative damage, it is clear that consumption of foods with high levels of phytochemicals that function as antioxidants is an effective way to promote health and fight disease. A large epidemiological study reported that a southern-United States dietary pattern, which specifically included okra, was associated with a lower risk of prostate cancer.

### Making the Most of Okra

The traditional ways of preparing okra, in soups and stews, do not diminish the antioxidant, mineral, and fat-soluble-vitamin content. For less gelatinous okra, select very young pods. Okra can also be boiled for a short time until tender, without concern for significant nutrient losses.

### What's in a Serving?

**COOKED OKRA
(1 cup/160 g)**
**Calories:** 35 (150 kJ)
**Protein:** 3 g
**Total fat:** 0.3 g
**Saturated fat:** 0.1 g
**Carbohydrates:** 7.2 g
**Fiber:** 4 g

### In a Nutshell

**Origin:** Africa and the Mediterranean
**Season:** Summer
**Why it's super:** High in vitamins C and K and fiber; good source of vitamins A and B6, folate, niacin, riboflavin, manganese, calcium, magnesium, copper, potassium, and antioxidants
**Growing at home:** Requires a long, frost-free season

BELOW For the best quality, select okra that has a strong green color, a smooth coat of fuzz, and is firm to the touch and blemish free.

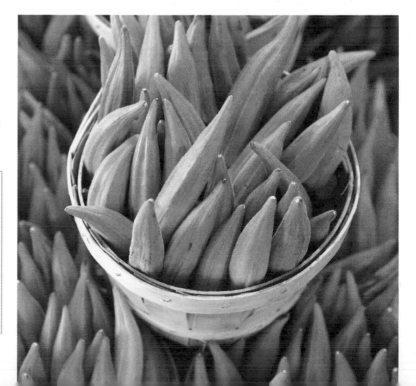

# Bell Pepper or Capsicum

❂ *Capsicum annuum*

BELOW Christopher Columbus first brought bell peppers to Europe, from the New World.

Bell pepper is part of the *Capsicum* genus, which also includes chili peppers (see p. 40). Usually bell-shaped, it grows in a variety of sizes, shapes, and colors—red, green, purple, brown, and even black—but all belong to the same species. Normally, bell peppers measure about 2–5 inches (5–12 cm) around and 2–6 inches (5–15 cm) long, and have three or four lobes at the bottom. The inside is hollow, with edible seeds and a white, spongy core. Bell pepper is called by many names: bell pepper in Canada and the United States; red or green pepper, or sweet pepper in Britain; and capsicum in Australia, New Zealand, and India.

The bright colors of bell peppers attract birds, which eat the pepper and disperse the seeds. Unlike most other members of the *Capsicum* genus, bell pepper does not produce capsaicin, the chemical that produces the "hot" or "spicy" flavor in chili, due to the presence of a recessive gene that eliminates it.

## FLOWER AND FRUIT

Bell pepper is native to the Americas, where it has been cultivated for thousands of years. Although it is a perennial, it is typically grown as an annual. The plant reaches 16–20 inches (40–50 cm) high and puts out a small white flower that produces the fruit, which is green and then may change color as it ripens. Botanically, the fruit is considered a berry.

Bell pepper is an outstanding source of vitamins C and A, the latter in the form of several antioxidants including beta-carotene, alpha-carotene, and beta-cryptoxanthin. It is

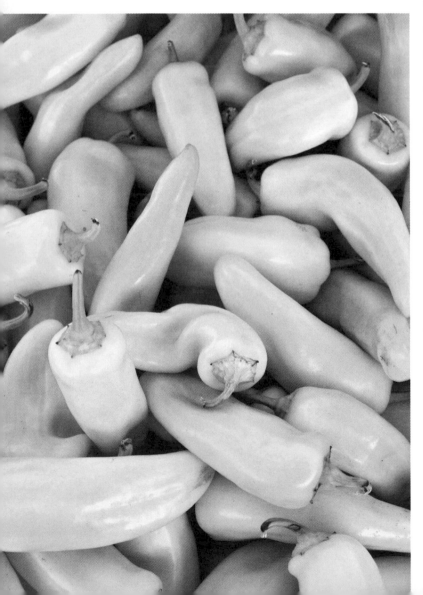

## Making the Most of Bell Peppers

An excellent way to retain the highest level of folate and vitamin C is to use raw peppers as a major ingredient in a fresh chopped-vegetable salad. Other chopped vegetables to add for texture and extra nutrients include carrots, tomato, romaine (cos) lettuce, and onion. Toss with a vinaigrette dressing.

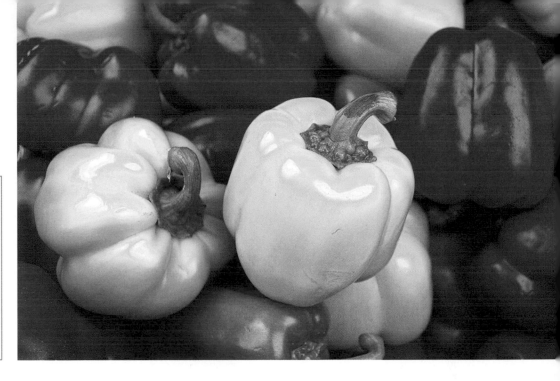

also an excellent source of vitamin B6, folate, and fiber, and a good source of vitamin E, riboflavin, niacin, thiamine, pantothenic acid, potassium, and manganese.

### THE HEALTHY EVIDENCE

A study published in the journal *Cancer Epidemiology, Biomarkers, and Prevention*, involving more than 60,000 adults, reported that those with the highest intake of foods

ABOVE The diverse hues of bell peppers can make for highly colorful dishes. Red, yellow, and orange bell peppers are generally sweeter than the green varieties. The sweetest of all are those ripened on the vine.

containing beta-cryptoxanthin had a 27 percent reduction in risk of lung cancer, and smokers following a similar diet had a 37 percent lower risk. In addition, while folate supplements have not been proven to lower the risk of heart disease, a 2009 review published in the journal *Archives of Cardiovascular Diseases* reported that higher intakes of the diet were associated with a lower risk, and a study in the journal *Metabolism* suggested that those with lower intakes of folate had a higher risk of cardiovascular events.

## How to Pick a Perfect Pepper

There are myriad culinary uses for peppers as well as in salads. They can be used in soups, egg dishes such as frittatas and omelettes, and they can be roasted and puréed. Additionally, they may be dried and ground for both paprika and pimiento. To ensure the freshest peppers, and therefore the highest nutrient content, select peppers that have taut, not wrinkled, skin and no blemishes. They should be firm and feel heavy for their size.

*One man yearns for fame, another for wealth, but everyone yearns for paprika goulash.*

Hungarian proverb

## In a Nutshell

**Origin:** Americas
**Season:** Late summer
**Why it's super:** High in vitamins C, A, and B6, folate, fiber, and antioxidants; good source of vitamin E, riboflavin, niacin, thiamine, pantothenic acid, potassium, and manganese
**Growing at home:** Easy to grow in the home garden

# Chili Pepper

✪ *Capsicum annuum*

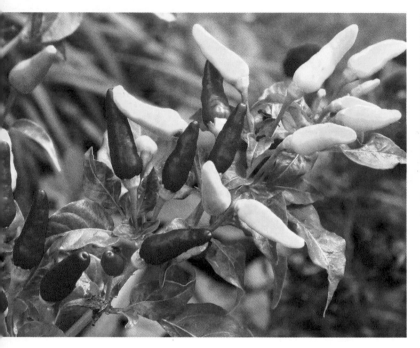

## Making the Most of Chili Pepper

The traditional ways of enjoying chili pepper are either in chili—a stew of ground meat, beans, and tomatoes—or in salsa. However, eating it raw will retain the high level of vitamin C: add a little chopped raw chili to whole-grain tortilla chips topped with melted low-fat cheese.

LEFT When chili peppers are consumed in moderation, their warmth can be an appetite stimulant as well as an aid to digestion.

Research has shown that capsaicin has significant potential health benefits, and it is widely used in topical ointments to relieve mild pain associated with arthritis, muscle aches, and pain associated with nerve conditions (neuropathies).

## THE HEALTHY EVIDENCE

A 2006 study in the journal *Cancer Research* reported that capsaicin used on human prostate cancer cells caused apoptosis, or cell suicide, leading the authors to suggest that it "may have a role in the management of prostate cancer." Studies published in the same journal two years earlier showed that capsaicin directly inhibited the growth of leukemic cells.

Chili pepper belongs to the same species as bell pepper (see p. 39), but contains capsaicin, the chemical that produces its hot or spicy flavor. The level of capsaicin varies widely, even in peppers from the same plant. It is unpleasant to most mammals and so deters consumption, while the bright colors attract birds, which are not affected by the capsaicin and consume the pepper and disperse its seeds. Capsaicin is not only spicy to taste, but can also irritate skin.

Just 3 tablespoons of chili pepper provide 67 percent of the Daily Value for vitamin C and are a good source of vitamins A, B6, and K. However, caution is advised when consuming chili as ingestion of large amounts by adults, or even small amounts by children, can cause nausea, vomiting, abdominal pain, and burning diarrhea.

## What's in a Serving?

**RAW CHILI PEPPER**
**(3 tablespoons/28 g)**
**Calories:** 11 (47 kJ)
**Protein:** 0.6 g
**Total fat:** 0.1 g
**Saturated fat:** 0 g
**Carbohydrates:** 2.7 g
**Fiber:** 0.4 g

## In a Nutshell

**Origin:** Americas
**Season:** Late summer
**Why it's super:** High in vitamin C and capsaicin; good source of vitamins A, B6, and K
**Growing at home:** Requires a long, frost-free season

# Summer Squash

✪ *Cucurbita pepo*

Summer squash, unlike their close relatives winter squash (see p. 42), are harvested when immature; if left on the plant too long they become fibrous and unappetizing. The best-known kind of summer squash is zucchini, also called courgette. Though these names come from Italy and France, respectively, summer squash most likely originated in Mexico and South America, where it has been cultivated for more than 5,000 years. Columbus brought it back to Europe, where it gained favor in the nineteenth century among the Italians, who then introduced it to France. Although most people eat only the fruit, the Italians and some other cultures also consume the yellow flowers.

Most home gardeners know the fruitful nature of the zucchini plant, and in fact are hard-pressed to devise new ways to eat the vegetable. However, they are not always aware of the vegetable's significant nutritional benefits. A 1-cup serving provides almost half of the day's need for vitamin A, and is a significant source of vitamins B6, C, and K, folate, thiamine, magnesium, manganese, potassium, and copper. It also provides a high level of the antioxidants beta-carotene, lutein, and zeaxanthin.

### Making the Most of Summer Squash

Most of the nutrients in summer squash hold up well to cooking, and those are the nutrients present in the largest amounts. The high water content and delicate flesh argue for rapid cooking with little or no liquid, such as roasting, sautéing, or simply placing in a covered dish in the microwave for a few minutes with no water added.

## THE HEALTHY EVIDENCE

An article published in the journal *Public Health Nutrition* reported that squash extracts reduced symptoms of a common condition affecting older men, benign prostatic hypertrophy. The high content of lutein may help protect against dementia associated with ageing, as suggested by a 2010 review article in the journal *Clinics in Geriatric Medicine*.

### In a Nutshell

**Origin:** Mexico and South America

**Season:** Summer

**Why they're super:** High in vitamin A and antioxidants; good source of vitamins B6, C, and K, folate, thiamine, magnesium, manganese, potassium, and copper

**Growing at home:** Easy to grow in the home garden

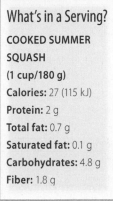

### What's in a Serving?

**COOKED SUMMER SQUASH**

**(1 cup/180 g)**

**Calories:** 27 (115 kJ)

**Protein:** 2 g

**Total fat:** 0.7 g

**Saturated fat:** 0.1 g

**Carbohydrates:** 4.8 g

**Fiber:** 1.8 g

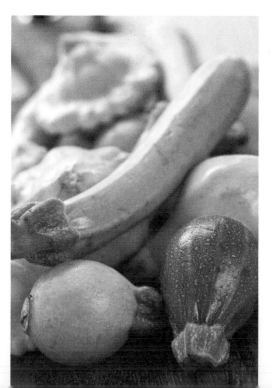

LEFT Summer squash must be consumed soon after picking or purchasing, unlike winter squash, which will keep for weeks or even months.

# Winter Squash or Pumpkin

✪ *Cucurbita maxima* Hubbard Squash, Pumpkin
✪ *Cucurbita moschata* Butternut Squash
✪ *Cucurbita pepo* Acorn Squash

BELOW Versatile and nutrient-rich, butternut squash has a sweet, nutty flavor. Its thick skin makes it an excellent storage vegetable.

Winter squash is the name for those members of the Cucurbitaceae family that are thick-skinned and are harvested as mature fruit in late autumn; thinner-skinned squashes that are harvested earlier in the season are known as summer squash (see p. 41). The winter squashes include butternut squash, acorn squash, Hubbard squash, pumpkin, and other varieties—the list grows every year as existing varieties cross-pollinate.

As well as thick skin, winter squashes usually have a mildly sweet and fine-grained flesh and a central cavity containing seeds. Their shapes and colors vary widely. Hubbard squash ranges from squat-shaped, colored either red or green, to a larger pear shape with bumpy green skin. Acorn squash resembles a large acorn, with dark green skin. The butternut varieties are pear-shaped and have smooth, pale yellow skin. Pumpkins are hugely varied, but typically have bright orange skin. Because of the hard shell, the flesh is protected and winter squash may last up to six months in storage.

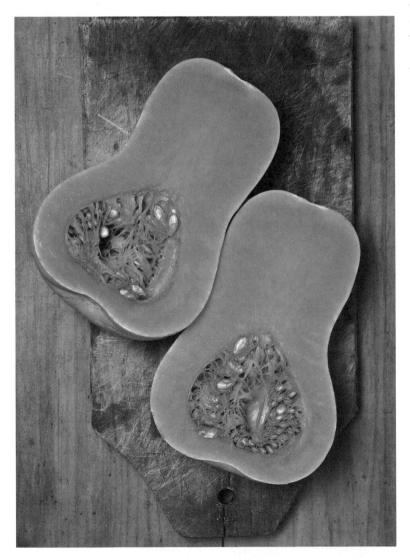

## In a Nutshell

**Origin:** South America
**Season:** Late autumn
**Why they're super:** High in vitamins A and C, fiber, manganese, potassium, and antioxidants
**Growing at home:** Easy to grow in the home garden

## What's in a Serving?

| COOKED BUTTERNUT SQUASH (½ cup/102 g) | COOKED HUBBARD SQUASH (½ cup/103 g) |
|---|---|
| **Calories:** 41 (173 kJ) | **Calories:** 51 (214 kJ) |
| **Protein:** 0.9 g | **Protein:** 2.5 g |
| **Total fat:** 0.1 g | **Total fat:** 0.1 g |
| **Saturated fat:** 0 g | **Saturated fat:** 0 g |
| **Carbohydrates:** 11 g | **Carbohydrates:** 11 g |
| **Fiber:** 5 g | **Fiber:** 3 g |

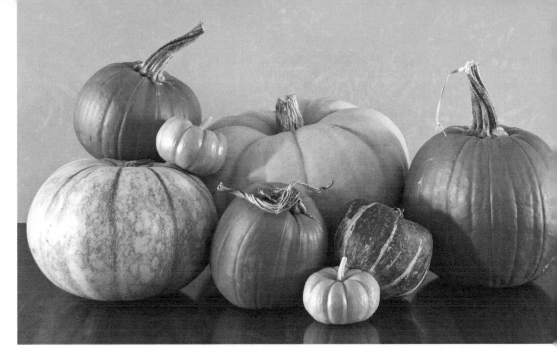

One of the most popular culinary uses for pumpkin in the United States and Canada is in pumpkin pie, served at Thanksgiving dinners. Winter squash can also be used in soups, or roasted, boiled, or mashed. The seeds are often roasted and eaten as a snack, and the flowers are edible as well: they are used as a garnish, or battered and deep-fried.

## JUDGING BY THE COLOR

Deep orange pigmentation is one of the hallmarks of beta-carotene content, and these foods live up to their colorful appearance. All contain beta-carotene, though pumpkin and butternut are superior in that regard, as well as in their content of two other anti-oxidant carotenoids, alpha-carotene and beta-cryptoxanthin; only pumpkin has a significant amount of lutein and zeaxanthin.

Of the three species of squash, acorn squash, which is the palest, has the lowest level of vitamin A, with 8 percent of the Daily Value in a ½-cup serving; butternut squash and Hubbard squash provide 230 percent and 140 percent, respectively. However, pumpkin exceeds all of the squashes, providing 380 percent of the Daily Value. All are also excellent sources of vitamin C, fiber, potassium, and manganese, although butternut has twice the level of vitamin C relative to the other types of squash, and pumpkin has the lowest level.

## THE HEALTHY EVIDENCE

As potent antioxidants, carotenoids help prevent diseases in which oxidative damage plays a role, such as cardiovascular disease and cancer. A 2009 study published in the journal *Cancer Research* reported that women with the highest blood levels of alpha-carotene, lutein, zeaxanthin, and beta-cryptoxanthin had as much as a 50 percent reduction in breast cancer risk. This was particularly true for women with high mammographic density, a common condition and a major predictor of breast-cancer risk.

ABOVE American colonists filled the insides of the pumpkin with honey and spices, then baked it, creating the original pumpkin pie.

### What's in a Serving?

| COOKED PUMPKIN (½ cup/122 g) | COOKED ACORN SQUASH (½ cup/123 g) |
|---|---|
| **Calories:** 24 (102 kJ) | **Calories:** 67 (282 kJ) |
| **Protein:** 0.9 g | **Protein:** 0.8 g |
| **Total fat:** 0.1 g | **Total fat:** 0.1 g |
| **Saturated fat:** 0 g | **Saturated fat:** 0 g |
| **Carbohydrates:** 6 g | **Carbohydrates:** 11 g |
| **Fiber:** 1.3 g | **Fiber:** 3.2 g |

### Making the Most of Winter Squash

During boiling, vitamin C seeps into the water, so baking or roasting is preferable; microwaving in a little water is another good option. The carotenoid antioxidants, however, are not lost in cooking liquid. Thus canned pumpkin is an excellent choice; in fact the canning process increases the concentration of carotenoids. Add canned pumpkin to soups, stews, and bread products, or to vanilla yogurt or dessert.

# Tomato

✪ *Lycopersicon esculentum*

The history of the tomato is an interesting case of mistaken identity, on at least a couple of counts. The misinformation began with a long-held belief, up until the sixteenth century, that the tomato was poisonous—this was based on its membership of the night-shade family, which includes infamous and toxic relatives such as poisonous nightshade (bittersweet) and black henbane. Confusion persists to the present with the widespread belief that tomato is a vegetable, even though it is classified botanically as a fruit.

The tomato originated in tropical regions of South and Central America, where the Aztecs first cultivated it. The Spanish brought it back to Europe, where it was treated with suspicion for many years before becoming a staple ingredient in Mediterranean cuisine. It was then taken back to America in the late 1700s and within the next 60 years widely cultivated, leading in turn to large-scale canning and bottling of various tomato products, including ketchup, now a staple of the Western diet.

## What's in a Serving?

**RAW TOMATO**
**(1 cup/180 g)**
**Calories:** 32 (135 kJ)
**Protein:** 1.6 g
**Total fat:** 0.4 g
**Saturated fat:** 0.1 g
**Carbohydrates:** 7 g
**Fiber:** 2.2 g

BELOW In 1893, the US Supreme Court ruled that the tomato is a vegetable, even though it is botanically a fruit.

## POWERFUL ANTIOXIDANTS

Though virtually all cultures have made use of tomatoes, the Italians have led the way. A basic tomato product from which many others emanate, tomato purée, is also known as passata. This is the Italian word from the phrase *passata di pomodoro*, which literally means that the tomato has passed through a sieve. The terms are not synonymous, however, as in the United Kingdom tomato purée refers to what Americans identify as tomato paste. These tomato products, and others including canned whole and diced tomatoes and tomato juice, are available today in reduced-sodium varieties.

Recently, the tomato has been in the spotlight for having the highest level of the carotenoid lycopene of any widely consumed food—the name lycopene actually derives from the first part of the tomato's scientific name. For decades, lycopene was largely ignored due to its lack of vitamin A activity—conversion of nutrients to vitamin A had long

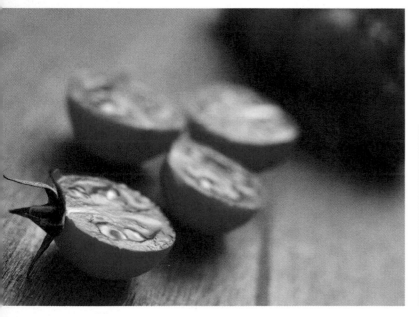

## Making the Most of Tomatoes

To obtain maximum vitamin C, eat tomatoes raw. However, the lycopene in tomatoes is best absorbed by the body from cooked tomato products, and the addition of fat, preferably in the form of a healthy oil such as canola or olive oil, increases lycopene absorption in the small intestine. When buying tomato products such as purée and canned tomatoes, choose those with reduced sodium, if available.

**In a Nutshell**

**Origin:** South and Central America

**Season:** Summer

**Why it's super:** High in vitamins A, C, and K and lycopene; good source of vitamin B6, folate, fiber, potassium, manganese, chromium, and the anti-oxidants beta-carotene, lutein, and zeaxanthin

**Growing at home:** Easy to grow in the home garden

been thought to be the only important role for the carotenoids. One scientist even labeled it as inert, saying, "So far as is known, lycopene is neither toxic nor beneficial, but is only an adventitious visitor to the body." But recent studies have shown that, far from being inert, it possesses superior antioxidant effects relative to other carotenoids.

Tomato is also an excellent source of vitamin C, with one serving providing more than half of the Daily Value, and of vitamins A and K. Tomato is, furthermore, a significant source of vitamin B6, folate, fiber, manganese, chromium, and potassium, and contains the antioxidants beta-carotene, lutein, and zeaxanthin.

## THE HEALTHY EVIDENCE

A 2008 review in the journal *Cancer Letters* reported studies of various types, including epidemiological and in-vitro experiments, showing that the more lycopene consumed the smaller the risk of prostate cancer. Other types of cancer may also be influenced by lycopene: a 2007 study in *Cancer Causes & Control* showed that cooked tomato consumption was associated with a lower risk of multiple myeloma, a form of bone cancer.

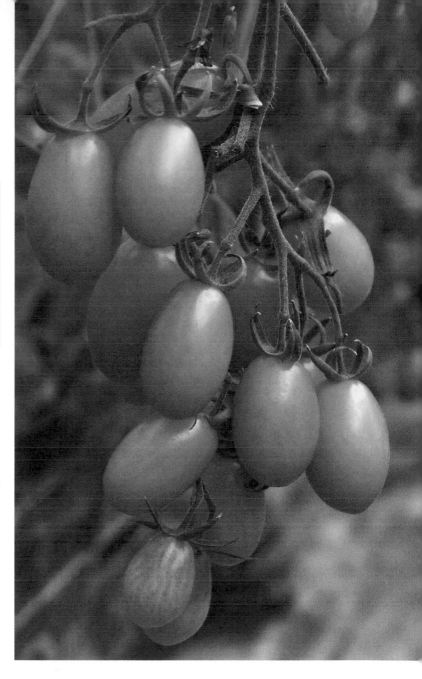

ABOVE In France, the tomato is traditionally known as the "apple of love." Not to be outdone, the Germans named it the "apple of paradise."

*It's difficult to think anything but pleasant thoughts while eating a homegrown tomato.*

Lewis Grizzard, Jr., US humorist (1946–94)

# Bitter Melon or Goya

✴ *Momordica charantia*

## What's in a Serving?

**COOKED BITTER MELON**

**(1 cup/180 g)**

**Calories:** 34 (142 kJ)

**Protein:** 1.5 g

**Total fat:** 0.3 g

**Saturated fat:** 0 g

**Carbohydrates:** 7.7 g

**Fiber:** 3.6 g

This food is aptly named, because bitter melon is one of the most bitter tasting of all vegetables. It is also known as bitter gourd, or by its Japanese name, goya. Though its precise origin is unknown, it is thought to be a tropical plant that spread throughout India, Asia, and the Caribbean. The vine grows up to 17 feet (5 m) tall, producing fruit that resembles a bumpy cucumber. Cutting the fruit lengthwise reveals a hollow central cavity with large flat seeds inside a thin layer of flesh.

Many cultures around the world consider bitter melon to have important medicinal properties, and scientists have identified one compound in the plant, momordicin, as having potential gastrointestinal benefits. The nutrient contained in the highest amount is vitamin C—a 1-cup serving of bitter melon provides an entire day's supply. Bitter melon is also high in folate, fiber, and potassium, and a good source of vitamin K, thiamine, riboflavin, and zinc.

### THE HEALTHY EVIDENCE

Canadian researchers published an article in the *Journal of Ethnopharmacology* reporting that extracts prepared from bitter melon showed high antiviral activity. A 2006 report in *Nutrition Reviews* pointed to studies of its ability to reduce insulin resistance, which can

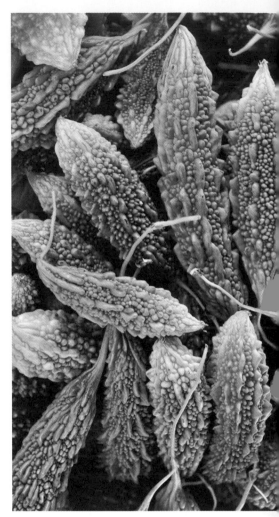

ABOVE An oddly shaped, knobbly skin conceals the fruit of the bitter melon. As it ripens, the fruit becomes increasingly bitter.

lead to type 2 diabetes. In addition, the abundance of vitamin C, fiber, and folate would suggest protection against cardio-vascular disease and cancer.

## In a Nutshell

**Origin:** Unknown

**Season:** Summer

**Why it's super:** High in vitamin C, folate, fiber, and potassium; good source of vitamin K, thiamine, riboflavin, and zinc

**Growing at home:** Easy to grow in the home garden

## Making the Most of Bitter Melon

The nutrient contained in the highest amount is vitamin C; restricting the cooking time will help preserve it. A most appropriate way, therefore, to cook bitter melon, and the most common way, is to incorporate the vegetable into a stir-fry.

# Sprouts

✪ *Phaseolus aureus* Mung Bean
✪ *Pisum sativum* var. *macrocarpon* Snap Peas, Snow Peas

Sprouts may be grown from seeds, grains, or beans. Beans may be sprouted in light or dark conditions. Those that are sprouted in the dark are crisper in texture and lighter in color, but have less nutritional content than those grown in partial sunlight. Commercially grown sprouts are usually raised in the dark.

Among the most popular sources of sprouts are mung beans and snap or snow peas. Mung beans come from India and the English word derives from the Hindi *moong*; mung bean sprouts are also referred to as "mongo" or "moong." The pea sprouts, also known as pea shoots, are harvested from the growing point of a plant and should be used at a young stage for optimal tenderness.

Mung sprouts are an excellent source of vitamins C and K and folate, and a significant source of vitamin B6, fiber, riboflavin, niacin, pantothenic acid, iron, manganese, copper, magnesium, and potassium. Pea sprouts have a similar nutrient profile and also contain high levels of vitamins A and E, with the vitamin A in the form of the carotenoid antioxidants.

## THE HEALTHY EVIDENCE

A study in *Critical Reviews in Food Science and Nutrition* reported that sprouting increases the activity of enzymes and levels of protein, fat, and B vitamins in the beans. Sprouts also contain antioxidants—as vitamin C in mung sprouts and as carotenoids and vitamin C in pea sprouts—so both offer protection against cardiovascular disease and cancer.

BELOW In East Asian cuisine, mung sprouts are used as a filling for Vietnamese spring rolls and frequently added to Chinese stir-fries.

### In a Nutshell

**Origin:** Mung beans: India; snow peas: southwestern Asia and India

**Season:** May be sprouted at any time of year

**Why they're super:** High in vitamins C and K and folate; good source of vitamin B6, fiber, riboflavin, niacin, pantothenic acid, iron, manganese, copper, magnesium, and potassium; pea sprouts are also high in vitamins A and E and antioxidants

**Growing at home:** Can easily be germinated at home

### What's in a Serving?

**MUNG SPROUTS**
**(2 cups/208 g)**
**Calories:** 62 (262 kJ)
**Protein:** 6.3 g
**Total fat:** 0.1 g
**Saturated fat:** 0.3 g
**Carbohydrates:** 12 g
**Fiber:** 3.7 g

**PEA SPROUTS**
**(2 cups/208 g)**
**Calories:** 298 (1,246 kJ)
**Protein:** 21 g
**Total fat:** 1.6 g
**Saturated fat:** 0.3 g
**Carbohydrates:** 65 g
**Fiber:** 0 g

### Making the Most of Sprouts

The optimal way to retain nutrients is to use the raw sprouts as salad ingredients. Serve a fresh mound of pea shoots with a squeeze of lemon juice and season with ground ginger. If using sprouts in a stir-fry, add near the end of cooking.

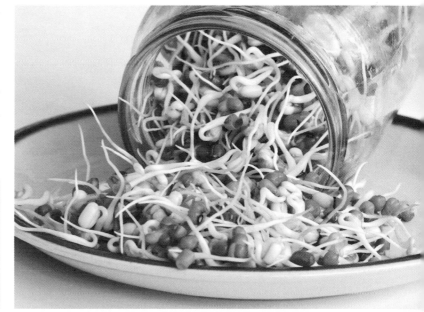

# Green Beans

✪ *Phaseolus coccineus* Runner Bean
✪ *Phaseolus vulgaris* Common Green Bean
✪ *Vigna unguiculata* Snake Bean

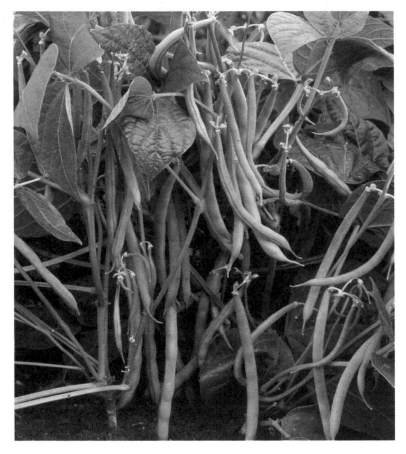

ABOVE So-called French beans are often slightly longer and narrower than other common beans, as with this cultivar, known as 'Verity'.

The term "green beans" refers to the unripe fruit of many types of beans, and includes more than 130 varieties of plant. The most widely grown, *Phaseolus vulgaris*, is usually known as the common green bean or common bean, though it has many aliases in the United States, such as string bean or snap bean. The haricot bean or *haricot vert* (French for "green bean") is the same species, but often slightly thinner and longer. The common green bean was first cultivated in Peru around 5000 BCE, and has been grown in Central America for 5,000 years.

## RUNNERS AND SNAKES

Runner bean, *Phaseolus coccineus*, is sometimes referred to as the scarlet runner because of its red flowers and the colored seeds of many of its varieties. It originated in the mountainous interior of Central America. Although it is a perennial plant, most growers use it as an annual. In the early growth stage, the pod tends to become fibrous, so that only the seeds within the pod are used.

Snake bean is also known as the yardlong bean, Chinese long bean, asparagus bean, and long-podded cowpea. Its scientific name, *Vigna unguiculata*, encompasses several

*What shall I learn
of beans or beans of me?
I cherish them, I hoe them, early
and late I have an eye for them;
and this is my day's work.*

Henry David Thoreau, US writer (1817–62)

## Making the Most of Green Beans

Short cooking methods such as steaming or roasting will best preserve the high vitamin C content. To enhance the body's absorption of the plentiful iron in the vegetable, add acidic ingredients such as lemon juice or diced tomato. Green beans are also a common ingredient in Asian-style stir-fries, where they work particularly well.

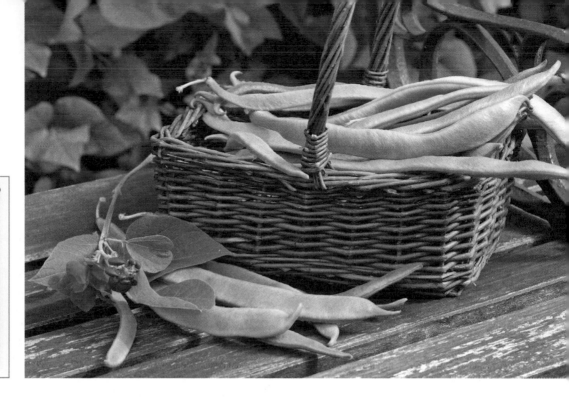

## In a Nutshell

**Origin:** Common bean: Peru and Central America; runner bean: Central America; snake bean: Africa and China

**Season:** Summer

**Why they're super:** High in vitamins A, C, and K, fiber, and manganese; good source of folate, niacin, riboflavin, potassium, iron, magnesium, copper, calcium, and antioxidants

**Growing at home:** Easy to grow in the home garden

varieties, including the black-eyed pea, and collectively the legumes from the pod are known as cowpeas. Most of the common names derive from the shape and length of the pod, which can grow to 14–30 inches (35–75 cm). Snake beans are a traditional African crop and widespread in Asia, though they are not well known elsewhere.

The nutrient found in green beans in the highest amount is vitamin C—a 1-cup serving provides a full day's supply. Green beans are also an excellent source of vitamins A and K, fiber, and manganese, and a good source of folate, niacin, riboflavin, potassium, iron, magnesium, copper, calcium, and the anti-oxidants beta-carotene, lutein, and zeaxanthin.

### THE HEALTHY EVIDENCE

A 2008 article in the *Journal of Food Science* reported that antioxidant content in frozen and cooked green beans was still excellent, although excessive boiling did reduce vitamin C content. The potassium, vitamin C, folate, carotenoids, and fiber all provide protection against heart disease and stroke. As part of a diet containing five specific vegetables, green beans reduced asthma symptoms in children, according to a 2007 study in *Pediatric Allergy and Immunology*. Feeding mice a diet containing green beans and three other vegetables inhibited atherosclerosis in a 2006 study.

### Selecting for Freshness

Purchase green beans loose rather than prepackaged, as then the best quality beans can be selected. Look for consistent coloration and avoid those with spots and bruises. Firmness is an indication of freshness and optimal vitamin content. If you break one of the pods, it should snap cleanly.

ABOVE Its striking scarlet blooms make the runner bean much treasured as an ornamental plant as well as a vegetable.

# Peas

✪ *Pisum sativum* Peas
✪ *Pisum sativum* var. *macrocarpon* Snap Peas, Snow Peas

The bane of many a child at the dinner table, the small green spheres known as peas are botanically a fruit, but usually eaten as a vegetable and enjoyed in many forms. The peas alone may be eaten, or peas and pod consumed whole, as with snow peas and snap peas (also known as sugar snap peas). These two peas are actually the same plant at different stages of growth: snow pea refers to the stage when the pod is flat, snap pea to the stage when it has matured further and is cylindrical. The French term *mangetout*, meaning "eat all," refers to both these peas. In addition, peas can also be dried and used to make a variety of dishes (see pp. 80, 88).

BELOW Norse peoples dedicated the pea to their god Thor, and only ate them on his day, Thursday.

## Choice Peas

When selecting snap peas, look for pods that are bright green with no blemishes and no wrinkles toward the ends of the pods. They should have a plump appearance, without demarcation of the peas within. Snow peas should also be bright green in color, and have flat, firm pods. Avoid those in which the peas inside appear large.

## AN ANCIENT, VITAL FOOD

Peas originated in the Mediterranean region and central Asia and were cultivated by many early cultures. Archaeologists have

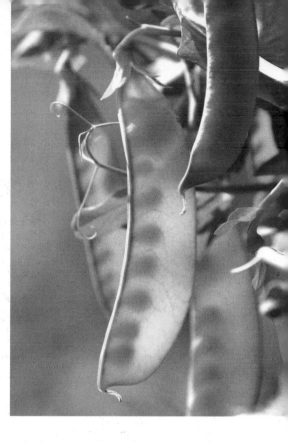

## Making the Most of Peas

Snap peas make an excellent addition to a raw vegetable tray, and eating them raw preserves the vitamin C, folate, and the B vitamins, which are sensitive to heat. Steaming and stir-frying are effective methods for limiting cooking time and using minimal liquid so that water-soluble nutrients are not lost into the cooking water. To boost nutrient content in soups and stews, add frozen green peas toward the end of the cooking time.

found them in ancient tombs, and discovered ancient treatises discussing the virtues of peas. Though dried peas were a staple in Europe from the Middle Ages on, Europeans did not start eating fresh peas until the late 1600s, when they became a fashionable delicacy.

Peas are an outstanding source of vitamins A, B6, C, and K, folate, fiber, protein, thiamine, niacin, and riboflavin, and a significant source of magnesium, potassium, iron, copper, and zinc. Peas also contain the antioxidant carotenoids beta-carotene, alpha-carotene, lutein, and zeaxanthin. Frozen peas maintain their nutrient levels, particularly if they are not exposed to long cooking times and excessive liquid. With modern canning processes, canned peas also retain their nutritive value.

## What's in a Serving?

**COOKED PEAS**
**(1 cup/160 g)**
**Calories:** 134 (563 kJ)
**Protein:** 8.6 g
**Total fat:** 0.4 g
**Saturated fat:** 0.1 g
**Carbohydrates:** 25 g
**Fiber:** 8.8 g

**COOKED SNAP PEAS**
**(1 cup/160 g)**
**Calories:** 67 (282 kJ)
**Protein:** 5.2 g
**Total fat:** 0.4 g
**Saturated fat:** 0.1 g
**Carbohydrates:** 11.3 g
**Fiber:** 4.5 g

ABOVE Bright color is a sign of a good snap pea. In the Middle Ages, pea purée often replaced gravy during Lent, when meat could not be eaten.

### THE HEALTHY EVIDENCE

In addition to the numerous cardio-protective nutrients, such as folate, vitamin B6, fiber, potassium, and the carotenoids, peas along with other non-soy legumes may help to lower blood cholesterol. A meta-analysis, which is a pooling of similar studies, published in a 2009 article in the journal *Nutrition, Metabolism, and Cardiovascular Diseases* reported that a diet high in peas and other legumes significantly lowered both total and LDL cholesterol in men and women.

## In a Nutshell

**Origin:** The Mediterranean and central Asia
**Season:** Late spring to mid-autumn
**Why they're super:** High in vitamins A, B6, C, and K, folate, fiber, protein, thiamine, niacin, and riboflavin; good source of magnesium, potassium, iron, copper, zinc, and antioxidants
**Growing at home:** Easy to grow in the home garden

*We lived very simply—but with all the essentials of life well understood and provided for—hot baths, cold champagne, new peas, and old brandy.*

Winston Churchill, British statesman (1874–1965)

# Eggplant or Aubergine

✪ *Solanum melongena*

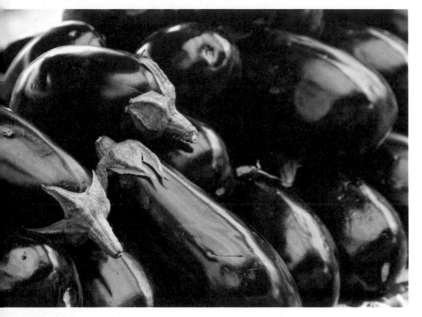

## Making the Most of Eggplant

Since most of the important nutrients and phytochemicals are resistant to cooking, eggplant can be cooked, puréed, or roasted. Asian cuisines often use eggplant in stir-fries, as well. To make the popular Mediterranean dip baba ghanoush, brush the eggplant with olive oil and roast; then remove the seeds, purée, add tahini and garlic, and season to taste.

LEFT The purple eggplant is the most widely recognized and eaten aubergine cultivar in the Western world. Salting eggplant before cooking will limit the amount of oil that is absorbed in cooking.

Eggplant, also known as aubergine and begun, is a member of the nightshade family and a close relative of the tomato. Because of its membership of this family, it was for a long time feared to be poisonous. Eggplant originated in India and was introduced to Europe by the Arabs during the Middle Ages, though it did not gain its current popularity among Mediterranean cultures until the fifteenth century. There are many varieties of eggplant, of different colors and shapes, although the most familiar is the oblong, dark purple variety.

Eggplant is a good source of vitamin B6, fiber, potassium, manganese, copper, and thiamine. More significantly, eggplant contains numerous phytochemicals, including antioxidant phenols, anthocyanins, and plant sterols, which lower blood cholesterol.

## What's in a Serving?

**COOKED EGGPLANT (1 cup/99 g)**
**Calories:** 35 (146 kJ)
**Protein:** 0.8 g
**Total fat:** 0.2 g
**Saturated fat:** 0 g
**Carbohydrates:** 8.6 g
**Fiber:** 2.5 g

## In a Nutshell

**Origin:** India
**Season:** Late summer to early autumn
**Why it's super:** High in plant sterols, phenols, and anthocyanins; good source of vitamin B6, fiber, potassium, manganese, copper, and thiamine
**Growing at home:** Easy to grow in the home garden

### THE HEALTHY EVIDENCE

A 2009 study published in the journal *Food and Chemical Toxicology* reported that purple eggplant had an excellent ability to scavenge free radicals, because of its level of antioxidants in the form of phenols and anthocyanins. One specific anthocyanin, nasunin, was also shown to have favorable effects on blood vessels in a 2005 study. Eggplant was part of a diet that helped to lower blood cholesterol as effectively as statin drugs in a study published in 2005 in the *American Journal of Clinical Nutrition*; the effect was assumed to be due to eggplant's content of plant sterols.

# Broad or Fava Bean

✪ *Vicia faba*

Broad beans are an ancient food with many common names, including fava, faba, field, bell, and tic bean. Although they originated in Africa, the Mediterranean, and southwestern Asia, they have been cultivated in many parts of the world for centuries, and are still a staple food in many countries. The plant is a hardy annual with large seed pods up to 12 inches (30 cm) in length. Most typically, the beans are shelled and cooked—young beans have a better flavor than older ones—but the Italians sometimes also eat the pods fresh while they are young and tender, and cook the more mature pods.

Broad beans are high in many nutrients, with a single serving of raw pods providing 47 percent of the Daily Value for folate, 42 percent for manganese, and 20 percent for protein. Broad beans are also a significant source of vitamins A and C, fiber, niacin, riboflavin, thiamine, iron, potassium, copper, and magnesium. In addition, they contain a high level of phytosterols, which have been shown to lower blood cholesterol.

## THE HEALTHY EVIDENCE

The excellent content of folate, fiber, potassium, and vitamins A and C suggests that broad beans will provide protection against cardiovascular disease. A review published in the *British Journal of Nutrition* reported on the cholesterol-lowering effect of the beans and recommended their daily inclusion in a diet for therapeutic benefit.

## In a Nutshell

**Origin:** Africa, the Mediterranean, and southwestern Asia
**Season:** Summer
**Why it's super:** High in protein, manganese, folate, and phytosterols; good source of vitamins A and C, fiber, niacin, riboflavin, thiamine, iron, potassium, magnesium, and copper
**Growing at home:** Easy to grow in the home garden

## Making the Most of Broad Beans

Broad beans contain a high level of folate, which is sensitive to heat, so it is best to keep any cooking time as short as possible. Try lightly cooking the beans in a microwave oven with only a small amount of water—just long enough for the beans to become slightly tender while retaining their crispness.

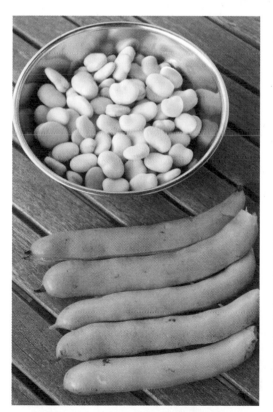

LEFT Fava beans, shown here in the pod and shelled, are rich in L-dopa, which helps control hypertension and Parkinson's disease.

## What's in a Serving?

**RAW BROAD BEANS
(1 cup/126 g)**
**Calories:** 111 (466 kJ)
**Protein:** 10 g
**Total fat:** 0.9 g
**Saturated fat:** 0.1 g
**Carbohydrates:** 22.2 g
**Fiber:** 5.5 g

## ROOT, BULB, AND TUBEROUS VEGETABLES

# Onion

✿ *Allium cepa*

The name "onion" comes from the Latin *unio*, which means "one." The onion is so named because it produces a single bulb, unlike its relative, garlic (see p. 154), each plant of which produces many bulbs. Onion bulbs may be red, white, or brown, and the flavor is determined by type. There are more than 1200 varieties of onions, but they fall into two broad categories: spring–summer onions and cold-climate storage onions.

Onions of the former group tend to be sweeter and milder. They include the cultivars

### A Potent Substance

The onion has a long and venerable history, dating back to ancient times. The Egyptians believed that its spherical shape and concentric rings were a symbol of eternal life—historical sources note that onion residue was placed in the eye sockets of Ramses IV, and other pharaohs were buried with onions. In ancient Rome, gladiators massaged themselves with onions, believing that it firmed the muscles.

BELOW So-called red onions are often purple in color. The color may disappear in cooking.

'Maui Sweet Onion' (in season spring to early summer), 'Vidalia' (late spring to early summer) and 'Walla Walla' (summer). Spring–summer onions don't store well and are available only at certain times of the year. The cold-climate varieties are typically dried for several months after harvest and have a dry, crisp skin; they are referred to by color: white, red, or brown.

### DISTINCTIVE VARIETIES

The shallot is a variety of onion that looks like garlic—with small, papery bulbs—and tastes a bit like an onion, but with a sweeter, milder flavor. Shallots tend to be more expensive than onions, especially in the United States. They can be stored for at least six months.

Another distinctive variety of onion is the scallion, also known as the spring onion,

### In a Nutshell

**Origin:** Uncertain; probably Asia

**Season:** Sweet onions available only during summer months, cold-climate varieties all year long

**Why it's super:** High in antioxidant flavonoids and phenols; good source of vitamins B6 and C, potassium, and manganese

**Growing at home:** Easy to grow in the home garden

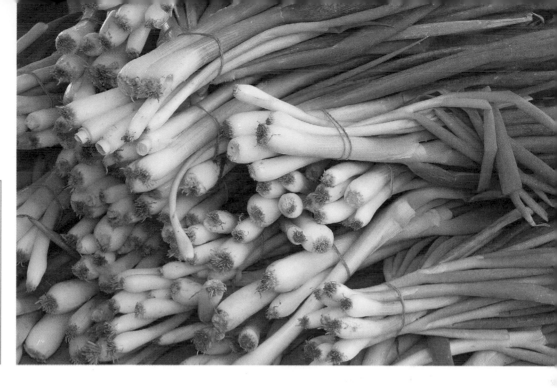

## What's in a Serving?

**COOKED ONIONS**

**(½ cup/105 g)**

**Calories:** 46 (193 kJ)

**Protein:** 1.4 g

**Total fat:** 0.2 g

**Saturated fat:** 0 g

**Carbohydrates:** 10.7 g

**Fiber:** 1.5 g

salad onion, or green onion. It has a hollow upper green portion and lacks a fully developed root bulb; its taste is milder than most onions.

Onions are a good source of vitamins C, B6, potassium, and manganese. Even more significantly, onions contain various phytochemicals that have been the focus of numerous studies related to health. These include a group of flavonoid compounds that function as antioxidants, notably quercetin, kaempferol, and myricetin. Studies have suggested that these compounds may play a role in cancer prevention. Quercetin has been shown to be a particularly powerful antioxidant, and it is found at high levels in many onion cultivars. All members of the onion family are good sources of the various flavonoids, but shallots contain the most and the 'Western White' onion the least.

### THE HEALTHY EVIDENCE

A 2006 study published in the *American Journal of Clinical Nutrition* reported that onion consumption was associated with a lower risk for head and neck cancers. A 2005 study reported that, in addition

### Making the Most of Onions

The nutritional benefits of the flavonoid and phenol compounds are not affected by cooking. Onions can be sliced and sautéed in a healthy oil and added to entrées and side dishes to boost health benefits. To save time during the week, sauté several onions at one time, place in a covered container, and use whenever needed.

to protection against cancer and cardiovascular disease (provided by the antioxidants), onion consumption was linked to a lower risk for developing osteoporosis in women, particularly in those at higher risk for the disease.

*The onion and its satin wrappings is among the most beautiful of vegetables and is the only one that represents the essence of things. It can be said to have a soul.*

Charles Dudley Warner, US novelist and essayist (1829–1900)

# Leek

✿ *Allium porrum*

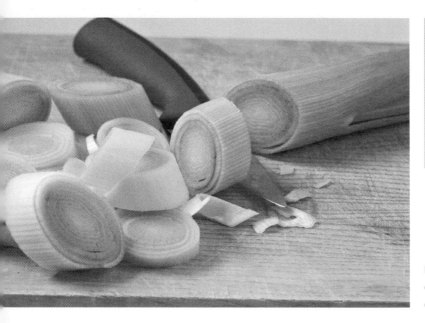

## In a Nutshell

**Origin:** Middle East, Mediterranean

**Season:** Summer through early winter

**Why it's super:** High in flavonoid compounds; good source of vitamins C and K and manganese

**Growing at home:** Relatively easy to grow in the home garden

LEFT It is the lower, paler part of the leek plant that is most commonly eaten. The leek is the symbol of Wales, and Welsh soldiers sport sprigs of leek in their caps on St. David's Day (March 1), the national day.

The leek is a member of the Alliaceae family and is related to onion (see p. 54) and garlic (see p. 154). Leeks were valued by the Greeks and Romans because of their purported beneficial effect on the throat. Aristotle attributed the clear voice of the partridge to a diet of leeks, and the Roman Emperor Nero ate leeks every day to strengthen his voice.

The leek plant reaches maturity in autumn and is adequately hardy to be harvested even during early winter. In addition to the white bulb, the bundle of sheaths of leaf, called the stem or stalk, can be eaten, although the outer dark green portion is less flavorful and usually discarded. The flavor of leek is similar to onion, though usually somewhat milder and sweeter.

Leeks are a good source of vitamins C and K and manganese. However, the more important nutritional benefits are those common to the family: all alliums appear to exert a cholesterol-lowering effect.

### THE HEALTHY EVIDENCE

A 2010 study published in the journal *Bioscience, Biotechnology and Biochemistry* reported that the addition of leeks to a high-fat and high-sugar diet fed to rats significantly lowered their elevated cholesterol levels. The effect was likely due to the high level of flavonoid compounds, including quercetin and kaempferol.

## Making the Most of Leeks

The benefits of the flavonoid compounds are not affected by cooking. Leeks are popular in soups and stews, where they enhance both nutritional value and flavor. For a larger serving of the vegetable on its own, try braising in olive oil or roasting in the oven.

## What's in a Serving?

**COOKED LEEKS**
(½ cup/52 g)

**Calories:** 16 (68 kJ)

**Protein:** 0.4 g

**Total fat:** 0.1 g

**Saturated fat:** 0 g

**Carbohydrates:** 4 g

**Fiber:** 0.5 g

# Beetroot or Beet

✪ *Beta vulgaris*

While many beets are grown for their leaves (see p. 17), others are cultivated primarily for their roots or tubers, most notably beetroot or beet. Beetroot originated along the Mediterranean and Atlantic coasts of Africa and Europe; selective breeding in the 1600s resulted in larger size of the cultivated beetroot in comparison to its wild counterpart. The leaves of the beetroot, beet greens, are also edible.

Beetroot is high in folate, with a serving providing 34 percent of the Daily Value, as well as 28 percent of the Daily Value of fiber and manganese. It is a good source of vitamins B6 and C, magnesium, potassium, and iron. Beetroot also contains phenols, which have antioxidant properties, and betalains, water-soluble plant pigments often used as food colorants, which also have beneficial effects on human health.

The beet greens are high in fiber, vitamins A, B6, C, K, and E, thiamine, and riboflavin, with the vitamin A present as beta-carotene, lutein, and zeaxanthin. They also contain high levels of the minerals magnesium, manganese, potassium, calcium, iron, and copper, and are a good source of folate, pantothenic acid, niacin, zinc, and phosphorus.

## In a Nutshell

**Origin:** Atlantic and Mediterranean coasts of Africa and Europe

**Season:** Summer and autumn

**Why it's super:** High in folate, fiber, manganese, and antioxidants; good source of vitamins B6 and C, magnesium, potassium, and iron

**Growing at home:** Easily grown in the home garden

## Making the Most of Beetroot

Beetroot can be boiled or roasted, but roasting may help preserve folate since no liquid is needed. Beet greens can also be roasted with a light drizzle of oil, or they can be sautéed; adding tomato juice for flavoring will also enhance iron absorption.

## THE HEALTHY EVIDENCE

A 2010 review in the journal *Plant Foods in Human Nutrition* reported that the betalain in beets has antioxidant, anti-inflammatory, and anti-cancer properties. A 2009 study in *Phytotherapy Research* reported that beetroot products (juice and chips) reduced oxidation and inflammation in obese women.

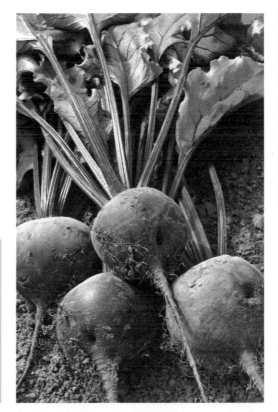

LEFT The first cultivated beetroots were paler than those today. Dark red beetroots were first recorded in the mid-seventeenth century.

## What's in a Serving?

**COOKED BEETROOT
(1 cup/170 g)**
**Calories:** 75 (313 kJ)
**Protein:** 2.9 g
**Total fat:** 0.3 g
**Saturated fat:** 0.1 g
**Carbohydrates:** 16.9 g
**Fiber:** 3.4 g

**COOKED BEET
GREENS
(1 cup/144 g)**
**Calories:** 39 (166 kJ)
**Protein:** 3.7 g
**Total fat:** 0.3 g
**Saturated fat:** 0.1 g
**Carbohydrates:** 7.9 g
**Fiber:** 4.2 g

# Turnips and Turnip Greens

✪ *Brassica napus* var. *napobrassica* Rutabaga, Swede Turnip
✪ *Brassica napus* var. *rapifera* Turnip

Turnips have been used as a nutritious food by virtually every culture since they originated in Europe around 4,000 years ago. Early on, they were seen as only good for animals and therefore associated with low social status; but during times of famine people abandoned this prejudice and the plant was grown more widely for food. Both the root and the leaves are edible, with some cultivars being grown only for their leaves or greens,

## Making the Most of Turnips

To preserve their vitamin C, turnips should be cut and cooked covered in the microwave, with a minimum of water, until just tender. The greens can be sautéed in a healthy oil with either garlic or onion—just long enough for them to become tender.

### What's in a Serving?

**COOKED TURNIP ROOT**
**(1 cup/156 g)**
**Calories:** 34 (142 kJ)
**Protein:** 1 g
**Total fat:** 0 g
**Saturated fat:** 0 g
**Carbohydrates:** 8 g
**Fiber:** 3 g

**COOKED TURNIP GREENS**
**(1 cup/156 g)**
**Calories:** 29 (121 kJ)
**Protein:** 2 g
**Total fat:** 0 g
**Saturated fat:** 0 g
**Carbohydrates:** 6 g
**Fiber:** 5 g

known as "tops" in the United Kingdom. Rutabaga, which first appeared in the 1600s, has a larger root with yellow flesh.

As one might expect of a member of the *Brassica* genus, turnips are highly flavored. More importantly, the family connection confers the same health-promoting nutrients, notably diindolylmethane (DIM) and sulforaphane. In addition, the turnip root is an excellent source of vitamin C and fiber, and a good source of vitamin B6, calcium, potassium, and manganese. The greens are more nutrient-rich, being high in vitamins A, B6, C, E, and K, folate, fiber, calcium, manganese, copper, and potassium.

## THE HEALTHY EVIDENCE

A 2009 study published in the journal *Biochemical Pharmacology* reported that DIM is a powerful modulator of the immune response that can protect against microbes, such as viruses and bacteria, as well as the development of cancer. Sulforaphane was shown to arrest the development of ovarian cancer cells in a 2010 study published in the journal *Molecular Cancer*.

### In a Nutshell

**Origin:** Europe
**Season:** Late summer
**Why they're super:** High in sulforaphane and DIM. Root high in vitamin C and fiber; good source of vitamin B6, calcium, potassium, and manganese. Greens high in vitamins A, B6, C, E, and K, folate, fiber, calcium, manganese, copper, and potassium
**Growing at home:** Easy to cultivate in the home garden

BELOW Turnips harvested immediately after the first frost of the year will have a sweeter taste than those harvested at an earlier stage.

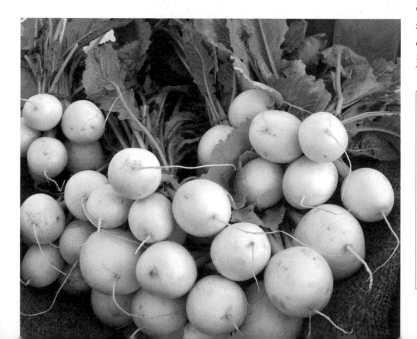

# Carrot

❁ *Daucus carota*

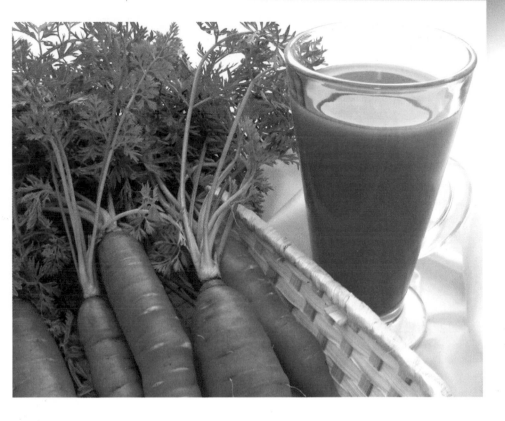

Carrots originated in Asia about 5,000 years ago. The ancient Greeks avoided them completely, but the Romans particularly enjoyed them. In the twelfth century, the Moors helped disseminate them in much of western Europe, from where they spread to Britain and thence to North America. They have since become a favorite vegetable worldwide.

Carrots can be used in a variety of ways: sliced, grated or chopped in salads; cooked in stocks, soups, and stews; or roasted, steamed, sautéed, or boiled as a side dish. As many people know, they are an outstanding source of vitamin A, with one serving providing 532 percent of the Daily Value. More importantly, the vitamin A is present as the antioxidant carotenoids beta-carotene, alpha-carotene, lutein, and zeaxanthin. Cooking and processing, such as puréeing, increases carotenoid absorption; for this reason, carrot juice is a particularly nutritious beverage. Carrots are, too, an excellent source of fiber and vitamin K and a good source of vitamins B6, C, and E, folate, thiamine, niacin, potassium, and manganese.

ABOVE Wild carrots are usually purple. Orange carrots were bred in the late Middle Ages for their superior taste and texture.

## In a Nutshell

**Origin:** Asia

**Season:** Late summer

**Why it's super:** High in vitamins A and K, fiber, and antioxidant carotenoids; good source of vitamins B6, C, and E, folate, thiamine, niacin, potassium, and manganese

**Growing at home:** Easy to cultivate in the home garden

## Making the Most of Carrots

Carrots are excellent eating on their own, and combine well with other flavors. Although cooking carrots will cause minor losses of vitamin C and folate, it will also increase the availability of the antioxidant carotenoids, as will the presence of even a small amount of fat. A vegetable stir-fry including carrots will therefore enhance carotenoid absorption and provide additional nutrients.

### THE HEALTHY EVIDENCE

A 2010 review published in the journal *Urology* reported that diets high in vegetables, and especially carrots, provide a protective effect against both the risk of bladder cancer and of its recurrence.

## What's in a Serving?

**COOKED CARROTS**
**(1 cup/156 g)**

**Calories:** 55 (229 kJ)

**Protein:** 1.2 g

**Total fat:** 0.3 g

**Saturated fat:** 0.1 g

**Carbohydrates:** 12.8 g

**Fiber:** 4.7 g

# Sweet Potato or Kumara

✿ *Ipomoea batatas*

The sweet potato, known as kumara in Polynesian cultures, belongs to a family of more than 1,000 species, many of which are poisonous. Native to Peru, sweet potatoes were cultivated in many New World areas, and Spanish explorers introduced them to the Polynesian islands, Africa, Asia, and Europe.

The plant's leaves are oval- to heart-shaped, lobed or toothed. The tubers, a staple food for many, have purple, red, or yellow skins, and orange or white flesh. One serving of sweet potato provides seven times the Daily Value for vitamin A, present almost exclusively as beta-carotene. Sweet potato is also an excellent source of vitamins B6 and C, fiber, thiamine, pantothenic acid, niacin, riboflavin, manganese, magnesium, potassium, and copper, as well as a good source of vitamin E, protein, calcium, and iron.

## THE HEALTHY EVIDENCE

The high level of two important antioxidants, beta-carotene and vitamin C, make sweet potato potentially effective in preventing cardiovascular disease and cancer. A 2008 study published in the journal *Diabetes, Obesity and Metabolism* reported that an extract of sweet potato, caiapo, improved insulin sensitivity and blood glucose levels in people with type 2 diabetes, which is the most common form of the disease.

### What's in a Serving?

**COOKED SWEET POTATO**
**(1 cup/200 g)**
**Calories:** 180 (756 kJ)
**Protein:** 4 g
**Total fat:** 0.3 g
**Saturated fat:** 0.1 g
**Carbohydrates:** 41.4 g
**Fiber:** 6.6 g

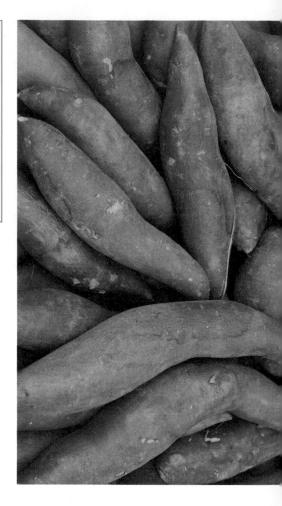

RIGHT Sweet potatoes have been an important food source in Asia and Africa, and have frequently proved reliable even when other crops have failed.

### In a Nutshell

**Origin:** Peru
**Season:** Autumn
**Why it's super:** High in beta-carotene, vitamins A, B6, and C, fiber, thiamine, niacin, riboflavin, pantothenic acid, manganese, magnesium, potassium, and copper; good source of vitamin E, protein, calcium, and iron
**Growing at home:** Easy to cultivate in the home garden

### Making the Most of Sweet Potato

Here's an excellent way to prepare sweet potato while retaining nutrients. Scrub the sweet potatoes well with a brush, leaving the skin intact. Slice into rounds ½ inch (12 mm) thick. Spread 2 tablespoons of olive oil on a baking sheet, place the slices on top, and bake until tender, turning at least once.

# Jicama

☼ *Pachyrhizus erosus*

The jicama, also known as yambean or Mexican turnip, is a leguminous tropical vine that is a common ingredient in Mexican cuisine. It is native to Central America and Mexico, and has been cultivated in South America for centuries. Jicama made its way to Asia and the Pacific Islands with Spanish explorers, who used it aboard ship because it stored well and did not require cooking.

The tuber is the edible component—other parts of the plant are actually poisonous. It is starchy and sweet in flavor, and is a common accompaniment to grilled fish. Reflecting jicama's popularity in both Mexican and

## Making the Most of Jicama

Because it is an excellent source of vitamin C, jicama is best eaten raw, although it can also be cooked. Add slices to fresh salads, and, to increase nutrient value, combine with vegetables with a high carotenoid content, such as carrots, red peppers (capsicums), and dark, leafy greens.

Asian cuisines, regularly used seasonings include chili powder and soy sauce.

A single serving of jicama slices provides 40 percent and 24 percent of the Daily Values for vitamin C and fiber, respectively. In addition, it is a good source of potassium.

### THE HEALTHY EVIDENCE

In 2002, researchers in Thailand reported that several compounds isolated from jicama demonstrated antiviral activity, specifically against the herpes simplex virus. Jicama's combination of nutrients—vitamin C, fiber, and potassium—is also likely to be effective in helping prevent various forms of cardiovascular disease.

## In a Nutshell

**Origin:** Central America and Mexico

**Season:** Late autumn

**Why it's super:** Low in calories, high in vitamin C and fiber; good source of potassium

**Growing at home:** Easy to grow in the home garden; allow pods to mature and use seeds for next planting

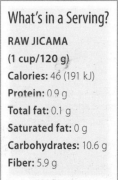

## What's in a Serving?

**RAW JICAMA**

**(1 cup/120 g)**

**Calories:** 46 (191 kJ)

**Protein:** 0.9 g

**Total fat:** 0.1 g

**Saturated fat:** 0 g

**Carbohydrates:** 10.6 g

**Fiber:** 5.9 g

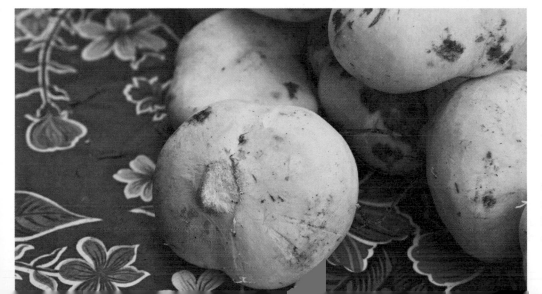

LEFT Cultivation of jicama has become popular in Asia, where it is used as the main ingredient in salads such as *rojak* and *yusheng*.

# SEA VEGETABLES

# Dulse

✪ *Palmaria palmata*

## What's in a Serving?

**RAW DULSE**
**(⅓ cup/7 g)**
**Calories:** 18 (75 kJ)
**Protein:** 2 g
**Total fat:** 0 g
**Saturated fat:** 0 g
**Carbohydrates:** 3 g
**Fiber:** 2 g

Dulse, grown on the northern coasts of the Pacific and Atlantic oceans, is an algae that can be collected when the tide is out. Other names for this nutritious and versatile food include dillisk, dilsk, red dulse, sea lettuce flakes, and creathnach. Its history can be traced as far back as 1,400 years ago to the coasts of Ireland and Scotland, where it was harvested by the monks of St. Columba and was an important supplement to their diet. Even today, dulse is a popular snack food

BELOW Dulse, seen here on sale in a Canadian market, is a highly versatile food. Notably, it adds an interesting flavor to pesto sauce.

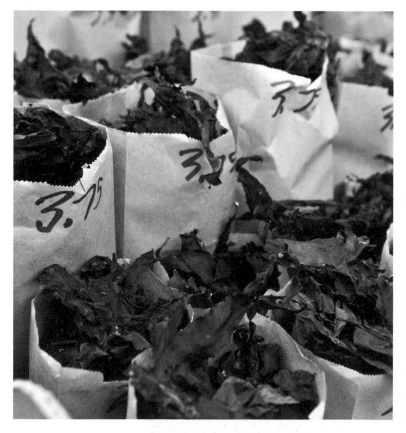

## Making the Most of Dulse

Dulse is easy to find in health food stores, where it is contained in a variety of products, and also in fish markets. It can be added to soups and stews, and makes an excellent addition to chili, because of its chewy texture.

in Iceland, Northern Ireland, and Canada. It can be eaten raw plucked directly off the rocks along the shore after the sun has dried it out, or it can be pan-fried, toasted, or even cooked in a microwave oven.

Dulse is an excellent source of vitamins B6 and B12, potassium, and iron, while adding a mere 18 calories per serving. It is also a good source of fiber, niacin, riboflavin, thiamine, and chromium. Of even greater importance for disease prevention, it is high in antioxidant polyphenols.

### THE HEALTHY EVIDENCE

A 2006 scientific study published in the journal *Food and Chemistry Toxicology* reported that, among three edible seaweeds, dulse demonstrated the highest level of antioxidant polyphenols and demonstrated the strongest anticancer effect.

## In a Nutshell

**Origin:** Northern Atlantic and Pacific coastal regions
**Season:** Summer to early autumn
**Why it's super:** Low in calories, high in vitamins B6 and B12, potassium, iron, and antioxidants; good source of fiber, niacin, riboflavin, thiamine, and chromium
**Growing at home:** Not applicable

# Nori

✿ *Porphyra* species

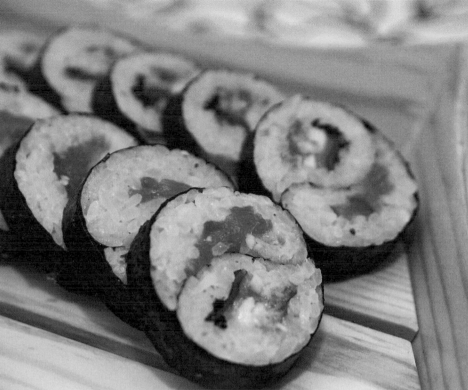

Nori is the Japanese term for several varieties of edible seaweed of the *Porphyra* genus, also known as laver. The word is mentioned in historical texts dating back to the eighth century. Nori was traditionally made into an edible paste, but today is more usually available in dried form in Asian markets.

Porphyra plants are cultivated in the sea, where they are grown on nets suspended near the surface of the water. Within 45 days of the initial cultivation, the plants are harvested by farmers working in boats. They are then pressed and dried to create black sheets as thin as paper. Quality varies greatly in nori products, as does cost, with high-end nori from the Japanese island of Kyushu commanding astronomical prices in the United States.

Nori is an excellent source of vitamins A, C, and K, folate, riboflavin, potassium, and antioxidants, as well as a good source of protein and magnesium. The antioxidants in nori are present in several forms, notably carotenoids, indicated by the significant content of vitamin A.

## What's in a Serving?

**DRIED NORI**
**(4 sheets/10 g)**

**Calories:** 20 (84 kJ)

**Protein:** 4 g

**Total fat:** 0 g

**Saturated fat:** 0 g

**Carbohydrates:** 1 g

**Fiber:** 4 g

ABOVE The principal use for nori in Japanese cuisine is to make sushi. Nori is a vitally important crop in Japan, with 230 square miles (600 sq km) of cultivation yielding a crop worth more than $1.5 billion dollars a year.

## THE HEALTHY EVIDENCE

In 2010, a study in the *Journal of Ethnopharmacology* reporting that nori extract was high in antioxidant phenols and demonstrated powerful anti-inflammatory effects. Nori's complement of other nutrients suggests potential benefits in both cancer and cardiovascular disease prevention.

## Making the Most of Nori

A common use for nori is as a wrap for sushi, but it can also be used as a nutritious wrap for less traditional contents. For example, in any recipe where lettuce is used as a wrap, try replacing it with nori. Nori also makes an excellent addition to soups.

## In a Nutshell

**Origin:** Japan

**Season:** Year-round

**Why it's super:** Low in calories, high in antioxidants, vitamins A, C, and K, folate, riboflavin, and potassium; good source of protein and magnesium

**Growing at home:** Not applicable

# Kombu

✪ *Saccharina japonica*

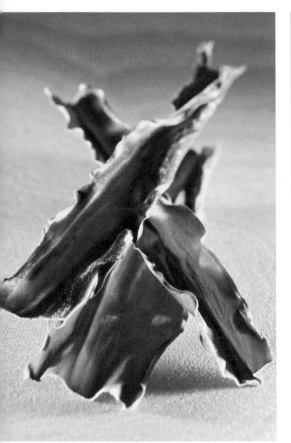

## What's in a Serving?

**RAW KOMBU**
**(½ cup/40 g)**
**Calories:** 17 (72 kJ)
**Protein:** 0.1 g
**Total fat:** 2.6 g
**Saturated fat:** 0.1 g
**Carbohydrates:** 3.8 g
**Fiber:** 0.5 g

## Making the Most of Kombu

An easy way to incorporate this health-promoting food into one's diet is to add it to soups and stews. Kombu can be purchased in many forms from Asian markets. If you buy it in dried form, place it in cold water and bring it to boil to soften it before adding it to other dishes.

LEFT Kombu contains iodine, which aids the body in producing thyroid hormones essential to human growth and development.

Kombu, a type of seaweed, is native to Japan but is also grown in China, Russia, France, and Korea. It is grayish-black or brown in color, and is usually sun-dried and folded into sheets. A staple of Japanese cuisine, kombu can be found dried, pickled, fresh, and frozen in many Asian markets.

When stored unopened in its original packaging in a dry place, kombu will keep indefinitely. Once opened, if it continues to be kept cool and dry, it will remain edible for up to six months. Kombu has a naturally occurring white powder coating that should not be washed off, since it is responsible for much of the flavor.

Kombu contains glutamic acid, an amino acid that produces *umami*, which, in addition to salt, sweet, bitter, and sour is one of the five basic tastes. Kombu is high in vitamin K, folate, magnesium, and antioxidants, and a good source of calcium and iron.

### THE HEALTHY EVIDENCE

A 2010 study published in the *International Journal of Biological Macromolecules* reported that extracts from kombu exhibited potent antioxidant activity and anticoagulant effects. Both could play key roles in the prevention of cardiovascular disease. Another study in 2009 reported that kombu lowered serum triglyceride levels in rats fed a high-fat diet and also showed anti-obesity effects.

## In a Nutshell

**Origin:** Japan
**Season:** Year-round
**Why it's super:** Low in calories; high in antioxidants, vitamin K, folate, and magnesium; good source of calcium and iron
**Growing at home:** Not applicable

# Wakame

✿ *Undaria pinnatifida*

An edible seaweed, wakame has been cultivated for centuries in Japan and Korea, and the name is Japanese in origin. Today it is also cultivated in France, off the coast of Brittany, and a wild form is harvested in Tasmania, Australia. Although wakame is highly nutritious, unfortunately the wild plant is also an aggressive, invasive species.

Wakame is an excellent source of omega-3 fatty acids, folate, and manganese, and a good source of calcium and magnesium. It also contains a high level of antioxidants and some intriguing compounds. Two, fucoidan and the carotenoid fucoxanthin, seem to have especially beneficial effects.

## THE HEALTHY EVIDENCE

Several studies have focused on the fucoidan in wakame. One 2010 study in the journal *Food and Chemical Toxicology* pointed to fucoidan's anticoagulant, antithrombotic, and antiviral properties. Another recent study published in the journal *Chemico-Biological Interactions* reported that fucoxanthin demonstrated a potent anticancer effect, particularly in liver cancer cells. Researchers at the University of South Carolina studied wakame's effect on markers of metabolic syndrome, a condition linked to cardiovascular disease and type 2 diabetes. Daily consumption of 4–6 grams of wakame for one month improved some of the markers, leading the authors to conclude that it "may be associated with low metabolic syndrome prevalence" seen in Japan.

---

### In a Nutshell

**Origin:** Japan

**Season:** All year

**Why it's super:** High in antioxidants, omega-3 fatty acids, folate, and manganese; good source of calcium and magnesium; contains fucoidan and fucoxanthin

**Growing at home:** Not applicable

---

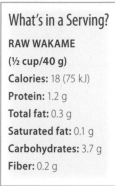

### What's in a Serving?

**RAW WAKAME**

**(½ cup/40 g)**

**Calories:** 18 (75 kJ)

**Protein:** 1.2 g

**Total fat:** 0.3 g

**Saturated fat:** 0.1 g

**Carbohydrates:** 3.7 g

**Fiber:** 0.2 g

---

## Making the Most of Wakame

One traditional use for wakame in Japan is in miso soup; another is in a dish of tofu cubes and scallions (spring onions), in either a vegetable or chicken broth. However, wakame makes a nutrient-rich addition to almost any kind of soup or stew, and is also an excellent addition to salads.

BELOW Wakame is dried on racks. The Japanese have a saying, "wakame is food and medicine in one"—testimony to its proven health benefits.

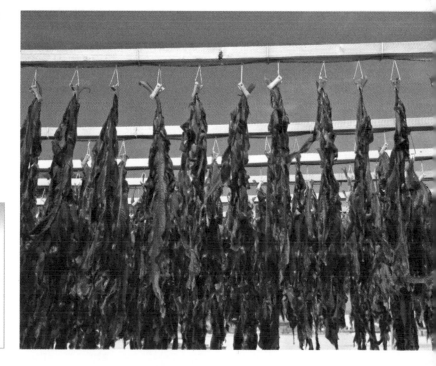

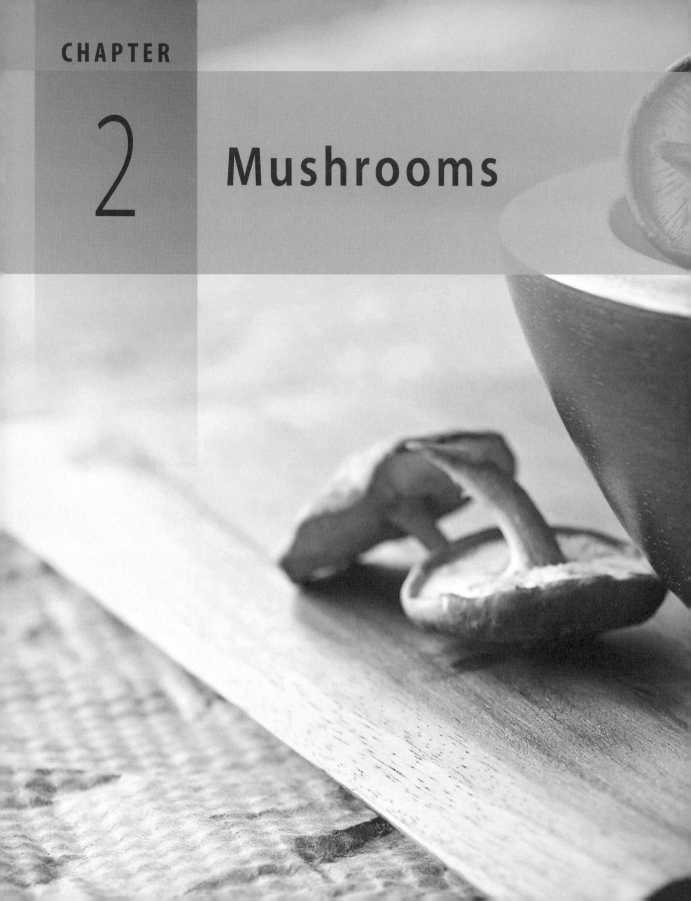

# Mushrooms

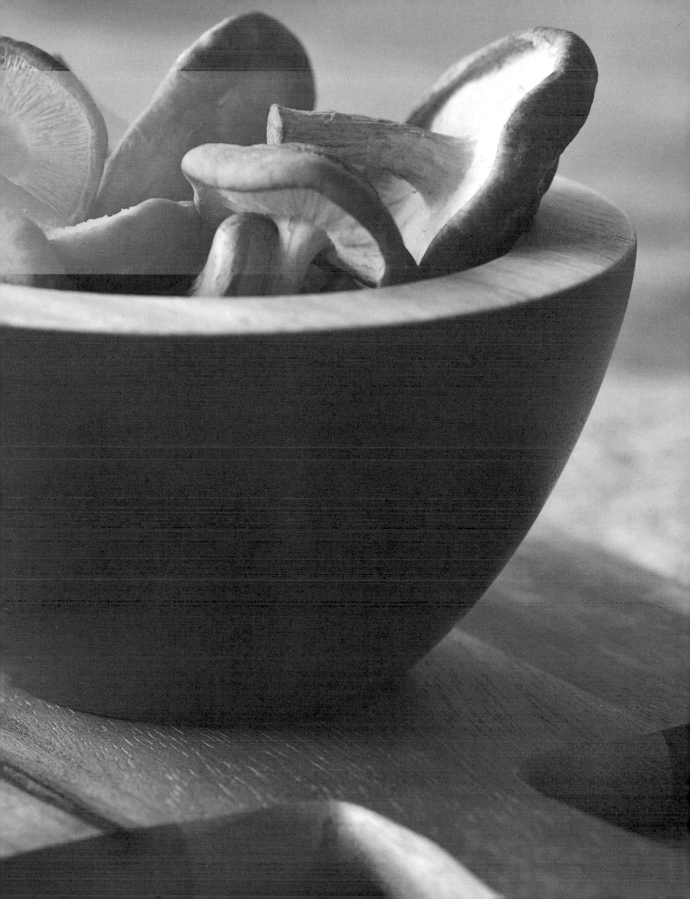

# White, Brown, and Field Mushrooms

✪ *Agaricus bisporus* White and Brown Mushrooms, Crimini Mushrooms
✪ *Agaricus campestris* Field Mushrooms

Mushrooms are the fruiting body of fungi, which reproduce by spores. Over the centuries, they have been prized for medicinal purposes and for their delicate flavor. Ancient Egyptian hieroglyphics dating back 4,600 years depict them as a symbol of immortality, and the pharaohs declared that only the royal family could eat mushrooms.

The most widely known mushrooms are the cultivated white and brown mushrooms *(Agaricus bisporus)* and the field mushroom

> ### What's in a Serving?
> **RAW MUSHROOMS**
> **(1 cup/72 g)**
> **Calories:** 16 (67 kJ)
> **Protein:** 1.8 g
> **Total fat:** 0.1 g
> **Saturated fat:** 0 g
> **Carbohydrates:** 3.1 g
> **Fiber:** 1.4 g

*(Agaricus campestris)*. The crimini (or cremini) mushroom, also known as Italian brown and Swiss brown, is a variety of brown mushroom that is darker in color and has a denser texture, due to the fact that it arises from a different spore strain. The portabella or portabello is a mature crimini. Its longer growth period accounts for its large cap, which can be 6 inches (15 cm) in diameter.

Mushrooms are an excellent source of riboflavin, niacin, pantothenic acid, selenium, copper, and potassium, as well as a good source of thiamine, zinc, and manganese. Research into the phytochemicals in mushrooms has shown many health-promoting effects.

Cultivating both species is difficult, though kits can be purchased for home-growing. Some varieties require association with a live tree, and are thus not suitable for cultivation.

### THE HEALTHY EVIDENCE

The authors of an article in *Critical Reviews in Biotechnology* concluded that mushrooms contain bioactive compounds that may influence human disease. In particular, they cited compounds known as lectins, which display anticancer and antiviral properties.

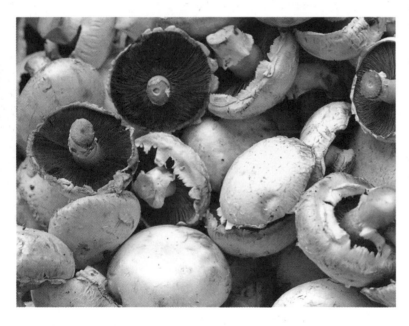

ABOVE Most commercially available mushrooms are grown on large farms. China is the world's largest producer.

## Making the Most of Mushrooms

Mushrooms are often relegated to serving as minor ingredients, which fails to optimize their content of nutrients and phytochemicals. An easy way to obtain a healthy dose is to sauté sliced mushrooms in canola oil, with onions and basil. Top with shredded cheese and serve as a main dish.

## In a Nutshell

**Origin:** Worldwide, but first cultivated in France
**Season:** Spring through autumn
**Why they're super:** High in riboflavin, niacin, pantothenic acid, selenium, copper, and potassium; good source of thiamine, zinc, and manganese; contain bioactive phytochemicals
**Growing at home:** Difficult to grow at home, though readymade kits can be purchased

# Porcini or Cep

✿ *Boletus edulis*

The porcini or cep mushroom is found throughout the Northern Hemisphere, but nowhere in the Southern Hemisphere. The common name, *porcini*, is Italian for "piglets"—a reference to their shape—and cep is derived from the Gascon French word *cep* for "tree trunk." The porcini cap can grow to a diameter of around 10 inches (25 cm) and weigh 2.2 lb (1 kg).

Porcini mushrooms are used as an ingredient in many dishes, in either raw or, more commonly, dried form—drying not only retains but intensifies the mushroom's flavor. In contrast to other fungi, porcini mushrooms are also available pickled.

Porcini are an excellent source of folate, protein, pantothenic acid, niacin, and zinc, and a good source of thiamine. In addition, they contain many bioactive phytochemicals, including antioxidants.

## THE HEALTHY EVIDENCE

A 2008 study published in the journal *Food Chemistry* reported on the high level of bioactive compounds in porcini and other wild mushrooms. Porcini had the highest level of antioxidants of all the mushroom samples, and the antioxidants were concentrated in the cap. As numerous other studies have shown, antioxidants are effective in combating cardiovascular disease and cancer.

| What's in a Serving? |
| --- |
| **RAW PORCINI** |
| **(1 cup/75 g)** |
| **Calories:** 61 (255 kJ) |
| **Protein:** 5.6 g |
| **Total fat:** 1.3 g |
| **Saturated fat:** 0.1 g |
| **Carbohydrates:** 6.9 g |
| **Fiber:** Not available |

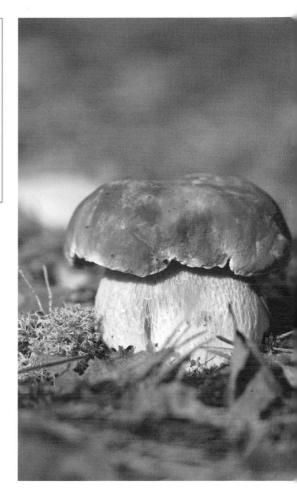

RIGHT Porcini mushrooms are excellent cooked on the grill and served with olive oil and parsley. They are sometimes referred to as "the poor man's steak."

## Making the Most of Porcini

To obtain the highest level of antioxidants, use raw porcini caps as a vegetable dish. Alternatively, slice the cap into strips and sauté with garlic and olive oil. Add diced fresh tomato to increase and vary the antioxidant content. Porcini can also be used as a major component of a stir-fry.

## In a Nutshell

**Origin:** Distributed throughout the Northern Hemisphere

**Season:** Summer to autumn

**Why it's super:** High in folate, protein, pantothenic acid, niacin, and zinc; good source of thiamine; contains bioactive phytochemicals including antioxidants

**Growing at home:** Difficult to grow at home

# Chanterelle or Girole

✪ *Cantharellus cibarius*

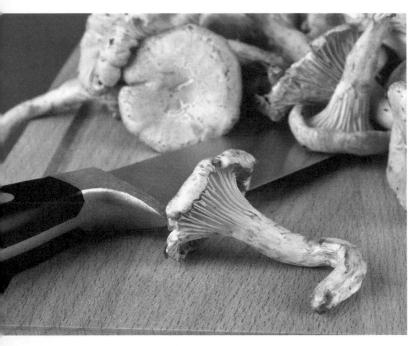

LEFT Chanterelles can be harvested from the same location year after year as long as care is taken not to disturb the area too much.

## Making the Most of Chanterelles

The important nutrients and phytochemicals stand up well to roasting, so this is an excellent method of cooking, which also enhances flavor. Slice 1 pound (455 g) of chanterelles into ⅓ inch (8 mm) slices and toss with 3 tablespoons of olive oil and thyme. Spread on a baking sheet and roast until tender. Add the chanterelles to cooked pasta.

## What's in a Serving?

**RAW CHANTERELLE**
**(1 cup/54 g)**
**Calories:** 17 (71 kJ)
**Protein:** 0.8 g
**Total fat:** 0.3 g
**Saturated fat:** 0 g
**Carbohydrates:** 3.7 g
**Fiber:** 2.1 g

Many fine restaurants have been named for the chanterelle or girole, though usually by its more descriptive name, the golden mushroom. Widely renowned as one of the best tasting wild mushrooms, it can be found in many regions of the world, including northern Europe, North America, Asia, and Africa.

### In a Nutshell

**Origin:** Northern Europe, North America, Asia, and Africa
**Season:** Summer to autumn
**Why it's super:** High in fiber, niacin, copper, iron, and potassium; good source of pantothenic acid; contains bioactive phytochemicals
**Growing at home:** Difficult to grow at home

The chanterelle is shaped like a funnel, with the cap inverted, and it can be either yellow or orange. Beneath the smooth cap, it has gills or lamellae, which run down the stem. Germans call the chanterelle *Pfifferling*, which refers to its mild peppery taste. It has also been described as having a pleasant apricot-like smell.

Chanterelles are high in fiber, niacin, copper, iron, and potassium, and a good source of pantothenic acid. They contain a high level of bioactive phytochemicals, which have been the subject of numerous studies related to health and disease.

### THE HEALTHY EVIDENCE

A 2007 study published in the journal *Chemistry & Biodiversity* reported that an extract of the chanterelle demonstrated potent antimicrobial and insecticidal activity. The extract was effective against bacteria, viruses, and yeasts. In another study published in the journal *Phytotherapy Research*, the extract inhibited a compound linked to cancer and inflammatory and autoimmune diseases.

# Enoki

*Flammulina velutipes*

The more correct name for these Japanese mushrooms is *enokitake*, also spelled *enokidake*, but the abbreviated form is widely used. The enoki is also known as golden needle mushroom, for its slender form, and wild enoki are sometimes called winter mushroom or velvet foot. The cultivated enoki varies from its wild counterpart in that the stems are considerably longer; in addition, because the cultivated enoki is grown without light, it is usually white in color, in contrast to the brown wild form.

When selecting enoki, look for firm texture and fresh white appearance, avoiding stalks that appear brown or slimy. Enoki should

## What's in a Serving?

**RAW ENOKI**
**(1 cup/65 g)**
**Calories:** 24 (99 kJ)
**Protein:** 1.7 g
**Total fat:** 0.2 g
**Saturated fat:** 0 g
**Carbohydrates:** 5.1 g
**Fiber:** 1.8 g

## In a Nutshell

**Origin:** Northern mountain ranges of Japan
**Season:** Summer to autumn
**Why it's super:** High in niacin and pantothenic acid; good source of potassium; contains bioactive phytochemicals including antioxidants
**Growing at home:** Difficult to grow at home

be refrigerated and used within a week of purchase for optimal freshness. The traditional Japanese use for enoki is in soups, most often miso soup; however, enoki are also used in salads and entrées.

Enoki are an excellent source of niacin and pantothenic acid, and a good source of potassium. Their beneficial phytochemicals, including antioxidants, have been the subject of some research.

### THE HEALTHY EVIDENCE

The *Journal of Food Science* published a 2010 study on the antioxidant potency of enoki extract and reported that it was more effective in preventing oxidation than compounds typically used in food processing. A National University of Singapore study concluded that the stalk of the mushroom contains a large quantity of a protein that helps in the regulation of immune function.

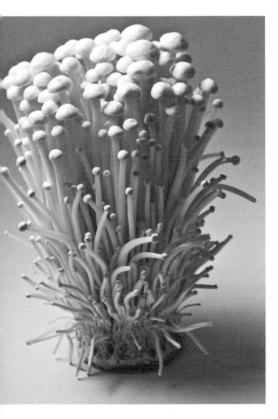

LEFT In Japan, the fragile, tasty, and slightly crunchy enoki mushroom is called the "snow-peak mushroom."

## Making the Most of Enoki

Enoki can be added to any dish to enhance antioxidant content, most typically soups and stir-fries. They also make an excellent addition to a fresh salad. Make an Asian-inspired salad by combining enoki, Asian greens, water chestnuts, fresh red peppers (capsicums), and carrots. Season with ginger, sesame oil, and soy sauce.

# Maitake

✪ *Grifola frondosa*

In nature, maitake mushrooms grow in clusters at the base of trees, often oak trees. The name is the Japanese word for "dancing mushroom"; other names for the fungus include hen of the woods, ram's head, and sheep's head—colorful descriptors of its brown-and-white bracket-shaped caps.

As a culinary ingredient, maitake is typically used in soups and stews, and is the feature of the Japanese dish *nabemono* or *nabe*. This consists of a one-pot meal shared by several people, and the word literally means "sitting around the pot."

Maitake is an excellent source of niacin, riboflavin, and copper, and a good source of thiamine and folate. The mushrooms have been studied for their content of phytochemicals, which appear to influence the immune system and may confer protection against cancer.

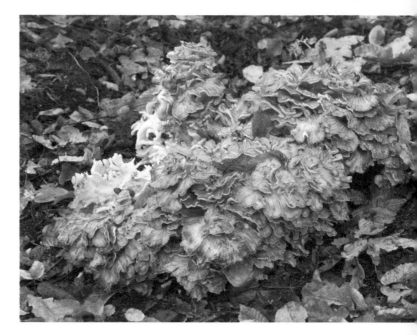

ABOVE The bizarre, large, and feathery form of certain varieties of maitake explains one of its traditional names: "hen of the woods."

## THE HEALTHY EVIDENCE

A 2010 study published in the *Journal of Medicinal Food* reported that a protein isolated from maitake enhanced the production of several cancer-fighting compounds. Mice in which colon cancer was induced showed significant inhibition of tumor growth when given the maitake protein. In a study published in the journal *Experimental and Molecular Medicine*, maitake extract significantly reduced the production of pro-inflammatory compounds associated with inflammatory bowel disease. The authors suggested that maitake might be a "valuable medicinal food for treatment."

### What's in a Serving?

**RAW MAITAKE**
**(1 cup/70 g)**
**Calories:** 22 (91 kJ)
**Protein:** 1.4 g
**Total fat:** 0.1 g
**Saturated fat:** 0 g
**Carbohydrates:** 4.9 g
**Fiber:** 1.9 g

### In a Nutshell

**Origin:** Northeastern Japan and North America
**Season:** Summer to autumn
**Why it's super:** High in niacin, riboflavin, and copper; good source of thiamine and folate; contains bioactive phytochemicals
**Growing at home:** Difficult to grow at home

### Making the Most of Maitake

Following the Japanese tradition of a one-pot meal, maitake can be used as the main ingredient of a nutritious vegetable stew. The addition of vegetables that bring along other nutrients will enhance the health benefits: try adding leafy greens, carrots, legumes, and tomatoes.

# Shimeji

✱ *Hypsizygus marmoreus*

The name "shimeji" is used to refer to a number of varieties of Japanese mushrooms, many of them wild mushrooms and some cultivated by Japanese companies (who often hold patents for their particular cultivation methods); however, strictly speaking it is the common name of the species called *Hypsizygus marmoreus*. In their natural environment, shimeji mushrooms grow in clusters high on trees, often beech trees, and another name for shimeji is beech mushroom. Shimeji is blotched pale brown to white in color; the stem, or stipe, is thick and up to 3 inches (8 cm) long. The flavor is often described as nut-like and mild, and the texture is firm. Shimeji is slow-growing, requiring up to 100 days before harvesting, and this may account for its strong flavor and firm texture.

Shimeji mushrooms are an excellent source of niacin, riboflavin, and potassium, and a good source of protein and thiamine. They also contain many phytochemicals, specifically the beta-glucan compounds.

## THE HEALTHY EVIDENCE

Researchers have studied beta-glucans for numerous purported health benefits, with the evidence suggesting a key role in enhancing immune function, which is important for warding off infections and inhibiting the development of cancer. A 2010 review published in the journal *Expert Review of Anti-Infective Therapy* describes their structure and how the compounds may modulate the immune response in both infections and cancer.

### Making the Most of Shimeji

Shimeji should be cooked because the raw mushroom tends to have a bitter flavor. They can be used in soups and sauces, but to obtain more of the health benefits use them in combination with other vegetables in a stir-fry.

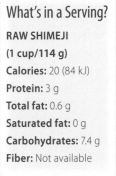

### What's in a Serving?

**RAW SHIMEJI**
**(1 cup/114 g)**
**Calories:** 20 (84 kJ)
**Protein:** 3 g
**Total fat:** 0.6 g
**Saturated fat:** 0 g
**Carbohydrates:** 7.4 g
**Fiber:** Not available

BELOW Shimeji mushrooms grow in clumps, with their stalks joined at the base and little space between the round, buttonlike heads.

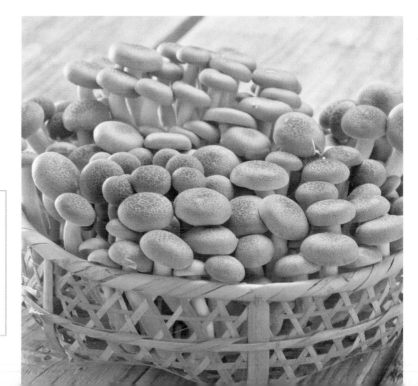

### In a Nutshell

**Origin:** Asia and North America
**Season:** Spring through late summer
**Why it's super:** High in niacin, riboflavin, and potassium; good source of protein and thiamine; contains bioactive phytochemicals
**Growing at home:** Difficult to grow at home

# Shiitake

*Lentinula edodes*

Native to various regions of Asia, shiitake mushrooms were likely first cultivated in 960 during the Song dynasty in China. However, the name is Japanese and means "mushroom"; the Chinese characters for the fungus translate to "fragrant mushroom." Early cultivation methods involved the use of natural oak logs and took up to four years to achieve adequate colonization and production. More efficient modern methods derived from a doctoral thesis in the 1970s by Dr. Gary Leatham, acknowledged as the "father of shiitake farming" in the United States.

Shiitake is an excellent source of pantothenic acid, copper, and selenium, and a good source of vitamin B6, riboflavin, niacin, zinc, and manganese. It is highly valued for its bioactive phytochemical content, which studies suggest may help prevent chronic diseases involving inflammation.

## THE HEALTHY EVIDENCE

A 2010 study published in the journal *Inflammation Research* reported that shiitake extract inhibited several pro-inflammatory compounds. A literature review presented in the journal *Nutrition Reviews* concluded that compounds known as beta-glucans, found at high levels in shiitake mushrooms, have shown anti-carcinogenic activity. The authors also noted that shiitake may be useful in reducing blood cholesterol levels and body weight.

## Making the Most of Shiitake

A great way to enjoy the flavor and health benefits of shiitake mushrooms is to sauté them with onions, snap peas, and thin strips of red pepper (capsicum). Season with powdered garlic and ginger, and serve over brown rice. The added vitamins from the vegetables and the protein and fiber from the rice make this a nutritious main dish.

BELOW Drying intensifies the flavor of the shiitake. The dried mushrooms will keep indefinitely, and can be reconstituted by adding water.

## What's in a Serving?

**RAW SHIITAKE**
**(1 whole piece/76 g)**
**Calories:** 26 (107 kJ)
**Protein:** 1.7 g
**Total fat:** 0.4 g
**Saturated fat:** 0 g
**Carbohydrates:** 5.2 g
**Fiber:** 1.9 g

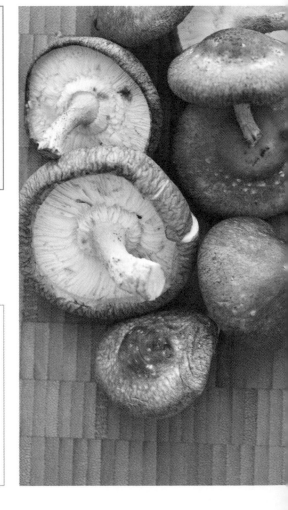

## In a Nutshell

**Origin:** East Asia

**Season:** Spring and autumn

**Why it's super:** High in pantothenic acid, copper, and selenium; good source of vitamin B6, riboflavin, niacin, zinc, and manganese; contains bioactive phytochemicals

**Growing at home:** Kits are available for growing shiitake on tree logs

# Morel

✿ *Morchella esculenta*

Many names have arisen for the morel mushroom, such as dryland fish, most likely because of its resemblance, when sliced, to a fish. It has also been called merkels and miracles, as well as hickory chickens in the state of Kentucky. Another name, sponge mushroom, describes the distinctive elongated cap, which has a honeycomb-like configuration on its surface. But the most common name, morel, is simply Latin for "brown."

Morels are ubiquitous, growing wild in many parts of Asia, Europe, and North America. They mature in spring, but may not necessarily grow in the same location the following year.

Morel is an excellent source of niacin, iron, copper, manganese, and a good source of riboflavin, potassium, and zinc. It is high in bioactive phytochemicals, and in particular a form of vitamin D, ergocalciferol, which has been studied with regard to chronic disease.

## THE HEALTHY EVIDENCE

The *Journal of Medicinal Food* published a study in 2010 reporting on the antimicrobial and antioxidant capabilities of various types of mushrooms. One of the strains of the *Morchella* mushrooms exhibited the greatest ability to scavenge free radicals. In a 2008 study published in the *Journal of Agricultural and Food Chemistry*, the authors concluded that, "On the basis of anticancer activity of ergocalciferol, it may be feasible to develop chemopreventive agents [drugs that help prevent cancer] from edible mushrooms."

ABOVE The dark, spongelike head of the morel is highly distinctive. Morels are difficult to cultivate commercially, and most of the morels for sale in shops and markets have been harvested in the wild.

### What's in a Serving?

**RAW MORELS**
**(1 cup/66 g)**
**Calories:** 20 (85 kJ)
**Protein:** 2.1 g
**Total fat:** 0.4 g
**Saturated fat:** 0.1 g
**Carbohydrates:** 3.4 g
**Fiber:** 1.8 g

### In a Nutshell

**Origin:** Asia, Europe, and North America
**Season:** Spring
**Why it's super:** High in niacin, iron, copper, and manganese; good source of riboflavin, potassium, and zinc; contains bioactive phytochemicals
**Growing at home:** Difficult to grow at home

### Making the Most of Morels

A favorite way to eat these mushrooms is simply to sautée them in a healthy oil (instead of in butter, the traditional French method of cooking morels). Make sure you avoid cooking the mushrooms too long, as this may reduce vitamin B content and adversely affect the delicate flavor.

# Oyster Mushroom

✿ *Pleurotus ostreatus*

## What's in a Serving?

**RAW OYSTER MUSHROOMS**
**(1 cup/86 g)**
**Calories:** 28 (120 kJ)
**Protein:** 2.9 g
**Total fat:** 0.4 g
**Saturated fat:** 0 g
**Carbohydrates:** 5.2 g
**Fiber:** 2 g

Oyster mushrooms are named for their distinctive appearance, similar to that of the bivalve mollusk. Its first Latin name, *Pleurotus*, describes its growth pattern, usually jutting sideways from a tree trunk, while the second, *ostreatus*, from the Latin for "oyster," points to its similarity to the mollusk. The oyster mushroom is also distinctive among fungi in that it is a carnivore, trapping and digesting nematodes for nitrogen.

### Making the Most of Oyster Mushrooms

Soups and stir-fries are ideal uses for oyster mushrooms, as any water-soluble nutrients will be eaten. Sautéeing oyster mushrooms in olive oil with leeks, sweet red pepper (capsicum), and tofu, and serving them over rice provides a protein-rich main dish.

### In a Nutshell

**Origin:** Throughout the Northern Hemisphere
**Season:** Spring through early autumn
**Why it's super:** High in niacin, pantothenic acid, iron, copper, and potassium; good source of vitamin B6, fiber, riboflavin, and zinc; contains bioactive phytochemicals such as beta-glucans and lovastatin
**Growing at home:** Difficult to grow at home

Germans were the first to cultivate the oyster mushroom, in the early 1900s. It is now cultivated throughout the world and remains a favorite wild mushroom. The flavor is mild, with a slight impression of anise, which may be due to its content of benzaldehyde.

Oyster mushrooms are an excellent source of niacin, pantothenic acid, iron, copper, and potassium. They are a good source of vitamin B6, fiber, riboflavin, and zinc. Oysters also contain numerous bioactive phytochemicals, including the beta-glucans.

### THE HEALTHY EVIDENCE

Beta-glucans have been shown to display significant anticarcinogenic activity. As reported in a 2009 article in *Nutrition Reviews*, they also stimulate the immune system and play a role in fat metabolism. This role may account for the mushroom's blood cholesterol-lowering effect. In addition, a study in 1995 reported that oyster mushrooms contain lovastatin, a well-known cholesterol-lowering agent.

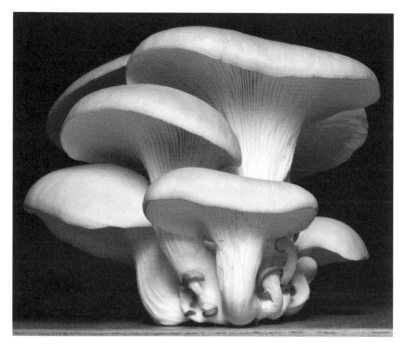

LEFT The broad cap of the oyster mushroom can measure up to 10 inches (25 cm) across. Young oyster mushrooms have the most desirable flavor; the older ones tend to become tough and have a more acrid taste.

# Straw Mushroom

✿ *Volvariella volvacea*

## What's in a Serving?

**RAW STRAW MUSHROOMS
(1 cup/182 g)**

**Calories:** 58 (242 kJ)
**Protein:** 7 g
**Total fat:** 1.2 g
**Saturated fat:** 0.2 g
**Carbohydrates:** 8.4 g
**Fiber:** 4.5 g

Straw mushrooms are indigenous to several regions of Asia, where cultivation began in the 1800s. Their name arises from the traditional method of cultivation, on rice-straw beds. The optimal growing conditions for straw mushrooms include a subtropical climate and high rainfall; the mushrooms are harvested when still immature, within four to five days, and prior to the opening of their caps.

Straw mushrooms are an excellent source of folate, iron, selenium, manganese, copper, and zinc, and a good source of potassium, pantothenic acid, and omega-3 fatty acids. They also contain various bioactive phytochemicals, including antioxidants. However, they are also high in sodium, with a serving meeting 47 percent of the recommended daily limit of 1500 milligrams.

### THE HEALTHY EVIDENCE

In an article in the *Journal of Chromatographic Science*, Chinese researchers compared the antioxidant content of various mushrooms.

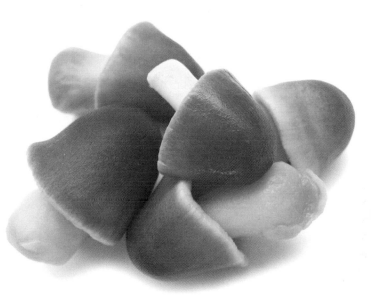

ABOVE Straw mushrooms are sometimes called paddy straw mushrooms. Commercial growers favor the straw mushroom because of its short growing time: a complete growing cycle is just 35 to 40 days.

Although the straw mushrooms did not have the highest levels of those tested during the study, they did contain significant levels of antioxidants. Furthermore, the authors pointed to the benefits of mushrooms generally, pointing out that "antioxidant activity is a very important property for disease prevention."

## In a Nutshell

**Origin:** Asia
**Season:** Summer
**Why it's super:** High in folate, iron, selenium, manganese, copper, and zinc; good source of potassium, pantothenic acid, and omega-3 fatty acids; contains bioactive phytochemicals and antioxidants
**Growing at home:** Difficult to grow at home

## Making the Most of Straw Mushrooms

To obtain the maximum benefit of the high folate content of straw mushrooms, eat them raw. If, however, straw mushrooms are only available in canned or dried form, add them to a soup, as that way the folate will be preserved in the cooking liquid and still consumed.

# Legumes

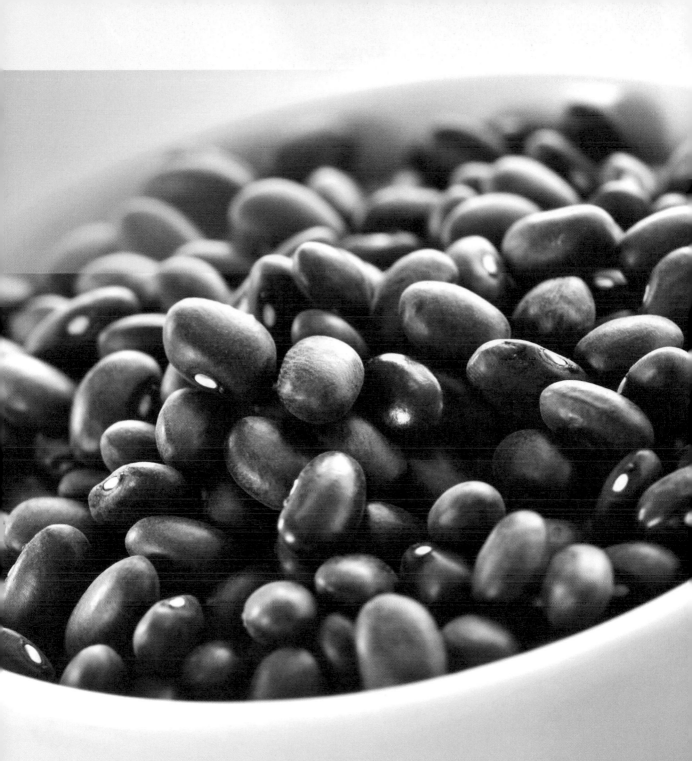

# Pigeon Pea

✪ *Cajanus cajan*

Pigeon pea is a perennial woody shrub grown mostly as an annual for the legume. It is also known as red gram and Congo pea. Pigeon pea is believed to be native to India and the Old World Tropics, where the peas are an ingredient in many traditional dishes and provide an important source of protein. As well as being used as dried peas, pigeon peas can be ground into flour. To improve their digestibility, the dried peas are sometimes sprouted before cooking—this reduces the levels of indigestible sugars.

Pigeon peas are notably high in folate, fiber, protein, thiamine, manganese, copper, magnesium, potassium, zinc, and iron. They are a good source of niacin, riboflavin,

## What's in a Serving?

**DRIED PIGEON PEAS
(1 cup/168 g)**
**Calories:** 203 (850 kJ)
**Protein:** 11.4 g
**Total fat:** 0.6 g
**Saturated fat:** 0.1 g
**Carbohydrates:** 39.1 g
**Fiber:** 11.3 g

## Making the Most of Pigeon Peas

To boost the antioxidant and vitamin A content, combine cooked pigeon peas with chopped carrots, diced tomatoes, green peppers (capsicums), and caramelized onions. Add a dressing of fresh lime juice, cumin, and olive oil, and serve with rice.

pantothenic acid, selenium, and calcium. They also contain a variety of antioxidant compounds, such as phenols.

### THE HEALTHY EVIDENCE

A 2009 article published in the *Journal of Environmental Biology* reported on the antioxidant content of the pigeon pea plant, citing the presence of several different antioxidants. Recent animal studies in China indicate that consuming pigeon pea lowers blood cholesterol. Another animal study published in 2008 in the *Journal of Ethnopharmacology* reported that pigeon pea extract protected the liver from alcohol-induced damage.

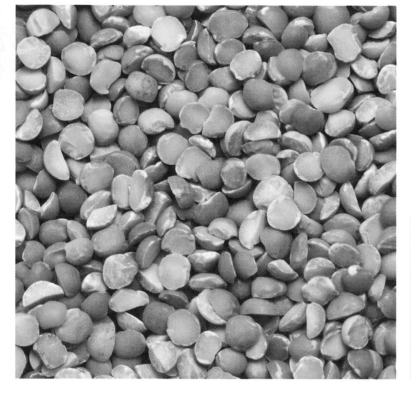

LEFT Pigeon peas are drought-resistant and can be grown on marginal land. They are therefore an important crop for resource-poor farmers.

## In a Nutshell

**Origin:** India and the Old World Tropics
**Season:** Autumn (for fresh pigeon peas)
**Why it's super:** High in folate, fiber, protein, thiamine, manganese, copper, magnesium, potassium, zinc, and iron; good source of niacin, riboflavin, pantothenic acid, selenium, and calcium; contains antioxidants
**Growing at home:** Easily grown in the home garden

# Chickpea or Garbanzo

✿ *Cicer arietinum*

Many people enjoy the food products made from chickpeas, such as hummus, falafel, and channa, without knowing that the main ingredient is this ancient legume. Chickpea evolved from a wild plant native to the Fertile Crescent of the Middle East, which was the first region to cultivate it, as early as 5000 BCE. It arrived in India approximately 2000 BCE, and is now the most important pulse there. Other common names for chickpeas include chichi bean, garbanzo, and Bengal gram.

Chickpeas are an excellent source of vitamin B6, folate, fiber, protein, thiamine, manganese, magnesium, iron, copper, zinc, and potassium. They are, too, a good source of vitamin K, pantothenic acid, calcium, and selenium. In addition, studies have shown they contain antioxidants.

## THE HEALTHY EVIDENCE

The journal *Experimental and Toxicologic Pathology* reported on an animal study showing that fiber from chickpeas protected the liver from a powerful dietary carcinogen, N-nitrosodiethylamine (NDEA). Part of the protective effect may be related to antioxidants in the chickpeas, as the authors stated that the fiber "reduced the peroxidative [cancer-causing] damage done by NDEA."

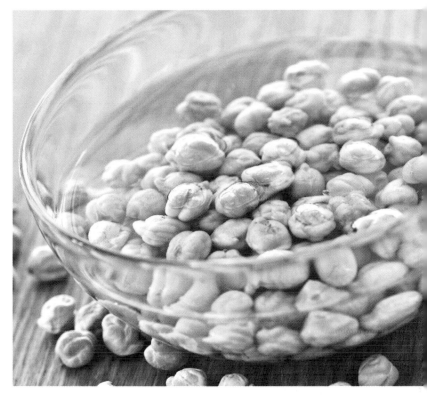

ABOVE Dry chickpeas are usually soaked in water before cooking. Chickpeas are among the oldest known cultivated vegetables, and are an important pulse in many cultures, notably in developing countries.

## Making the Most of Chickpeas

To make a low-fat hummus, use a food processor to purée 2 cups (400 g) of cooked chickpeas. Add 1 tablespoon of olive oil, crushed garlic, fresh lemon juice, and salt to taste. For extra antioxidants and vitamins A and C, add diced red pepper (capsicum).

## What's in a Serving?

**COOKED CHICKPEAS (1 cup/164 g)**

**Calories:** 264 (1125 kJ)
**Protein:** 14.5 g
**Total fat:** 4.3 g
**Saturated fat:** 0.4 g
**Carbohydrates:** 45 g
**Fiber:** 12.5 g

## In a Nutshell

**Origin:** Middle East
**Season:** Late summer (for fresh chickpeas)
**Why it's super:** High in vitamin B6, folate, fiber, protein, thiamine, manganese, magnesium, iron, copper, zinc, and potassium; good source of vitamin K, pantothenic acid, calcium, and selenium; contains antioxidants
**Growing at home:** Can be grown in the home garden; requires 100 days to mature, so start indoors

# Soybean

✪ *Glycine max*

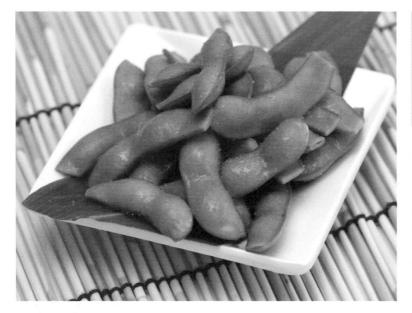

LEFT Fresh baby soybeans boiled with salt and served in the pod is a popular dish in eastern Asian cuisines, known as edamame.

## What's in a Serving?

**COOKED SOYBEANS (1 cup/180 g)**

**Calories:** 254 (1062 kJ)

**Protein:** 22.2 g

**Total fat:** 11.5 g

**Saturated fat:** 1.3 g

**Carbohydrates:** 20 g

**Fiber:** 7.6 g

The soybean, or soya bean, is one of the most important legumes in the world today. Native to China, it arrived in the United States in 1915, as the result of a weevil infestation that devastated cotton crops. It has gradually replaced cottonseed oil as a major edible fat throughout the world. Prominent among the huge variety of soy-based products are tofu and tempeh. Tofu is made by coagulating the liquid from soybeans to form a curd. It is high in protein, but the fiber content is low compared to whole soybeans. Tempeh, which originated in Indonesia, is made from fermented soybeans; it retains the high protein and fiber of the whole soybean.

Soybeans are an excellent source of vitamin K, folate, fiber, protein, thiamine, riboflavin, manganese, copper, magnesium, potassium, zinc, iron, selenium, and calcium. They are also a good source of vitamin C, niacin, and pantothenic acid, and contain bioactive compounds, notably isoflavones.

## THE HEALTHY EVIDENCE

Recent research has pointed to a preventive role for soy in counteracting diseases including cardiovascular disease, diabetes, cancer, and osteoporosis. Much of the focus has been on its isoflavones, polyphenols that act as antioxidants and weak estrogens. In a 2009 review published in *Molecular and Cellular Endocrinology*, the authors concluded that "there is a suggestive body of evidence that soy favorably alters glycemic control, improves weight and fat loss, and lowers triglycerides and cholesterol."

## In a Nutshell

**Origin:** China

**Season:** Early summer (for fresh soybeans)

**Why it's super:** High in vitamin K, folate, fiber, protein, thiamine, riboflavin, manganese, copper, magnesium, potassium, zinc, iron, selenium, and calcium; good source of vitamin C, niacin, and pantothenic acid; contains bioactive compounds, notably isoflavones

**Growing at home:** Easy to grow in the home garden

# Lentil

✿ *Lens culinaris*

Lentils originated in the Mediterranean region, were domesticated as early as 8000 BCE, and were used by ancient civilizations in, among other places, Egypt, Syria, Greece, and Turkey. They played a starring role in the Old Testament, when Esau gave up his birthright for a dish of red pottage made from lentils.

The plant is an erect to sprawling annual that yields a small flat pod containing the familiar convex seeds. Varieties include the familiar brown lentil; the red lentil, which may be whole or split; and the green lentil. A traditional dish from India, dal, or dahl, consists of lentils and/or other legumes puréed and incorporated into a thick creamy stew with onions and various spices.

Lentils are high in vitamin B6, folate, fiber, protein, pantothenic acid, thiamine, manganese, iron, copper, potassium, and zinc. They are a good source of vitamin C, niacin, riboflavin, and selenium. Additionally, they contain antioxidants.

## THE HEALTHY EVIDENCE

A 2009 meta-analysis (a summary of related studies) published in the journal *Diabetologia* reported that lentils, among other pulses, improved blood glucose control in people with diabetes.

### Making the Most of Lentils

Enhance the level of nutrients and antioxidants by combining lentils with kidney beans in a tomato base to make a nontraditional chili without meat. Replacing the meat with legumes also lowers the fat and saturated-fat content of the chili.

### In a Nutshell

**Origin:** Mediterranean

**Season:** Late summer (for fresh lentils)

**Why it's super:** High in vitamin B6, folate, fiber, protein, pantothenic acid, thiamine, manganese, iron, copper, potassium, and zinc; good source of vitamin C, niacin, riboflavin, and selenium; contains antioxidants

**Growing at home:** Easy to grow. Requires up to 110 days to mature, so start indoors.

### What's in a Serving?

**COOKED LENTILS
(1 cup/198 g)**

**Calories:** 230 (964 kJ)

**Protein:** 17.9 g

**Total fat:** 0.8 g

**Saturated fat:** 0.1 g

**Carbohydrates:** 40 g

**Fiber:** 15.6 g

BELOW High in protein, lentils are often a common part of the diet where animal protein is scarce or not eaten for religious or ethical reasons.

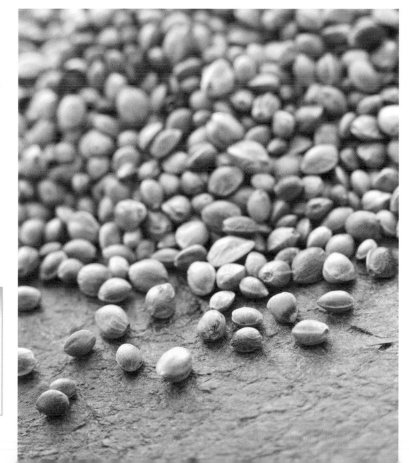

# Beans

✪ *Lupinus* species
✪ *Phaseolus* species

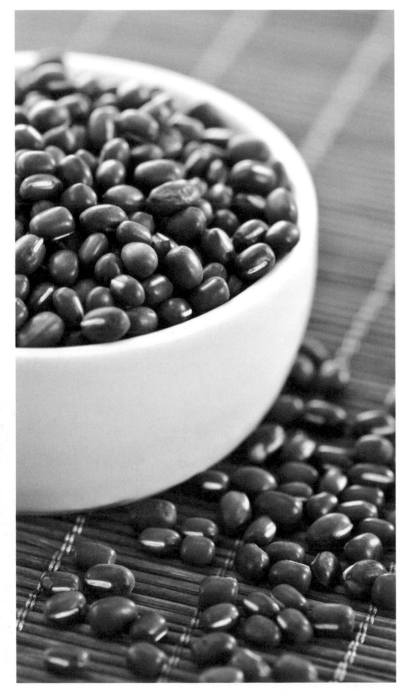

The beans of the *Phaseolus* genus include numerous types, many with an ancient lineage. Thought to have originated in Central America, *P. vulgaris* was cultivated as early as 5000 BCE in the Andes. Now it is grown worldwide, although individual countries tend to favor particular varieties, which include black, borlotti, cannellini, kidney, navy, and pinto beans. The adzuki bean, *P. angularis*, is native to tropical Asia, while the lima bean, *P. lunatus*, originated in South America. Lupins belong to the related *Lupinus* genus.

The high nutrient content of these beans has elevated them to the status of staple foods in the diets of many people around the world. In the past few decades, nutrition research focusing on chronic disease and diet has suggested that they also have a role to play in protecting against cardiovascular disease, diabetes, and cancer. However, it is the protein content of beans that has meant the difference between life and death for millions of people throughout history. When other protein sources were scarce, such as animal products, beans have often taken up the slack.

LEFT Adzuki beans have a nutty, sweet flavor. In Eastern cuisines they are boiled with sugar to make red bean paste, an ingredient in cakes and sweets.

## In a Nutshell

**Origin:** Central America

**Season:** Summer (for fresh beans)

**Why they're super:** High in folate, fiber, protein, thiamine, magnesium, manganese, iron, potassium, copper, and zinc; good source of riboflavin, calcium, and omega-3 fatty acids

**Growing at home:** Easy to grow in the home garden

The protein in beans is of lower quality, based on its ability to support growth, than that found in foods such as meat and dairy products, because it lacks the full complement of essential amino acids. However, in a mixed diet other foods can make up for this deficiency. Early peoples discovered this accidentally by supplementing beans (lacking in the amino acid methionine) with grains (lacking in the amino acid lysine), to provide the full complement of amino acids needed to form a complete protein. Examples of these traditional combinations include dal (a dish of puréed beans or lentils) and rice in India, and corn tortillas and beans in Mexico. One noted botanist, Charles B. Heiser, Jr., referred to this as a "happy accident," since early peoples had no way of knowing about proteins and the individual amino acids from which they arise.

## STORAGE AND PREPARATION

Beans can be stored for long periods of time without it affecting quality or nutrient content. The typical preparation involves soaking the beans overnight, or for at least five hours. Cooking time varies, depending on the soaking duration, but generally requires one or more hours. Beans can of course also be purchased in canned form. Canned beans retain their nutrients, but manufacturers typically add sodium or salt, which may be a problem for those on a restricted sodium diet.

The nutritive value of the various varieties of beans is broadly similar, aside from minor variations due to the different volumes of the beans in a serving. Common beans are generally an excellent source of folate, fiber, protein, thiamine, magnesium, manganese, iron, potassium, copper, and zinc, and a

> ### What's in a Serving?
> **COOKED BLACK BEANS**
> **(1 cup/172 g)**
> **Calories:** 227 (949 kJ)
> **Protein:** 15.2 g
> **Total fat:** 0.9 g
> **Saturated fat:** 0 g
> **Carbohydrates:** 40.8 g
> **Fiber:** 15 g

BELOW Black beans are popular for use in stews, soups, and sauces, especially in Central and South America and the United States.

good source of riboflavin, calcium, and omega-3 fatty acids. The fiber is present partly as soluble fiber, which has particular benefits in controlling blood glucose.

## POPULAR VARIETIES

Among the most popular and nutritious varieties of common bean are the following:

### Adzuki Bean

Also called azuki or aduki, this bean is most familiar as a small red bean, but other cultivars may be black, gray, white, or have a mottled appearance. Adzuki may have originated in the Himalayas, although it is now widespread throughout Asia and second only to the soya bean in Japan.

### Black Bean, Turtle Bean

Particularly popular in Latin American cuisine, this small black bean is often known

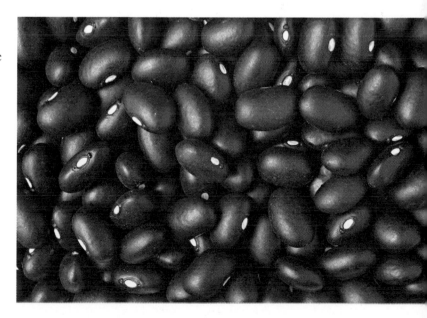

*Beans are practically indestructible ...
and thus have provided critical insurance
against times of famine.*

Ken Albala, US author (1964–)

simply as the black bean, but more properly should be called the black turtle bean to avoid confusion with other black beans. One of the most popular dishes featuring this legume is black bean soup.

### Borlotti Bean
The borlotti bean, also known as the romano bean, is a variety of the cranberry bean, which originated in Colombia. The borlotti was cultivated in Italy, where it is very popular and an ingredient in several traditional dishes. The fresh bean, which is also eaten, has a long curved pod that is bright magenta in color with white mottling.

### Cannellini Bean
This elongated variety of white bean is related to the kidney bean. It is particularly

### Eliminating Toxins
Many varieties of beans contain toxic compounds, phytohemagglutinins, with kidney beans having the highest level. The toxin is destroyed during the typical long cooking time needed for dried beans, as long as the temperature exceeds boiling point (212°F/100°C) for at least ten minutes. However, slow cooking the dried beans does not bring the temperature to this level, and cases of poisoning have occurred when this method has been used. To avoid the potential for toxicity, soak beans for five hours, and always bring to the correct temperature.

popular in Italy, from where the name derives (it means, literally, "little tubes"), especially in soups and pasta dishes.

### Kidney Bean
The distinctive deep red skin and resemblance to the human organ make the kidney bean one of the most familiar of the beans. It is used in the United States in the popular chili con carne dish, and also in the Creole specialty of red beans and rice. Kidney beans are also an important part of the cuisine of northern India.

### Lima Bean, Butter Bean
The lima bean was first cultivated around 2000 BCE in the Andes and takes its name from the city in Peru. It is also known as the butter bean. A favorite way to serve lima beans is boiled and dabbed with butter.

### Lupin
The ancient Romans spread cultivation of the lupin throughout their empire, and the name, which derives from the Latin word for "wolf," has persisted. The beans remain popular in the Mediterranean, notably in Italy. Pale yellow in color, and large and flat, lupins are often

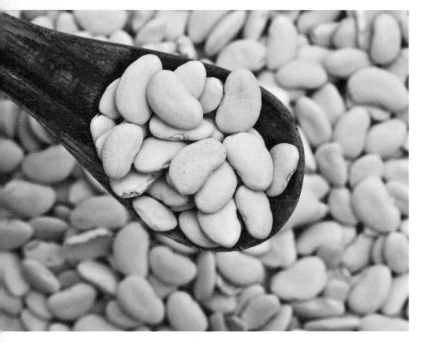

BELOW The Lima bean was important to the ancient Moche people of northern Peru and often appears in their art.

pickled in salty brine and eaten as a condiment, in a similar way to pickles and olives.

### Navy or Haricot Bean, Great Northern Bean

The navy bean, as it is known in the United States, or haricot bean, as it is known in the United Kingdom, is a variety of white bean. It is the bean most often used in recipes in which the bean name is not specified, such as baked beans. The great northern bean is a variety of white bean that is shaped like a lima bean but is larger. It is popular in stews.

### Pinto Bean

Its mottled appearance provides this bean with its common name, which is Spanish for "painted." It also causes some confusion as it is similar in appearance to the borlotti bean and other cranberry beans. Texans know these beans as "cowboy beans," because they were a staple food for cowboys. Pinto is the usual choice for the dish known as refried beans.

### THE HEALTHY EVIDENCE

Researchers at the Food and Nutrition Research Institute conducted a study, published in the *British Journal of Nutrition*, to determine the health effects of ten legumes, mostly beans. They measured blood cholesterol in subjects with and without high cholesterol, and blood glucose and insulin in subjects with and without diabetes. They concluded that legumes are useful as a low glycemic index food and have the potential to lower cholesterol levels, and that this is a "scientific basis for considering legumes as functional foods [foods with health-promoting effects]." The benefits were thought to derive from the high content of soluble fiber in beans.

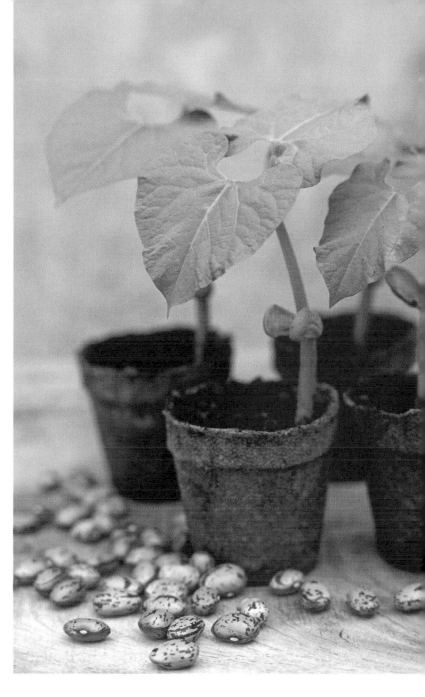

### Making the Most of Common Beans

The time-honored use of beans as a main course, in combination with a grain, makes the best use of its nutrients. In addition, this ensures an adequate serving to maximize health benefits. Season cooked kidney beans with chili powder and cilantro, and add fresh diced tomatoes. Serve over brown rice.

ABOVE 'Lingua di fuoco', meaning "tongue of fire," is a popular cultivar of the borlotti bean. Both its pods and its beans have bright red markings.

# Split Pea

✪ *Pisum sativum*

Though *Pisum sativum* is native to the Mediterranean, archaeologists have found indications that peas were grown in Switzerland around 3000 BCE. The cultivation of peas was common in ancient Greece, Rome, and India, and reached China by the seventh century CE. During the Middle Ages, dried peas were a vital part of the diet of impoverished Europeans. Peas were introduced to the United States in the early colonial period.

The pea plant produces pods containing between five and nine round seeds or peas, and they may be yellow or green. The pea pods are harvested when fully mature and then dried. After drying, when the skins are removed, the peas split naturally. If the pods are allowed to dry in the field, the peas are known as marrowfat peas.

Split peas are an excellent source of vitamin K, folate, fiber, protein, thiamine, pantothenic acid, manganese, potassium, magnesium, copper, iron, and zinc. They are also a good source of vitamin B6, niacin, and riboflavin. In addition, peas contain significant levels of flavonoids, which research has shown to help prevent chronic diseases.

## THE HEALTHY EVIDENCE

A 2010 study published in the journal *Molecular Nutrition and Food Research* reported that a protein isolated from peas had a significant blood-cholesterol-lowering effect. Studies have also reported that flavonoids function as antioxidants and anti-inflammatory agents, suggesting that higher dietary intake may lower risk of heart disease and cancer.

### Making the Most of Split Peas

Try this healthy method to introduce more nutrients and antioxidants to split pea recipes: Bring 2 cups (400 g) of peas in 8 cups (2 l) of water to the boil, and then simmer for 40 minutes. Drain the excess water; add 1 teaspoon each of turmeric and ginger, 3 bay leaves, 2 tablespoons of olive oil, and salt to taste.

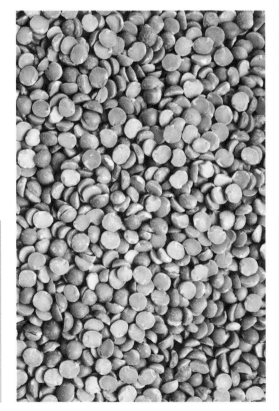

LEFT The Chinese consumed split peas at least as early as 2000 BCE. Peas were not widely consumed fresh until the 1600s.

### In a Nutshell

**Origin:** Mediterranean region

**Season:** Summer (for fresh peas)

**Why it's super:** High in vitamin K, folate, fiber, protein, thiamine, pantothenic acid, manganese, potassium, magnesium, copper, iron, and zinc; good source of vitamin B6, niacin, and riboflavin; contains flavonoids

**Growing at home:** Easy to cultivate in the home garden

### What's in a Serving?

**COOKED SPLIT PEAS
(1 cup/196 g)**

**Calories:** 231 (968 kJ)

**Protein:** 16.4 g

**Total fat:** 0.8 g

**Saturated fat:** 0.1 g

**Carbohydrates:** 41.4 g

**Fiber:** 16.3 g

# Black-eyed Pea

✪ *Vigna unguiculata*

## What's in a Serving?

**COOKED BLACK-EYED PEAS**

**(1 cup/172 g)**

**Calories:** 200 (832 kJ)

**Protein:** 13.3 g

**Total fat:** 0.9 g

**Saturated fat:** 0.2 g

**Carbohydrates:** 35.7 g

**Fiber:** 5.7 g

Although it is also grown for its immature seed pods, black-eyed pea is more usually cultivated for its dried beans. The beans are also known as cowpeas and have been a staple food in the southern United States for centuries. Black-eyed peas originated in Africa and were first domesticated in West Africa around 3000 BCE. They spread from Africa 1,500 years later to India and Southeast Asia, but did not reach the New World until Spanish and Portuguese explorers took them there in the sixteenth century.

The plant can be shrublike, erect, vining, or take other forms, and the flowers range from white to deep purple. Similar variation occurs in the coloration and shape of the pods and seeds. The most familiar is the distinctive pale yellow bean with the black spot on one side.

Black-eyed peas are high in folate, fiber, protein, thiamine, manganese, iron, magnesium, zinc, copper, and potassium. They are a good source of vitamin B6, riboflavin, pantothenic acid, and selenium.

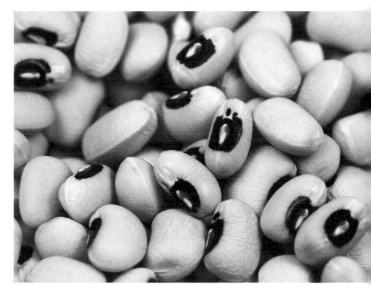

ABOVE In the southern United States, eating dishes incorporating black-eyed peas on New Year's Day is said to bring good luck.

## Making the Most of Black-eyed Peas

Here's a way to make a healthy version of a traditional southern United States recipe, quick Hoppin' John soup. Combine cooked or canned black-eyed peas with chicken or vegetable stock, add diced tomatoes, chopped onions and carrots, and cooked wild brown rice. Simmer for approximately 30 minutes.

## In a Nutshell

**Origin:** Africa

**Season:** Summer (for fresh black-eyed peas)

**Why it's super:** High in folate, fiber, protein, thiamine, manganese, iron, magnesium, zinc, copper, and potassium; good source of vitamin B6, riboflavin, pantothenic acid, and selenium

**Growing at home:** Easy to grow in the home garden

## THE HEALTHY EVIDENCE

A 2009 review published in the *American Journal of Clinical Nutrition* pointed to the benefits of a vegetarian diet based on higher levels of the nutrients contained in black-eyed peas. The author noted that vegetarians tend to be "thinner, have lower serum cholesterol, and lower blood pressure, thus reducing their risk of heart disease."

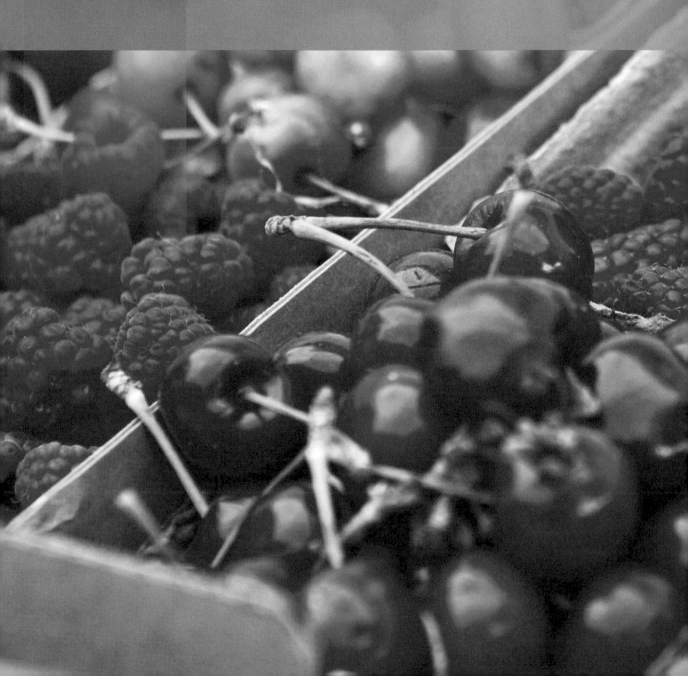

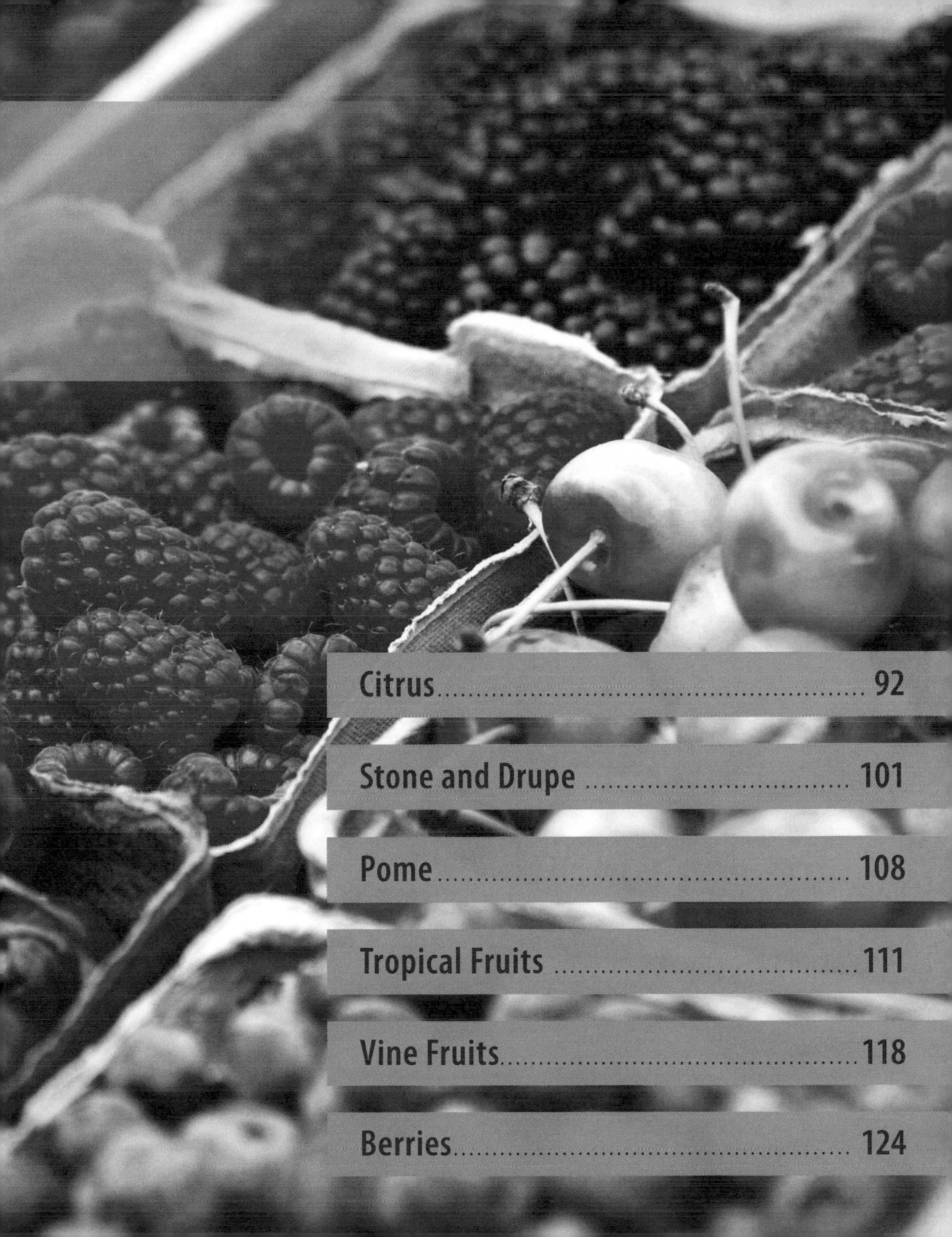

## CITRUS

# Limes

- ✪ *Citrus aurantifolia* Lime, Key Lime
- ✪ *Citrus hystrix* Kaffir Lime
- ✪ *Citrus latifolia* Persian Lime, Tahitian Lime

<table>
<tr><td colspan="2">What's in a Serving?</td></tr>
<tr><td colspan="2">FRESH LIME</td></tr>
<tr><td colspan="2">1 peeled</td></tr>
<tr><td colspan="2">(2.4 ounces/67 g)</td></tr>
<tr><td>Calories:</td><td>20 (84 kJ)</td></tr>
<tr><td>Protein:</td><td>0.5 g</td></tr>
<tr><td>Total fat:</td><td>0 g</td></tr>
<tr><td>Saturated fat:</td><td>0 g</td></tr>
<tr><td>Carbohydrates:</td><td>7.1 g</td></tr>
<tr><td>Fiber:</td><td>2 g</td></tr>
</table>

The most common lime species, *Citrus aurantifolia*, likely originated in southern India or the northern end of the Persian Gulf. In the Middle Ages, Arabs took limes to western areas of conquest, and Columbus carried them to the island of Hispaniola. In 1747, a British physician determined that limes could prevent scurvy—vitamin C deficiency—which had claimed the lives of many sailors; British sailors soon became known as "limeys" for their cargo of limes.

The less familiar species, the Persian or Tahitian lime, did not arrive in the West until the 1800s, when it was introduced by the Persians. Another species, the kaffir lime, is used in Southeast Asian cuisine, notably Thai cookery, which also makes use of the leaves.

BELOW The smallest of the true citrus, limes are particularly important in Latin American, Southeast Asian, and Caribbean cuisines.

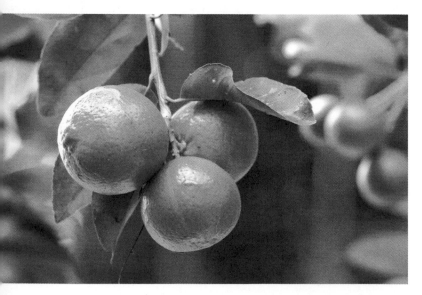

### In a Nutshell

**Origin:** Southern India or northern Persian Gulf
**Season:** Year-round
**Why they're super:** High in vitamin C; good source of fiber; contain flavonoids and liminoids
**Growing at home:** Difficult to grow and requires a tropical climate

Limes are an excellent source of vitamin C, with a single lime providing 32 percent of the Daily Value, as well as a good source of fiber. Limes also contain the compounds flavonoids and liminoids, which may protect against cancer and other diseases.

### THE HEALTHY EVIDENCE

A 2009 study published in the *Journal of Agricultural and Food Chemistry* reported that lime juice inhibited the growth of pancreatic cancer cells in two ways: the liminoids, which include limonexic acid, isolimonexic acid, and limonin, inhibited the growth process of the cells, and the flavonoids, which include rutin, neohesperidin, hesperidin, and hesperitin, acted as antioxidants to fight cancer, while also restricting cancer cell growth.

### Making the Most of Limes

For optimal benefits, consume the juice (usually 1–2 tablespoons per lime), which is only missing the fiber. Limes at room temperature are easier to juice. Combine the juice with olive oil and seasonings, and use as a fresh salad dressing.

# Kumquat

✿ *Citrus japonica*

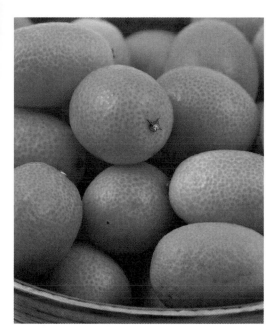

LEFT Because it is more resistant to cold than other citrus, the kumquat is often crossed with other citrus species to produce hybrid fruit.

Oval to round in shape, the kumquat is the smallest member of the citrus family. It originated in China, where literary references to the fruit date back to the twelfth century. It was first taken to Europe in 1847, when a renowned British plant collector, Robert Fortune, brought it home from China—the genus, *Fortunella*, is still named for him. From Britain, the kumquat was transported to Florida, where it is still popular as a miniature ornamental plant.

The kumquat cultivars include 'Nagami', 'Marumi', 'Meiwa', and 'Hong Kong Kumquat', although this last is not edible. 'Nagami', which has oval-shaped and somewhat bitter fruit, is the cultivar that Robert Fortune brought from China and later exported to Florida. Both 'Marumi' and 'Meiwa' hail from Japan, and 'Meiwa' has become the most popular kumquat because of its sweet flesh.

Kumquats are an excellent source of vitamin C and a good source of fiber—the peel is edible. They also contain numerous phytochemicals, including several flavonoids, which are powerful antioxidants.

## THE HEALTHY EVIDENCE

A 2009 study published in the journal *Plant Foods for Human Nutrition* reported on an analysis of kumquat composition. It found a rich supply of various antioxidants, including flavonoids, which encompass several thousand compounds and are a type of polyphenol. The authors concluded that the kumquat "peel may be regarded as a rich source of potentially bioactive polyphenols."

### In a Nutshell

**Origin:** China
**Season:** Late fall through winter
**Why it's super:** High in vitamin C; good source of fiber; contains antioxidant flavonoids
**Growing at home:** Can be grown at home in warm climates. Will tolerate cold better than most other citrus trees.

### What's in a Serving?

FRESH KUMQUAT
**2 whole kumquats
(1.3 ounces/38 g)**
**Calories:** 26 (112 kJ)
**Protein:** 0.8 g
**Total fat:** 0.4 g
**Saturated fat:** 0 g
**Carbohydrates:** 6 g
**Fiber:** 2.4 g

# Oranges

- ✿ *Citrus aurantium* Seville Orange, Bitter Orange
- ✿ *Citrus aurantium* subsp. *bergamia* Bergamot Orange
- ✿ *Citrus reticulata* x *Citrus sinensis* Florida Orange, Tangor
- ✿ *Citrus sinensis* Sweet Orange

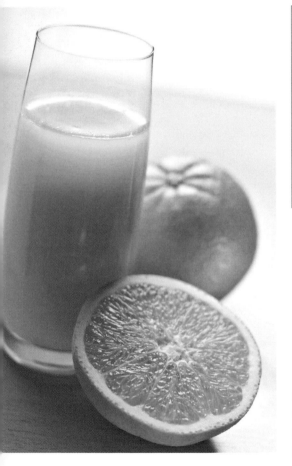

## What's in a Serving?

**FRESH ORANGE**

**1 peeled**

**(5 ounces/141 g)**

**Calories:** 65 (271 kJ)

**Protein:** 0.1 g

**Total fat:** 0.3 g

**Saturated fat:** 0 g

**Carbohydrates:** 16.3 g

**Fiber:** 3.4 g

LEFT Freshly squeezed orange juice is richer in nutrients than other popular fresh juices, such as apple, pineapple, and grape juices.

## In a Nutshell

**Origin:** Southeast Asia

**Season:** Late autumn

**Why they're super:** High in vitamin C, thiamine, and dietary fiber; good source of vitamins A and B6, folate, pantothenic acid, calcium, magnesium, and potassium; contain numerous antioxidants

**Growing at home:** Can be grown at home in warm (subtropical) climates

Although the orange is one of the most familiar, widely available, and popular of all fruits, it is actually a hybrid of other citrus fruits, most likely a cross between the pummelo or pomelo *(Citrus maxima)* and the tangerine *(C. reticulata)*. Of the major varieties, the sweet orange, which is also known as the Portuguese or China orange, is the most widely enjoyed, followed by the Seville orange. The Florida or tangor orange is a hybrid of the sweet orange and the tangerine (also known as mandarin; see p. 99), the word "tangor" deriving from "tang" from tangerine and "or" from orange. A subspecies of the Seville, the bergamot orange is popular in Italy for its fragrance and is used in the perfume industry; it is also an ingredient in Earl Grey tea.

### SWEET AND FRAGRANT

Both the sweet orange and the Seville orange originated in Southeast Asia. Although it is unclear which arrived first, the Seville was the first to be widely cultivated in Europe. It was imported by Arabs during the conquest of the Iberian peninsula, where the tree became highly prized for its beauty and fragrant blossoms and leaves. In 1500, Vasco Da Gama introduced the sweet orange to Europe from India. The first Spanish colonists to settle in southern Florida took the sweet orange to the United States about 60 years later, and missionaries spread the plant to California within the next three decades. In the early nineteenth century, the orange traveled from Brazil to Australia.

Oranges are an excellent source of vitamin C, thiamine, and fiber, most of which is

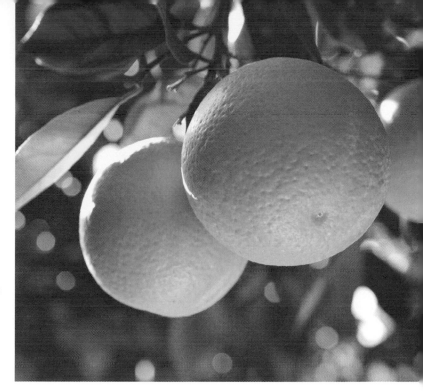

soluble fiber, the type most associated with lowering cholesterol and regulation of blood glucose. In addition, oranges are a good source of vitamins A and B6, folate, pantothenic acid, calcium, magnesium, and potassium. They also contain numerous phytochemicals, including a variety of antioxidants such as beta-cryptoxanthin, lutein, and zeaxanthin.

## THE HEALTHY EVIDENCE

By itself, vitamin C is a significant anti-oxidant, but in oranges it works even more effectively by combining with other anti-oxidants, and together these can protect against oxidative damage that leads to cardiovascular disease, cancer, and ageing. This effect was demonstrated by a study described in the *British Journal of Nutrition*, which reported that a vitamin C supplement did not confer the same antioxidant benefits as consuming orange juice. The Italian researchers found that, while vitamin C alone provided some protection against oxidative damage, other compounds in oranges were more important, including cyanidin-3-

*I got the blues thinking of the future, so I left off and made some marmalade. It's amazing how it cheers one up to shred oranges and scrub the floor.*

D. H. Lawrence, British poet, novelist, and essayist (1885–1930)

glucoside, flavanones, and carotenoids, though the researchers noted, "how they are interacting is still anyone's guess."

In a major report, "The Health Benefits of Citrus Fruits," Australia's federal government scientific research body, the CSIRO (Commonwealth Scientific and Industrial Research Organisation), reviewed 48 studies on citrus fruits. They concluded that citrus fruits were especially beneficial in warding off esophageal, laryngeal, and stomach cancer, with a risk reduction approaching 50 percent. One large study included in the review reported a 19 percent risk reduction in stroke, resulting from the addition of just one daily serving of citrus fruit.

### Making the Most of Oranges

The most effective way to derive the benefits of all the nutrients in orange is to eat a fresh orange or drink the juice. The juice will have higher levels of almost all the nutrients, because of its concentration from the fruit. However, a serving of juice contains double the calories and 85 percent less fiber.

# Lemons

✪ *Citrus ichangensis* Ichang Lemon
✪ *Citrus limetta* Sweet Lemon
✪ *Citrus limon* Lemon
✪ *Citrus x meyeri* Meyer Lemon

Lemons originated in India and China, arriving in the Middle East in the twelfth century. On his second voyage to the New World, Columbus took lemons to the West Indies, and by the sixteenth century they had made their way to Florida via Haiti. Lemons are hardy plants that thrive in an arid sub-tropical climate. Their popularity has been such that the cuisines of virtually every human culture rely on their aromatic flavor and acidic quality.

## VARIETIES AND ORIGINS

*Citrus limon* most likely represents a mutation of the citron *(Citrus medica)* rather than a separate citrus species. Other important species of lemon include the Meyer lemon, the Ichang lemon, and the sweet lemon. The Meyer, grown in California and other parts of the world, has a thin peel and sweet juicy flesh. The Ichang Lemon, which probably derives its name from the city of Yichang in China, is native to East Asia; it is a slow-growing cultivar and extremely hardy. The sweet lemon, also known as the sweet lime, has a round shape and sweet flesh.

Lemons are an excellent source of vitamin C and fiber. They contain numerous phyto-chemicals, many of them antioxidants,

| What's in a Serving? |
|---|
| **FRESH LEMON** |
| **1 peeled** |
| **(3 ounces/84 g)** |
| **Calories:** 24 (102 kJ) |
| **Protein:** 1 g |
| **Total fat:** 0.3 g |
| **Saturated fat:** 0 g |
| **Carbohydrates:** 7.8 g |
| **Fiber:** 2.4 g |

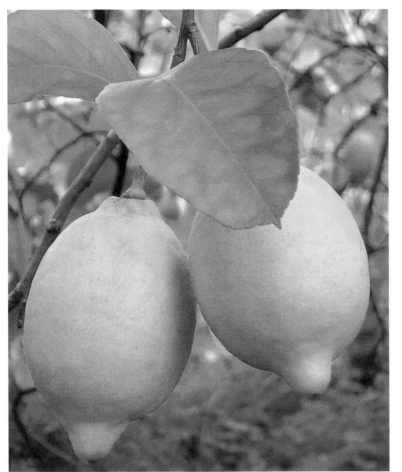

LEFT Lemon is highly versatile. Not only the fruit, but also the juice, the rind or zest, and the seeds can be used in cuisine.

## In a Nutshell

**Origin:** India and China
**Season:** Year-round
**Why they're super:** High in vitamin C and fiber; contain phytochemicals, such as limonin and limonene
**Growing at home:** Can be grown at home in warm (subtropical) climates

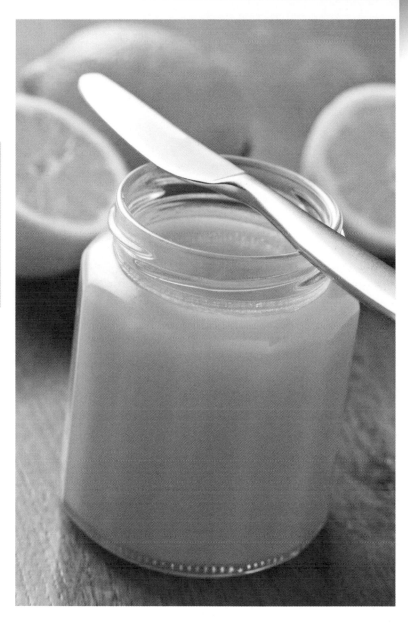

ABOVE Lemons can be preserved or incorporated in jams and curds. Lemon curd is traditionally used as an alternative to jam, and served on breads or in tarts.

## Making the Most of Lemons

Traditional lemonade provides the best supply of nutrients and phytochemicals. Make sure the lemons are at room temperature for most effective juicing. Wash the lemons well, then use a juicer to extract juice and some pulp. Add sliced lemons and sugar or other sweetener to taste, then cover, refrigerate, and use quickly to avoid loss of vitamin C.

which can help fight disease. Some of the antioxidants, notably limonin and limonene, appear to have an anticancer effect.

### THE HEALTHY EVIDENCE

A 2010 article in the *Journal of Pharmaceutical and Biomedical Analysis* highlighted the health-promoting nutrients and phytochemicals in lemons, such as phenols, essential oils, and other antioxidants. One group of phenols, the liminoids, has been shown in both animal and human cell studies to combat viruses and bacteria, as well as cancer. A study published in the journal *Nutrition and Cancer* reported on the anticancer effects of one particular liminoid contained in lemons, limonin, as well as other liminoids, against two human cancer cell types, neuroblastoma and colon cancer cells. The compounds exerted more than one effect to combat the cancer cells.

A 2009 study published in the *Journal of Carcinogenesis* reported on another compound high in lemons, limonene. The authors found that in prostate cancer cells it enhanced the anticancer effect of a chemotherapy drug without damaging normal cells. They concluded that limonene could be combined with other treatments to improve outcomes.

## The Lemon Cure?

First popularized 50 years ago and still touted on the Internet as a way to lose weight, the "Lemon Detox Diet" involves consuming a solution of water, lemon juice, cayenne pepper, and maple syrup, referred to as the "Master Cleanse." However, although lemons contain a bevy of potent phytochemicals, no studies to date have supported the claims that eating lemons promotes weight loss.

# Grapefruit

✪ *Citrus x paradisi*

The grapefruit differs from other citrus species in that it is the only citrus indigenous to the New World. It's a hybrid of the pummelo *(Citrus maxima)* and the sweet orange, and it first appeared in Barbados in the early 1800s. The seedless 'Marsh' grapefruit is the main cultivar, and it descended from the oldest cultivar, the 'Duncan'. The latter is named for A. L. Duncan, who in 1892 began cultivating the plant in Florida. The 'Marsh' grapefruit may be white, or pink-fleshed; in contrast, the 'Star Ruby' cultivar grown in Texas has deep red flesh. The perception that the pink or red grapefruit is sweeter than the white is unfounded, although only pink and red contain significant vitamin A.

Grapefruit is an excellent source of vitamin C, fiber, and potassium, and pink and red grapefruits are high in vitamin A. It is also a good source of vitamin B6, pantothenic acid, thiamine, magnesium, copper, and selenium. Grapefruit contains phytochemicals, notably the antioxidant phenols; pink and red grapefruits also contain high levels of antioxidant carotenoids.

## Making the Most of Grapefruit

Eat a fresh grapefruit or drink grapefruit juice to obtain the highest level of nutrients. One serving of the juice is higher in most nutrients due to the increased concentration relative to the fruit, but significantly lower in fiber.

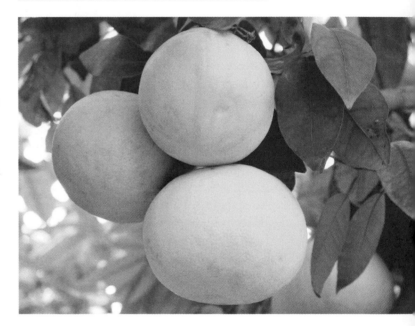

## In a Nutshell

**Origin:** Jamaica

**Season:** Late autumn to early winter

**Why it's super:** High in vitamin C, potassium, and fiber (pink and red are also high in vitamin A); good source of vitamin B6, pantothenic acid, thiamine, magnesium, copper, and selenium; contains antioxidant phenols

**Growing at home:** Easy to grow at home in warm (subtropical) climates

ABOVE In a good year, a single grapefruit tree can produce 1300–1500 pounds (591–682 kg) of fruit. In the United States, approximately 40 percent of the harvest is used for juice and the rest is sold fresh.

### THE HEALTHY EVIDENCE

A 2007 study published in the *Journal of Agricultural and Food Chemistry* evaluated the antioxidant potency of various fruit juices by analyzing their content of the antioxidant phenols. Of the 13 juices studied, grapefruit was among the highest in phenol content and antioxidant potency.

## What's in a Serving?

**FRESH GRAPEFRUIT**
**Segments with juice**
**(1 cup/230 g)**
**Calories:** 76 (317 kJ)
**Protein:** 1.59 g
**Total fat:** 0.2 g
**Saturated fat:** 0 g
**Carbohydrates:** 19.3 g
**Fiber:** 2.5 g

# Tangerine, Mandarin, or Clementine

✿ *Citrus reticulata*

The tangerine is also known as a mandarin orange or Clementine. Hybridization has given rise to the many varieties of this species. They all tend to have thin skins, which are easy to peel, and sweet flesh. Early species were taken from China to Japan in CE 500, but the fruit did not arrive in the United States until the mid-1800s. A popular variety, the Clementine, derives its name from a French missionary, Father Clément Rodier, who developed it in Oran, Algeria, in 1902.

Tangerines are an excellent source of vitamins A and C and fiber, and a good source of vitamin B6, thiamine, calcium, folate, magnesium, and potassium. Tangerines also contain antioxidant carotenoids, such as alpha-carotene, beta-carotene, beta-cryptoxanthin, lutein, and zeaxanthin, as well as many flavonoids, including tangeretin (also spelled tangeritin) and nobiletin.

## THE HEALTHY EVIDENCE

The numerous and diverse types of anti-oxidants, including both phytochemical and essential nutrients, make tangerines a small powerhouse in fighting chronic disease. A 2010 study published in the journal *Biochemical Pharmacology* reported that nobiletin improved blood glucose control in obese diabetic mice. Research also suggests that tangeretin may help to protect against cardiovascular disease, cancer, and Parkinson's disease. A study published in the journal *Agricultural and Food Chemistry* reported that the compound lowered blood cholesterol in hamsters with high levels of cholesterol.

### What's in a Serving?

**FRESH TANGERINE**
Sections (1 cup/195 g)
**Calories:** 103 (435 kJ)
**Protein:** 1.6 g
**Total fat:** 0.6 g
**Saturated fat:** 0.1 g
**Carbohydrates:** 26 g
**Fiber:** 3.5 g

### In a Nutshell

**Origin:** China
**Season:** Late autumn to early winter
**Why it's super:** High in vitamins A and C and fiber; good source of vitamin B6, thiamine, calcium, folate, magnesium, and potassium; contains antioxidant carotenoids and flavonoids
**Growing at home:** Moderately difficult to grow at home (takes five to seven years to produce fruit)

### Making the Most of Tangerines

Tangerines are best enjoyed raw and make a highly nutritious addition to a fresh salad. To boost the variety of nutrients and antioxidants, combine tangerine segments with fresh leaf spinach, water chestnuts, thinly sliced sweet red pepper, and shredded carrots. Toss with a sesame-based dressing.

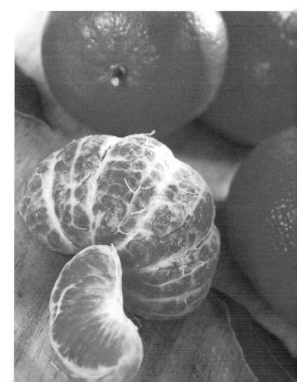

RIGHT Clementines are small, juicy, and sweet, and less acidic than oranges. Their skin generally peels off easily, which makes them popular with children.

# Tangelo

✿ *Citrus x tangelo*

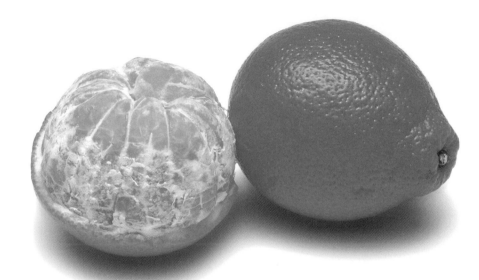

ABOVE Easy to peel, the tangelo is extremely juicy. It has a slightly sharp taste, closer to that of a tangerine than an orange.

Citrus hybrids arise without human assistance, and the tangelo is one of these "happy accidents," having originated in China 2,500 years ago. It is a cross between either a pummelo *(Citrus maxima)* or grapefruit and a tangerine, and normally closer in size to its larger progenitor. Two popular cultivars are the 'Honeybell' and the 'Minneola', both developed by researchers in Florida in 1930.

Tangelos are an excellent source of vitamin C and fiber, as well as a good source of folate and potassium. They also contain a wide range of flavonoids, including naringin, a powerful antioxidant.

## In a Nutshell

**Origin:** China

**Season:** Late autumn through winter

**Why it's super:** High in vitamin C and fiber; good source of folate and potassium; contains flavonoids

**Growing at home:** Can be grown at home in warm (subtropical) climates

## What's in a Serving?

**FRESH TANGELO**

**Sections (1 cup/99 g)**

**Calories:** 47 (196 kJ)

**Protein:** 0.9 g

**Total fat:** 0.1 g

**Saturated fat:** 0 g

**Carbohydrates:** 11.8 g

**Fiber:** 2.4 g

## Making the Most of Tangelos

Tangelos are excellent in salads, where they add significantly to the nutrients in other ingredients. Combine lettuce with peeled segments and chopped walnuts, and toss with a honey and poppy seed dressing (grate the peel and add 1–2 tablespoons of honey, 2 tablespoons of tangelo juice, 1 tablespoon canola oil, and 1 teaspoon poppy seeds).

## THE HEALTHY EVIDENCE

Tangelos contain high levels of vitamin C, an essential nutrient that functions as an antioxidant, as well as numerous other antioxidants that protect against chronic diseases. A 2010 study published in the journal *Toxicology* reported that while many types of citrus fruits contain similar flavonoids, tangelos contain the highest level of naringin. This flavonoid metabolizes to another compound, naringenin. Studies have shown that both flavonoids may inhibit the growth of cancer cells and lower blood cholesterol levels.

# STONE AND DRUPE

# Avocado

✿ *Persea americana*

Native to areas of South and Central America, the avocado is also known as butter pear and alligator pear. The name for the tree and the fruit comes from the Aztec word *ahuacatl*, meaning "testicle," a reference not only to the fruit's shape but also to its propensity to hang from the tree in pairs. The avocado spread to Indonesia by 1750, to California by 1850, and to Australia 50 years later.

Avocados are an excellent source of vitamins B6, C, E, and K, folate, fiber, pantothenic acid, riboflavin, niacin, magnesium, potassium, copper, and manganese, and a good source of thiamine, iron, phosphorus, and zinc. They also contain the antioxidant carotenoids lutein and zeaxanthin, as well as healthy fatty acids, including alpha-linolenic acid and oleic acid.

## THE HEALTHY EVIDENCE

In a study published in the *Journal of Nutritional Biochemistry*, avocado extract was shown to inhibit the development of prostate cancer cells. The combination of carotenoids and vitamin E, and perhaps other nutrients, is thought to provide the anticancer benefit. The healthy fatty acids also ensure that these fat-soluble compounds are readily absorbed.

## In a Nutshell

**Origin:** South and Central America

**Season:** Winter to late summer, depending on variety

**Why it's super:** High in vitamins B6, C, E, and K, folate, fiber, pantothenic acid, riboflavin, niacin, magnesium, potassium, copper, manganese; good source of thiamine, iron, phosphorus, and zinc; contain antioxidant carotenoids lutein and zeaxanthin, and healthy fatty acids

**Growing at home:** Can be grown from seeds and transplanted outdoors in warm climates; in cooler climates, keep indoors until weather warms

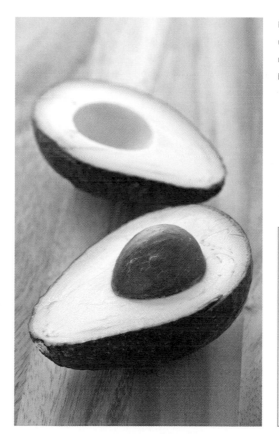

LEFT Ripe avocados will dent under gentle pressure. To speed up ripening, place the avocado in a brown paper bag with an apple.

## Making the Most of Avocados

An excellent way to maximize the nutrients is to mash fresh avocados together with chopped onion, diced tomato, and seasonings to make a dip. For even more nutrients, eat with fresh vegetables such as baby carrots, sweet red pepper, or sugar snap peas.

## What's in a Serving?

**FRESH AVOCADO**

**1 cut in cubes
(1 cup/150 g)**

**Calories:** 240 (1005 kJ)

**Protein:** 3 g

**Total fat:** 22 g

**Saturated fat:** 3.2 g

**Carbohydrates:** 12.8 g

**Fiber:** 10 g

# Date

✿ *Phoenix dactylifera*

The date palm originated in the lands around the Persian Gulf and in ancient times was abundant between the Nile and Euphrates rivers. Archaeological evidence suggests it was cultivated in eastern Arabia in 4000 BCE, where it was regarded as a symbol of fertility. The name comes from the Greek word *daktulos*, meaning "finger," a reference to its shape.

Arabs took the date palm to parts of Asia, northern Africa, Spain, and Italy, where dates were widely eaten fresh, dried, pressed into cakes, and even made into wine. By 1765,

## What's in a Serving?

**PITTED DATES**
**3 whole**
**(2.6 ounces/72 g)**
**Calories:** 199 (835 kJ)
**Protein:** 1.3 g
**Total fat:** 0.1 g
**Saturated fat:** 0 g
**Carbohydrates:** 54 g
**Fiber:** 4.8 g

## Making the Most of Dates

Fresh dates make an excellent snack and will retain nutrients even when cooked. Chop them and add them to cereals, breads, muffins, and other grain products, or use them to add fiber and other nutrients to meat and rice dishes.

Spanish missionaries had transported the date to Mexico and California.

More than 1,500 cultivars of date exist, among the most popular of which is the 'Medjool'. It is marketed as a deluxe date in California, because of its large size, soft texture, and rich flavor.

Dates are an excellent source of fiber, potassium, copper, and manganese, and a good source of vitamin B6, niacin, pantothenic acid, and calcium. They also contain phenols, which function as antioxidants.

### THE HEALTHY EVIDENCE

A 2009 study published in the *Journal of Agricultural and Food Chemistry* reported on the effects of the 'Medjool' and 'Hallawi' dates in human subjects. Both were high in phenols and exhibited significant antioxidant activity. They also reduced blood triglyceride levels, elevated levels of which are a risk factor for heart disease.

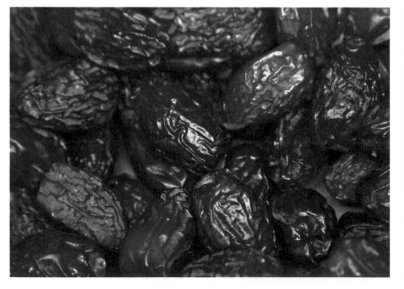

## In a Nutshell

**Origin:** Around the Persian Gulf
**Season:** Autumn to early winter
**Why it's super:** High in potassium, copper, manganese, and fiber; good source of vitamin B6, niacin, pantothenic acid, and calcium; contains phenols
**Growing at home:** Can be grown in warm climates, but may take several years to fruit

LEFT Most dates sold commercially in Western countries are dried dates, which are high in sugar. They can be added to sweet foods such as cakes, desserts, and milk shakes, but will also effectively complement the flavors of certain savory foods including breads, cheeses, and meats.

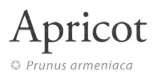

# Apricot

✪ *Prunus armeniaca*

## What's in a Serving?

**FRESH APRICOT**

Slices (1 cup/165 g)

**Calories:** 79 (332 kJ)

**Protein:** 2.3 g

**Total fat:** 0.6 g

**Saturated fat:** 0 g

**Carbohydrates:** 18.4 g

**Fiber:** 3.3 g

The apricot is native to Armenia and was cultivated in ancient times; its scientific name, which means "Armenian plum," acknowledges its land of origin. The apricot was also cultivated in ancient Persia, and Alexander the Great may have introduced the fruit to Greece, from where it spread quickly throughout Europe. English settlers took apricots to the New World, and later Spanish missionaries carried seedlings to California, now a major source of the fruit. Apricots are also grown from western Asia to Japan, and in southern Europe, northern and southern Africa, and Australia (notably South Australia's Riverland).

Apricots are an excellent source of vitamins A and C, potassium, and fiber, and a good source of vitamins E and K, protein, niacin, copper, and manganese. They also contain antioxidant carotenoids such as beta-carotene, beta-cryptoxanthin, lutein, and zeaxanthin.

### THE HEALTHY EVIDENCE

Apricots can combat the oxidative damage that occurs in many diseases, as indicated by the *Iowa Women's Health Study*, conducted

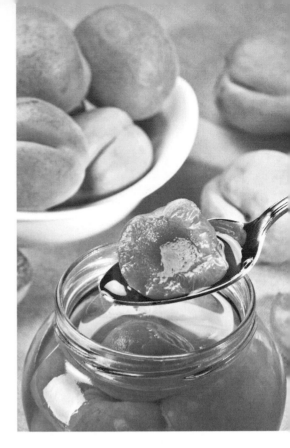

ABOVE Apricots are sweet and naturally high in pectin, which makes them an excellent choice for jams and other kinds of preserves.

by the University of Minnesota Cancer Center, which found that higher intakes of carotenoids and vitamins C and E were associated with a lower risk of gastrointestinal cancers. A 2009 study published in the *British Journal of Nutrition* reported that apricots significantly reduced liver damage in rats exposed to liver toxins. The authors concluded that "Dietary intake of apricot can reduce the risk of liver damage caused by free radicals."

### In a Nutshell

**Origin:** Armenia

**Season:** Spring through mid-summer, depending on climate

**Why it's super:** High in vitamins A and C, fiber, and potassium; good source of vitamins E and K, protein, niacin, copper, and manganese; contains antioxidant carotenoids

**Growing at home:** Easy to grow, but may take three years to fruit

### Making the Most of Apricots

Fresh apricots are the best choice for preserving the water-soluble and heat-sensitive nutrients. They can be sliced and added to either fruit salads or a green salad. The antioxidants and minerals are retained even when the fruit is dried, making dried apricots an excellent snack.

# Cherries

✪ *Prunus avium* Sweet Cherry
✪ *Prunus cerasus* Sour Cherry

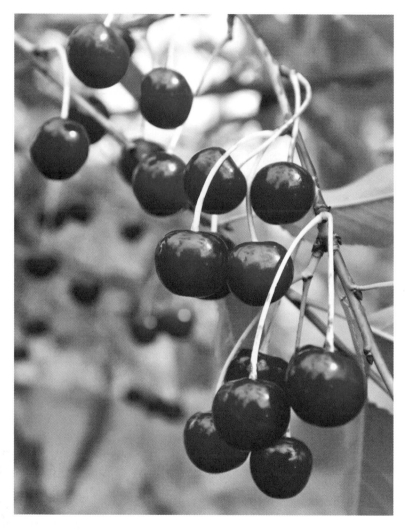

Cherry stones have been found at prehistoric sites in Switzerland, and ancient texts indicate that the cherry was first cultivated in Greece around 300 BCE. Roman conquerors carried the cherry to all parts of their empire, including England, where it later was, reputedly, one of Henry VIII's favorite fruits. The name derives from the ancient Roman site from which it was first spread through Europe, Cerasus, which became *cérise* in French, *cereza* in Spanish, and, later, "cherry" in English.

Today, there are over 1,000 cultivars of both sweet and sour, or tart, cherries, with sweet outnumbering sour three to one. Favorite sweet cultivars include the 'Bing' and 'Rainier', while among sour cultivars the 'Montmorency' is particularly popular. The major producers are Iran, Turkey, and the United States.

Sweet cherries are an excellent source of vitamin C, fiber, and potassium, and a good source of copper and manganese. They contain numerous phytochemicals, including

## Making the Most of Cherries

Eating cherries fresh will retain the vitamin C, which is heat-sensitive and water-soluble. Drinking fresh cherry juice is another excellent way to obtain maximimum nutrients and antioxidants. Using dried cherries in salads, baked goods, and grain dishes will boost the antioxidant and mineral content of those foods.

ABOVE Make sure you pick only ripe cherries from the tree, as the fruit will not ripen any further once off the tree. It is best to pick and store cherries with their stems on.

## Cherry Juice

In a study of the effects of cherries on obesity-prone rats, researchers at the University of Michigan (a state famed for sour cherry production) found that sour cherry juice reduced risk factors for heart disease and diabetes. The lead researcher, Steven Bolling, MD, also a cardiac surgeon, stated, "these new findings are very encouraging, especially in light of what is becoming known about the interplay between inflammation, blood lipids, obesity in cardiovascular disease, and diabetes." To derive the benefit, one need drink only 1½ cups daily.

## In a Nutshell

**Origin:** Near the Caspian Sea

**Season:** Early summer

**Why they're super:** Sweet cherries: high in vitamin C, fiber, and potassium; good source of copper and manganese; contain anthocyanin and other flavonoids. Sour cherries: high in vitamins A and C and fiber; good source of potassium, copper, and manganese; contain anthocyanin and other flavonoids and antioxidant carotenoids

**Growing at home:** Can be grown at home, but may take up to five years to produce fruit

*Life is just a bowl of cherries,*
*Don't take it serious, it's too*
*mysterious.*

"Life is Just a Bowl of Chrerries," Lew Brown,
US lyricist (1893–1958)

## What's in a Serving?

**FRESH CHERRIES**

**Sweet**

**(1 cup/154 g)**

**Calories:** 97 (405 kJ)

**Protein:** 1.6 g

**Total fat:** 0.3 g

**Saturated fat:** 0.1 g

**Carbohydrates:** 24.7 g

**Fiber:** 3.2 g

**Sour**

**(1 cup/155 g)**

**Calories:** 78 (324 kJ)

**Protein:** 1.6 g

**Total fat:** 0.5 g

**Saturated fat:** 0.1 g

**Carbohydrates:** 18.9 g

**Fiber:** 2.5 g

anthocyanin and other flavonoids. Sour cherries are an excellent source of vitamins A and C and fiber, and a good source of potassium, copper, and manganese; they also contain anthocyanin and other flavonoids, and are high in antioxidant carotenoids.

## THE HEALTHY EVIDENCE

A study from Cornell University analyzed several cherry cultivars for phenols and reported that both sweet and sour cherries contain high levels of seven phenols, which help fight disease. Another study, published in the journal *Experimental and Toxicologic Pathology*, reported that rutin, a phytochemical found in sour cherries, was a powerful anti-inflammatory agent (inflammation plays a major role in several chronic diseases, particularly in cardiovascular disease).

A 2008 study published in the *Journal of Medicinal Food* reported on the effects of sour cherries on the development and markers of metabolic syndrome (MetS), a condition in which higher levels of blood pressure, blood

cholesterol, insulin, and blood glucose predict a risk for cardiovascular disease, gall bladder disease, and diabetes. The researchers fed sour cherries to rats that were susceptible to insulin resistance and high blood cholesterol, and found that the cherries had beneficial effects with regard to combating MetS; they also produced a high antioxidant capacity in the blood. The researchers concluded that sour cherries "may represent a whole food research model of the health effects of anthocyanin-rich foods and may possess nutraceutical value against risk factors for metabolic syndrome."

BELOW English king Henry VIII not only loved cherries, but is credited with introducing new cultivars and raising the quality of the fruit in his realm.

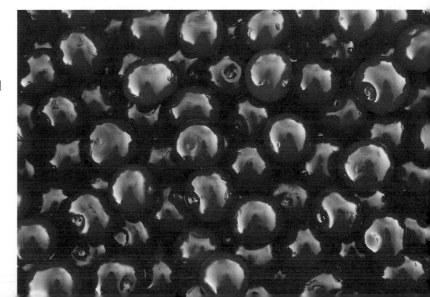

# Plums

- *Prunus* x *domestica* European Plum
- *Prunus institia* Damson
- *Prunus nigra* Canadian Plum

- *Prunus salicina* Japanese Plum
- *Prunus spinosa* Blackthorn, Sloe

The writings of Confucius contain several references to plums, most likely the damson and the Japanese plum, which, despite its name, is actually native to China. In first-century CE Rome, Pliny the Elder also made reference to plums in his writings. The European or prune plum is native to central Europe, and plums were cultivated in England from the Middle Ages onward, with many new cultivars being developed in the 1800s. The first American colonists initially made use of wild plums, although the European

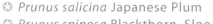

### Making the Most of Plums

Plums are best used fresh to retain vitamin C, and they make a nutritious addition to salads. Prunes can be chopped and added to a variety of baked goods to boost nutritive value—use them in rice dishes to add antioxidants and minerals.

plum subsequently became the most popular plum there. Plums are also popular in their dried form, known as the prune.

Plums are an excellent source of vitamins A, C, and K and fiber, and a good source of potassium and copper. They also contain anthocyanins and the antioxidant carotenoids beta-carotene, lutein, and zeaxanthin.

### THE HEALTHY EVIDENCE

Plums contain nutrients and antioxidants that may help fight chronic disease. In addition, they may be of benefit to people who are trying to lose weight. A 2010 study published in the journal *Appetite* reported that, compared to other common snack choices, prunes resulted in lower rises in blood glucose, insulin, and hormone levels. This effect led to subjects reporting less hunger for up to two hours after eating the prunes.

### In a Nutshell

**Origin:** China

**Season:** Early spring until autumn, with the peak harvest in late summer

**Why they're super:** High in vitamins A, C, and K and fiber; good source of potassium and copper; contain anthocyanins and antioxidant carotenoids

**Growing at home:** Easy to grow at home

BELOW The white coating on plums is called "wax bloom." It is a harmless, naturally occurring substance that is easily removed.

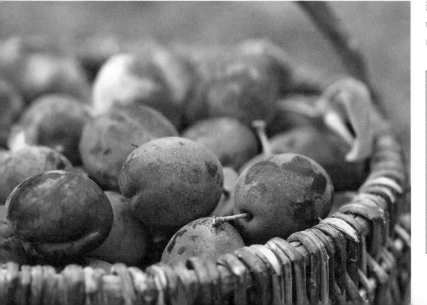

### What's in a Serving?

| FRESH PLUMS | PRUNES |
| --- | --- |
| Sliced (1 cup/165 g) | Whole (¼ cup/44 g) |
| **Calories:** 76 (317 kJ) | **Calories:** 104 (438 kJ) |
| **Protein:** 1.2 g | **Protein:** 1 g |
| **Total fat:** 0.5 g | **Total fat:** 0.2 g |
| **Saturated fat:** 0.1 g | **Saturated fat:** 0 g |
| **Carbohydrates:** 18.8 g | **Carbohydrates:** 27.8 g |
| **Fiber:** 2.3 g | **Fiber:** 3.1 g |

# Nectarine and Peach

✿ *Prunus persica*

Nectarine and peach are the same species, and some studies suggest that the only difference between them is the gene responsible for the fuzzy skin of the peach, which generally predominates. The peach originated in China and has been cultivated there for 3,000 years, although its scientific name refers to the belief that it originated in Persia. It was mentioned in ancient Greek writings in 300 BCE, and referred to by Pliny the Elder in the first century CE. The origins of the nectarine are obscure: a French term *brugnon*, meaning "fuzzless peach," emerged in the Middle Ages, but the word "nectarine" did not appear in England until the 1600s, when it was used to describe several cultivars. The nectarine reached the United States in 1906.

Both fruits are an excellent source of vitamins A and C and fiber, as well as a good source of vitamin E, potassium (especially high in peach), niacin, and copper; peach is also a good source of vitamin K and manganese. Both fruits are high in anti-oxidant carotenoids and flavonoids, although white-fleshed varieties of both fruits are lower in carotenoids.

## What's in a Serving?

**FRESH NECTARINE**
1 large
(5.5 ounces/156 g)
Calories: 69 (289 kJ)
Protein: 1.7 g
Total fat: 0.5 g
Saturated fat: 0 g
Carbohydrates: 16.5 g
Fiber: 2.7 g

**FRESH PEACH**
1 large
(6.2 ounces/175 g)
Calories: 68 (289 kJ)
Protein: 1.6 g
Total fat: 0.4 g
Saturated fat: 0 g
Carbohydrates: 16.7 g
Fiber: 2.6 g

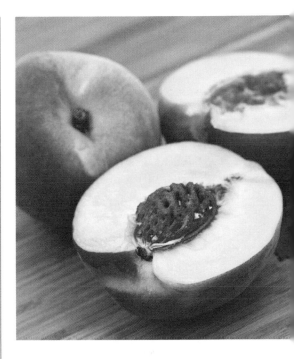

ABOVE Peaches and nectarines may have white or yellow flesh. They are classified as either "freestone," meaning that the fruit separates easily from the pit, or "clingstone," meaning that the fruit adheres to the stone.

## THE HEALTHY EVIDENCE

A 2009 study published in the *Journal of Agricultural and Food Chemistry* found the peach extract was a potent inhibitor of human breast cancer cells. Of the various phytochemicals present, the most potent was a type of anthocyanin, called procyanidin.

## In a Nutshell

**Origin:** China
**Season:** Late summer
**Why they're super:** Nectarine: high in vitamins A and C and fiber; good source of vitamin E, potassium, niacin, and copper. Peach: high in vitamins A and C, potassium, and fiber; good source of vitamins E and K, niacin, copper, and manganese; both contain antioxidant carotenoids and flavonoids
**Growing at home:** Easy to grow at home

## Making the Most of Nectarines and Peaches

Fresh nectarines and peaches provide the maximum nutritional benefits. Slice fresh fruit and add to cold cereal, green salads, fruit salads, or vanilla yogurt. Canned nectarines and peaches are lower in vitamin C but retain the antioxidants. Choose canned fruit preserved in juice rather than syrup.

POME

# Japanese Persimmon

*✿ Diospyros kaki*

The genus name, *Diospyros*, is an ancient Greek word meaning "fruit of the gods," while the word "persimmon" comes from the Native American Algonqian language and means "dry fruit." Persimmons have long been eaten by Native Americans, but compared to the Japanese persimmon the native American persimmon *(Diospyros virginiana)* is of low nutritional value. Although its name would indicate otherwise, the Japanese persimmon is native to China. It spread to other parts of Asia and reached Europe, California, and South America in the nineteenth century. Following its introduction to the United States, it quickly overtook the native persimmon in popularity.

Japanese persimmons are typically yellow-orange to dark red-orange in color, and vary in size from ½–3½ inches (1.5–9 cm) in diameter. They are an excellent source of vitamins A and C, fiber, and manganese, and a good source of vitamins B6, E, and K, potassium, and copper. They are also high in antioxidant carotenoids, including lycopene, beta-carotene, beta-cryptoxanthin, lutein, zeaxanthin, and phenols.

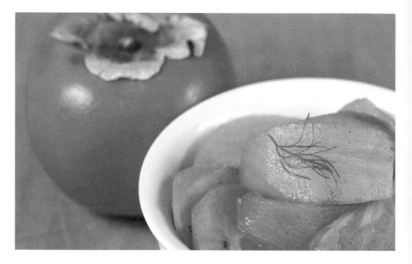

ABOVE Persimmons can be either astringent or nonastringent. The latter should be eaten when firm, the former only once ripe and soft.

## In a Nutshell

**Origin:** China

**Season:** Late autumn and early winter

**Why it's super:** Japanese persimmon: high in vitamins A and C, fiber, and manganese; good source of vitamins B6, E, and K, potassium, and copper; contains antioxidant carotenoids and phenols

**Growing at home:** Easy to grow in moderate (temperate) climates

## Making the Most of Persimmons

Aside from vitamin C, most of the key nutrients and phytochemicals are retained during cooking. To add persimmon to your diet, make a persimmon sauce for use with roasted poultry or pork. Blanch 12 persimmons in boiling water for 5 minutes, then peel and dice. Add lemon zest, ¼ cup (60 ml) of canola oil, 1 cup (200 g) of sugar, 2 tablespoons of chopped fresh ginger, and ½ cup (60 g) of dried cranberries. Bring to a boil and simmer for 40 minutes until thickened.

## THE HEALTHY EVIDENCE

A study published in the *Journal of Agricultural and Food Chemistry* found that, in addition to the nutrients that protect the heart, such as fiber, vitamins C and E, and potassium, Japanese persimmons contained a high level of a variety of phenols. The researchers concluded that "the relatively high contents of fiber, total and major phenolics, main minerals, and trace elements make persimmon preferable for an anti-atherosclerotic diet."

## What's in a Serving?

**FRESH JAPANESE PERSIMMON**

**1 whole (5.9 ounces/168 g)**

**Calories:** 118 (492 kJ)

**Protein:** 1 g

**Total fat:** 0.3 g

**Saturated fat:** 0 g

**Carbohydrates:** 31.2 g

**Fiber:** 6 g

# Apple
*Malus x domestica*

The old saying "eat an apple a day to keep the doctor away" lost favor in recent times, but contemporary studies have rekindled interest in the apple's health benefits. The tree originated in several parts of the world, including Europe, Asia, and North America—Alexander the Great is said to have brought the dwarf apple tree to Europe from Asia Minor. American colonists took apples with them to North America, and the first US orchard was planted near Boston in the early 1600s. Popular products made from apples include cider and juice, as well as dried apples.

Apples are an excellent source of fiber, and a good source of vitamins C and K and potassium. They contain several important flavonoids that help fight cancer.

## THE HEALTHY EVIDENCE
Although many fruits are higher in vitamins and minerals, studies show that apples contain important antioxidant phytochemicals. Korean researchers published a study in the journal *Biofactors*, which analyzed the phytochemicals in apples. They found apples contained high levels of flavonoids such as

### Making the Most of Apples
Cooking apples does not diminish the important antioxidant flavonoids. Drinking apple juice and cider are excellent ways to obtain a concentrated level of these compounds. Dried apples also retain the antioxidants, fiber, and minerals.

quercetin, epicatechin, and procyanidin. The researchers concluded, "Our results indicate that the cancer chemopreventive activity of apples is associated with the combined antioxidant capacity and antitumor-promoting activities of diverse antioxidants."

### What's in a Serving?
**FRESH APPLE**
1 whole
**(6.4 ounces/182 g)**
Calories: 95 (397 kJ)
**Protein:** 0.5 g
**Total fat:** 0.3 g
**Saturated fat:** 0 g
**Carbohydrates:** 25.1 g
**Fiber:** 4.4 g

### In a Nutshell
**Origin:** Europe, Asia, and North America
**Season:** Autumn
**Why it's super:** High in fiber; good source of vitamins C and K and potassium; contains flavonoids
**Growing at home:** Easy to grow at home

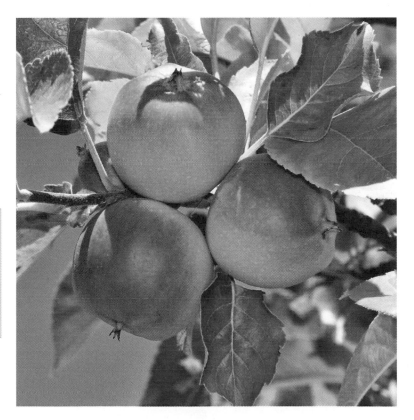

RIGHT Apple is one of the most commonly consumed and widely grown fruits in the world. Worldwide, about 7,500 different varieties are cultivated; about 2,500 kinds are grown in the United States alone.

# Pears

✿ *Pyrus communis* Pear, European Pear, Wild Pear
✿ *Pyrus pyrifolia* Asian Pear, Nashi Pear

Pears originated in the coastal and temperate regions of Europe and western Asia. The Asian or nashi pear has been cultivated in Asia for over 4,000 years; it is more round in shape and has a grainier texture than the more familiar European pear.

## In a Nutshell

**Origin:** Europe and western Asia

**Season:** Autumn

**Why they're super:** High in fiber; good source of vitamins C and K, potassium, and copper; contain antioxidant phenols

**Growing at home:** Easily grown at home

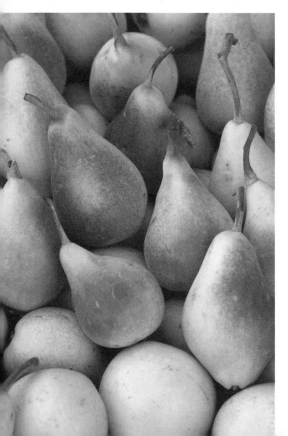

Pears are cultivated and propagated in much the same way as apples, and the two fruits are related and can even be similar in appearance—some pears resemble apples and the only difference is in the texture of the flesh. The flesh of pears contains stone cells, often called "grit."

Pears are an excellent source of fiber as well as a good source of vitamins C and K, potassium, and copper. They also contain antioxidant phenols.

### THE HEALTHY EVIDENCE

A 2009 study published in the *European Journal of Nutrition* reported on the health benefits of chlorogenic acid, a phenol found in pears (and some other fruits) at a high level. They tested the compound on human endothelial cells and found that it exhibited potent anti-inflammatory effects and countered some of the other processes involved in atherosclerosis, an underlying cause of cardiovascular disease. The chlorogenic acid also functioned as a powerful antioxidant. The authors concluded that these effects "suggest that chlorogenic acid could be useful in the prevention of atherosclerosis."

LEFT 'Forelle' is a popular European pear cultivar. The *Pyrus* genus includes 20 or so species, but *P. communis* and *P. pyrifolia* are the most common.

## What's in a Serving?

**FRESH PEAR**
1 medium
**(6.3 ounces/178 g)**
**Calories:** 103 (431 kJ)
**Protein:** 0.7 g
**Total fat:** 0.2 g
**Saturated fat:** 0 g
**Carbohydrates:** 27.5 g
**Fiber:** 5.5 g

## Making the Most of Pears

The important antioxidants in pears and the high level of fiber will be retained in cooking. This makes pears versatile from a nutritional standpoint, in that their health benefits can be incorporated into flavorful entrées and desserts. A pear treat that also includes other health-promoting ingredients is roasted pears drizzled with a mixture of honey, fresh lemon juice, and cinnamon.

# TROPICAL FRUITS

# Pineapple

✪ *Ananas comosus*

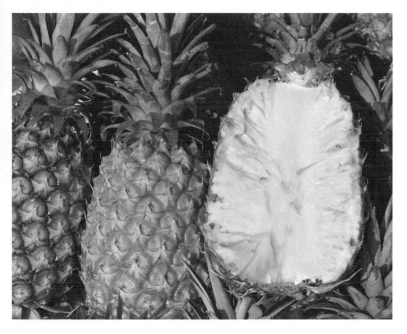

## Making the Most of Pineapples

Pineapple is best eaten fresh to capitalize on all the nutrients, but many important minerals and antioxidants will be present in canned pineapple, too. Choose products packed in 100 percent juice, and be sure to use the liquid to obtain all the water-soluble nutrients.

LEFT When Columbus first saw the pineapple, he described it as "in the shape of a pine cone, twice as big, which fruit is excellent and it can be cut with a knife, like a turnip, and it seems to be wholesome."

## What's in a Serving?

**FRESH PINEAPPLE**
**(1 cup/165 g)**
**Calories:** 82 (345 kJ)
**Protein:** 0.1 g
**Total fat:** 0.2 g
**Saturated fat:** 0 g
**Carbohydrates:** 21.7 g
**Fiber:** 2.3 g

Pineapple is a multiple fruit, in that it forms as the fruits (drupelets) of individual flowers on the plant merge and grow together. Pineapple is most often associated with Hawaii, but was not introduced there until 1813. It is in fact native to Paraguay and southern Brazil, and the indigenous peoples of those regions

## In a Nutshell

**Origin:** Brazil and Paraguay
**Season:** Year-round
**Why it's super:** High in vitamin C and manganese; good source of vitamin B6, folate, thiamine, magnesium, potassium, and copper; contains antioxidant flavonoids
**Growing at home:** Can be grown at home; pineapples do well in containers in warm climates

spread it throughout South America and the Caribbean. Spanish explorers took the pineapple back to Europe, where it became wildly popular and, notably in painting and sculpture, a symbol of all things exotic.

Pineapple is an excellent source of vitamin C, with one serving providing 131 percent of the Daily Value, and manganese. It is also a good source of vitamin B6, folate, thiamine, magnesium, potassium, and copper. In addition, pineapple contains several antioxidant flavonoids that may help combat chronic diseases.

### THE HEALTHY EVIDENCE

A 2009 study published in the journal *Food and Chemical Toxicology* reported on the analysis of the antioxidant compounds in pineapple. The results showed that the antioxidant potency of pineapple extract was high, and either similar to or higher than that of other fruits and vegetables. In addition to the abundant vitamin C, an antioxidant nutrient, they found important flavonoids such as quercetin.

# Papaya

✪ *Carica papaya*

The papaya is native to the tropical regions of the Americas, and its cultivation has been traced to Mexico in the centuries before the familiar Mesoamerican cultures appeared in those regions. The plant is large with a single stem or trunk that can grow more than 30 feet (9 m) high, and has a scarred exterior. The fruit is pear-shaped and large, growing up to 12 inches (30 cm) in diameter. When ripe, the skin color is amber to orange. Papaya gained fame when it became the first fruit tree for which botanists mapped the genome.

Fresh papayas are an excellent source of vitamins A, C, E, and K, folate, fiber, and potassium. They are also a good source of thiamine, riboflavin, niacin, pantothenic acid, calcium, and magnesium. Furthermore,

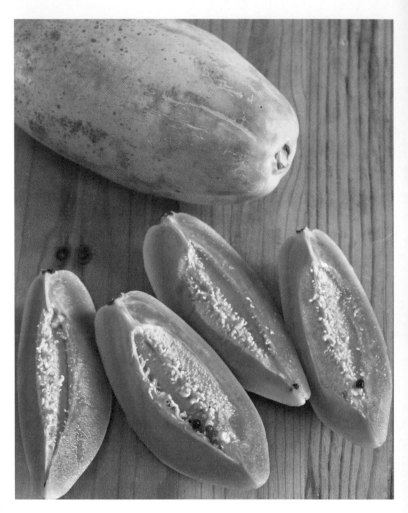

ABOVE Smooth and silky, papaya flesh has a slightly tart flavor; the seeds can be but are seldom eaten. Green papaya fruit and the latex from the papaya tree contain papain, which is an effective meat tenderizer.

## Making the Most of Papaya

Eating papaya fresh will maximize the nutritional benefits. Combine the fruit with a low-fat yogurt, and rolled whole oats for a quick and complete meal packed with essential nutrients and disease-fighting antioxidants.

## In a Nutshell

**Origin:** Most likely Central America

**Season:** Early summer and autumn

**Why it's super:** High in vitamins A, C, E, and K, folate, fiber, and potassium; good source of thiamine, riboflavin, niacin, pantothenic acid, calcium, and magnesium; contains antioxidant carotenoids and phenols

**Growing at home:** Can be grown outdoors in warm (subtropical) climates

papayas contain a high level of antioxidant carotenoids and phenols.

### THE HEALTHY EVIDENCE

A 2009 study in the *International Journal of Food Sciences and Nutrition* compared the effects of various plant foods commonly eaten in Mexico on the growth of breast cancer cells. Of 14 plant foods analyzed, only the papaya extract significantly inhibited cellular proliferation. This effect was independent of the antioxidant capacity, which was also high because of the content of phenols.

## What's in a Serving?

**FRESH PAPAYA**

**1 medium**

**(10.7 ounces/304 g)**

**Calories:** 119 (496 kJ)

**Protein:** 1.9 g

**Total fat:** 0.4 g

**Saturated fat:** 0.1 g

**Carbohydrates:** 29.8 g

**Fiber:** 5.5 g

# Acai Berry

✿ *Euterpe oleracea*

Acai berries grow on the acai palm, a Central and South American member of the palm tree family. The name, which is the English version of an indigenous South American word meaning "fruit that cries or expels water," is pronounced "ah-sah-ee." The acai berry is similar to a grape but smaller and less pulpy, with a large seed that makes up 80 percent of the fruit. Given the large size of the seed, which makes eating the fruit difficult, and the fruit's high fat content (present in the seeds), which makes it highly perishable, it tends to be exported and sold overseas only as juice or extract.

Acai berry juice and extracts are an excellent source of vitamins C and E and iron. They are also a good source of potassium and contain a high level of various antioxidant phenolic compounds.

## THE HEALTHY EVIDENCE

A 2008 study published in the *Journal of Agricultural and Food Chemistry* reported on an analysis of the antioxidant compounds in acai that isolated six different phenols. An earlier study in the same journal found that these and other compounds in acai resulted in an up to 86 percent reduction in the proliferation of leukemia cells. The authors concluded that their study "demonstrated that acai offers a rich source of bioactive polyphenolics."

---

### In a Nutshell

**Origin:** Central and South America

**Season:** Available year-round

**Why it's super:** High in vitamins C and E and iron; good source of potassium; contains anti-oxidant phenols

**Growing at home:** Can be grown in a warm climate

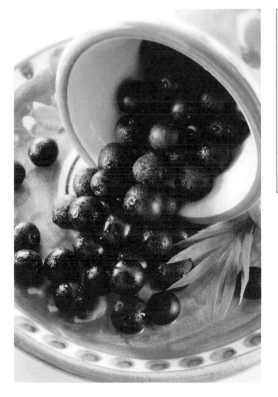

### What's in a Serving?

**ACAI BERRY JUICE BLEND (1 cup/235 ml)**

**Calories:** 111 (462 kJ)

**Protein:** 0 g

**Total fat:** 0 g

**Saturated fat:** 0 g

**Carbohydrates:** 27 g

**Fiber:** 0 g

---

### Making the Most of Acai Berries

For the maximum benefit, purchase juice rather than extract. Juice that is 100 percent acai is hard to find, partly because the flavor is so overpowering. Look for juices that say "100 percent juice" on the label and show acai as the first ingredient.

ABOVE Acai is the fruit of the acai palm tree, which grows in the Amazon rain forest. It is used not only to make juices and nutritional supplements but is also added to wines and liqueurs

# Mango
✿ *Mangifera indica*

Although the mango is indigenous to India, it is widely cultivated in many tropical and subtropical countries and also widely distributed. Indeed, mango is one of the most widely consumed fruits of all, with, worldwide, three mangoes being eaten for every banana and ten for every apple. The leaves are important in several cultures, being used in weddings and other public celebrations, as well as religious ceremonies. Mango cultivars can be yellow, orange, red, or green in color, but all have a flat, oblong pit.

The fruit is an excellent source of vitamins A, B6, C, E, and K, fiber, and copper, and a good source of folate, thiamine, niacin, riboflavin, magnesium, and potassium. Mangoes also contain antioxidant phenols and beta-carotene, and an antioxidant unique to the fruit, a xanthone known as mangiferin.

## THE HEALTHY EVIDENCE
A 2010 study published in the *Journal of Agricultural and Food Chemistry* reported on the antioxidants in mangoes. It reviewed numerous studies highlighting the anticancer properties of mango extracts in cancer cell lines, including leukemia, lung, breast, prostate, and colon cancer cells. While all mango varieties demonstrated anticancer effects, the 'Haden' and 'Ataulfo' "possessed superior chemopreventive activity."

RIGHT Mangoes were introduced to Africa about 1,000 years ago. The British brought mangoes back home from India in the 1800s, and the fruit made its way to Florida soon after. India is the world's largest producer.

---

### In a Nutshell

**Origin:** Southeast Asia, most likely Myanmar (Burma) and eastern India

**Season:** Summer

**Why it's super:** High in vitamins A, B6, C, E, and K, fiber, and copper, and a good source of folate, thiamine, niacin, riboflavin, magnesium, and potassium; contains antioxidant phenols and beta-carotene

**Growing at home:** Will only produce fruit in a tropical climate

---

### What's in a Serving?
**FRESH MANGO**
**1 whole**
**(7.3 ounces/207 g)**
**Calories:** 135 (563 kJ)
**Protein:** 1.1 g
**Total fat:** 0.6 g
**Saturated fat:** 0.1 g
**Carbohydrates:** 35.2 g
**Fiber:** 3.7 g

---

### Making the Most of Mangoes
Although they are available in canned and dried form, mangoes are best eaten fresh to obtain the highest levels of the plentiful water-soluble vitamins. The skin color is not an indication of ripeness or nutritional value. Mangoes are ready to eat when they emit a faint fragrant scent and are slightly soft to the touch.

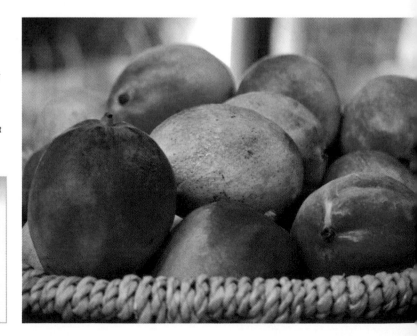

# Noni

✦ *Morinda citrifolia*

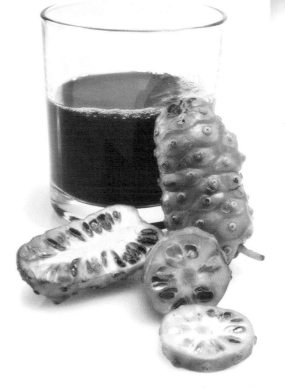

## What's in a Serving?

**NONI JUICE**
**100 percent noni**
**(2 ounces/60 ml)**

**Calories:** 14 (59 kJ)
**Protein:** 0.4 g
**Total fat:** 0 g
**Saturated fat:** 0 g
**Carbohydrates:** 3.4 g
**Fiber:** 0.2 g

The noni plant, *Morinda citrifolia*, is also known as the great morinda, Indian mulberry, or, in Hawaii, noni. A member of the coffee family, it is native to Southeast Asia, from where it spread throughout India, the Pacific islands, and Central America. Tahiti is now the largest cultivator of the tree.

Other names for the fruit reflect its bitter flavor and strong smell: cheese fruit, vomit fruit. Another, starvation fruit, refers to the fact that in several cultures noni fruit has been a significant food source during famines. More recently, noni has been touted as a health food, and websites selling the juice and products made from the powdered pulp have proliferated.

Noni is a good source of vitamin C and zinc, and in addition contains a wide range of phytochemicals, many of which are antioxidants.

ABOVE Traditional Asian folk medicine recommended the noni fruit, leaves, and root as a highly effective treatment for menstrual cramps, bowel problems, and urinary-tract infections.

### THE HEALTHY EVIDENCE

In a 2010 study, Indian researchers noted noni's longstanding medicinal uses in Southeast Asia and found that *Morinda citrifolia* extract exhibited several effects that may account for its apparent effectiveness in treating hypertension. In another 2010 study,

## Making the Most of Noni

Potentially health-promoting phytochemicals are fairly concentrated in noni juice, so even a small amount may be beneficial. Choose a product that is pure noni juice and combine 1–2 ounces (30–60 ml) with other pleasant-flavored juices.

## In a Nutshell

**Origin:** Southeast Asia
**Season:** Year-round
**Why it's super:** Good source of vitamin C and zinc; contains antioxidants and other phytochemicals
**Growing at home:** Can be grown in tropical and subtropical climates

researchers from Nihon University in Tokyo, Japan, reported on the plant extract's ability to inhibit the development of melanoma cells, a form of skin cancer that accounts for 75 percent of skin cancer deaths. And in a 2010 study among smokers published in *Nutrition and Cancer*, drinking 1–4 ounces (30–120 ml) of noni juice daily for one month significantly reduced a marker for lung cancer.

# Banana

✪ *Musa acuminata*

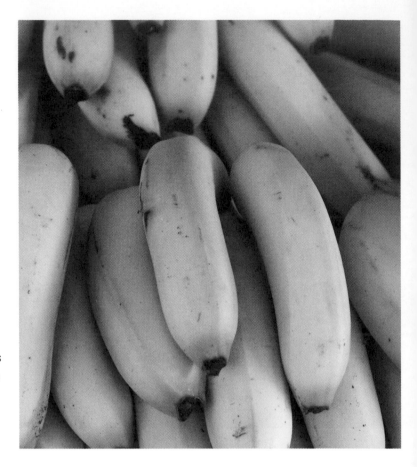

The familiar banana comes from a herbaceous plant, meaning that it does not possess a woody stem. In the wild state, bananas have hard, large seeds, but all bananas grown for consumption have small edible seeds, visible as black specks in the middle of the fruit. These bananas are called "dessert" bananas, the main cultivar being the 'Cavendish'. Bananas are usually yellow, but they can also be purple or red when ripe. Green bananas, and their relative, the plantain, are used mainly in cooking.

Bananas are an excellent source of vitamins B6 and C, fiber, potassium, manganese, and a good source of folate, riboflavin, magnesium, and copper. In addition, they contain antioxidant phenols. Bananas are a particularly good choice for those who wish to increase their consumption of potassium.

## THE HEALTHY EVIDENCE

A 2009 study published in the *International Journal of Cancer* reported on the comparative effects of various fruits and vegetables and breast cancer risk among Chinese women. It found that bananas were one of eight specific fruits and vegetables associated with a lower

ABOVE Before recorded history, early Filipinos most likely spread the banana east to the islands of the Pacific, including the Hawaiian Islands. The fruit moved westward following the major trade routes.

risk of the disease. An earlier study conducted in Uruguay and published in the journal *Nutrition and Cancer* found that a high intake of bananas was the strongest predictor for protection against colorectal cancer.

### What's in a Serving?

**FRESH BANANA**
**1 medium**
**(4.2 ounces/118 g)**
**Calories:** 105 (438 kJ)
**Protein:** 1.3 g
**Total fat:** 0.4 g
**Saturated fat:** 0 g
**Carbohydrates:** 27 g
**Fiber:** 3.1 g

### In a Nutshell

**Origin:** Southeast Asia

**Season:** Year-round

**Why it's super:** High in vitamins B6 and C, fiber, potassium, and manganese; good source of riboflavin, folate, magnesium, and copper; contains antioxidant phenols

**Growing at home:** Moderately difficult: climate must be warm or tree will not produce fruit

### Making the Most of Bananas

The high content of the heat-sensitive and water-soluble vitamins B6 and C means that fresh bananas are the best choice—vitamin B6 may decline by 50 percent when heated. For added nutrients, combine sliced bananas with a fruit high in vitamin A, such as mango or peach, and mix in low fat cottage cheese to add protein.

# Guavas

- *Psidium guajava* Common Guava, Yellow Guava, Apple Guava
- *Psidium littorale* Strawberry Guava

Guavas originated in Central and northern South America and are thought to have spread naturally, by drifting across the seas, to the Caribbean and regions of Southeast Asia and Africa. International demand for the fruit has resulted in widespread cultivation in tropical countries and in some subtropical regions, as well.

The common guava that is familiar to most people is also known as the yellow guava or apple guava. The less well-known strawberry guava has a characteristic red skin. Both are an excellent source of vitamins A and C, folate, fiber, potassium, copper, and manganese, as well as a good source of vitamins B6, E, and K, protein, thiamine, niacin, pantothenic acid, magnesium, and phosphorus. Guavas are also high in lycopene and antioxidant phenols.

## THE HEALTHY EVIDENCE

A 2006 study published in the *Journal of Agricultural and Food Chemistry* reported on an analysis of various tropical fruits with regard to their antioxidant content and activity. Of the 14 fruits tested, guava

RIGHT When Spanish explorers first visited the Americas, they found guavas growing from Mexico to Peru. European settlers in North America wrote of Seminole Indians growing the trees in Florida in 1816.

### Making the Most of Guavas

Although guavas are used to make jellies and jams, the high level of folate and vitamin C makes fresh guava the best choice. Guava juice will also provide a high level of nutrients and phytochemicals, but much of the fiber will be lost.

### In a Nutshell

**Origin:** Common guava: Central America; strawberry guava: Brazil

**Season:** Late summer through early spring

**Why they're super:** High in vitamins A and C, folate, fiber, potassium, copper, and manganese; good source of protein, vitamins B6, E, and K, thiamine, niacin, pantothenic acid, magnesium, and phosphorus; contain antioxidants including lycopene and phenols

**Growing at home:** Can be grown outdoors in warm climates, and indoors in temperate climates

### What's in a Serving?

**FRESH GUAVA**
**(1 cup/165 g)**
**Calories:** 112 (470 kJ)
**Protein:** 4.2 g
**Total fat:** 1.6 g
**Saturated fat:** 0.4 g
**Carbohydrates:** 23.6 g
**Fiber:** 8.9 g

had the highest antioxidant activity, which was thought to be due to the presence of phenols and other compounds. In 2007, researchers in India reported that guava peel extract exhibited antidiabetic effects in rats with the disease.

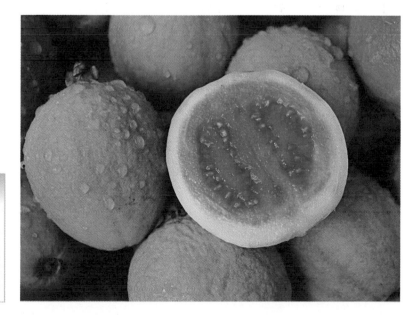

## VINE FRUITS

# Kiwi Fruits

✪ *Actinidia arguta* Hardy Kiwi
✪ *Actinidia chinensis* Golden Kiwi Fruit
✪ *Actinidia deliciosa* Kiwi Fruit

Kiwi fruits, or kiwis, are usually about the size of a chicken egg and have dull brownish-green skin and bright green or golden flesh. They originated in China and reached New Zealand in the early 1900s. When the fruits began to be exported from New Zealand in the 1950s, they were renamed kiwi fruits, for the small flightless bird indigenous to New Zealand. The green-fleshed kiwi fruit *(Actinidia deliciosa)* is the most familiar and widely available of the three species. The golden kiwi fruit has yellowish flesh and less hairy skin; the hardy kiwi fruit is quite small and can be eaten without peeling.

All kiwi fruits are an excellent source of vitamins C, K, and E, folate, fiber, potassium, and copper. They are also a good source of vitamin B6, calcium, magnesium, phosphorus, and manganese. In addition, kiwi

### What's in a Serving?

**FRESH KIWI FRUIT**
**Sliced (1 cup/180 g)**
**Calories:** 110 (459 kJ)
**Protein:** 2.1 g
**Total fat:** 0.9 g
**Saturated fat:** 0 g
**Carbohydrates:** 26.4 g
**Fiber:** 5.4 g

### Making the Most of Kiwi

Eating fresh kiwi fruit will make the most of the high content of water-soluble nutrients. To benefit from more fiber, wash the kiwi and eat with the skin. Add kiwi to fruit salads, where its vibrant color complements other fruits, nutritionally and visually.

fruits contain the carotenoids lutein and zeaxanthin, and they are an excellent source of alpha-linolenic acid (ALA), which may protect against heart disease.

### THE HEALTHY EVIDENCE

A study published in the journal *Platelets* reported on the effect of eating kiwi on platelets, cells in the blood that clot. The researchers fed subjects two to three kiwi fruits daily for 28 days and found it lowered platelet aggregation or clumping (a cause of heart attacks and strokes) by 18 percent and blood triglyceride levels (also a contributor to heart disease) by 15 percent. They concluded that "consuming kiwi fruit may be beneficial in [combating] cardiovascular disease."

BELOW The Chinese picked and ate wild kiwi for thousands of years, but never domesticated the plant.

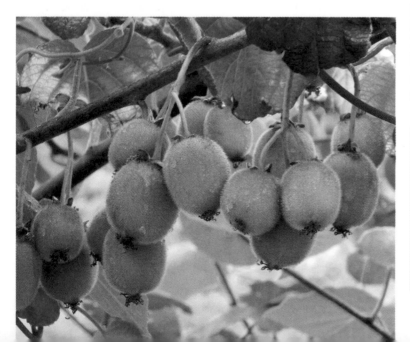

### In a Nutshell

**Origin:** China
**Season:** Late summer to early autumn
**Why they're super:** High in vitamins C, K, and E, folate, fiber, potassium, and copper; good source of vitamin B6, calcium, magnesium, phosphorus, and manganese; contain antioxidant carotenoids and ALA
**Growing at home:** Easy to grow at home

# Watermelon

✿ *Citrullus lanatus*

## What's in a Serving?

**FRESH WATERMELON**
1 wedge
(10 ounces/286 g)
**Calories:** 86 (363 kJ)
**Protein:** 1.7 g
**Total fat:** 0.4 g
**Saturated fat:** 0 g
**Carbohydrates:** 21.6 g
**Fiber:** 1.1 g

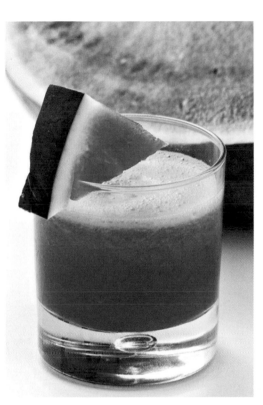

RIGHT The cultivation of watermelon began in China in the tenth century, and today that country is the world's largest producer of the fruit.

## In a Nutshell

**Origin:** Africa
**Season:** Summer
**Why it's super:** High in vitamins A and C; good source of vitamin B6, fiber, thiamine, magnesium, potassium, and copper; contains the carotenoid lycopene, and phenols
**Growing at home:** Easy to grow in the home garden

Watermelon is a member of the Cucurbitaceae family, so it is closely related to cantaloupe, squash, and pumpkin. Watermelon is believed to have originated in Africa, and was held in such high regard by the ancient Egyptians that they placed watermelons in the tombs of Egyptian kings. Like its relatives, the plant grows as a ground vine, producing fruit that is usually round, oblong, or spherical in shape (though Japanese botanists developed a method to cultivate cube-shaped watermelons, so that they would be easier to stack).

Watermelon is an excellent source of vitamins A and C, as well as a good source of vitamin B6, fiber, thiamine, magnesium, potassium, and copper. Watermelon also contains the antioxidant carotenoids beta-carotene, beta-cryptoxanthin, and lycopene (in which it is especially high), as well as a range of phenols.

### THE HEALTHY EVIDENCE

In a 2008 review published in the journal *Cancer Letters*, the author reported on the various effects of lycopene that may help combat cancer. He cited numerous studies suggesting that lycopene might confer protection against prostate cancer. This was mainly due to its antioxidant activity, although it also inhibits the growth of cells and induces apoptosis, or cell death, in cancer cells but not normal cells.

## Making the Most of Watermelon

Eating the fruit fresh is the best way to enjoy it and benefit from its nutrients. However, lycopene is most easily absorbed when heated and combined with fat, but cooking the fruit is not recommended and the lycopene content is so high that the difference is not significant anyway.

# Cantaloupe or Rockmelon

✪ *Cucumism melo* var. *cantalupensis*

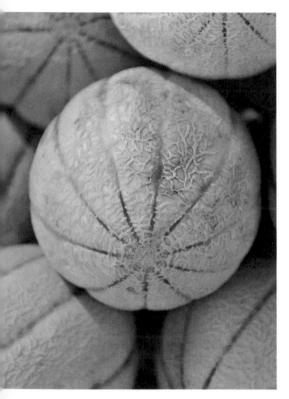

LEFT Most cultivars of cantaloupe have a scent similar to musk, which is the source of the fruit's other common name, muskmelon.

## What's in a Serving?

**FRESH CANTALOUPE
(1 cup/177 g)**
**Calories:** 60 (250 kJ)
**Protein:** 1.5 g
**Total fat:** 0.3 g
**Saturated fat:** 0 g
**Carbohydrates:** 14.4 g
**Fiber:** 1.6 g

## Making the Most of Cantaloupe

To get the most benefit of the high vitamin C, use fresh cantaloupe. Try the traditional Italian pairing of melon with thinly sliced prosciutto and a sampling of low-fat cheese for a high nutrient antipasto course.

Cantaloupes or rockmelons are orange-fleshed melons. The most common types are the European, with green-ribbed and netted skin, and the North American, with netted skin and no ribbing. Another name for the cantaloupe is muskmelon.

The cantaloupe originated in the region encompassing Egypt, Iran, and northwest India thousands of years ago. In the early fifteenth century, these orange-fleshed melons were introduced to Europe and within the next 100 years they had reached England. The name comes from the Italian word for the papal village where it was first cultivated on a large scale in the eighteenth century, Cantalupo, a name that translates as "wolf cry." Columbus took cantaloupe seeds to Haiti, and from there the fruit spread to Central and North America.

Cantaloupes are an excellent source of vitamins A and C, with one serving providing more than the entire day's requirement for both nutrients. They are also a good source of vitamins B6 and K, folate, niacin, thiamine, potassium, and magnesium. In addition, cantaloupes contain the antioxidant beta-carotene and various phenols.

### THE HEALTHY EVIDENCE

The high level of vitamin C and beta-carotene provides a two-pronged antioxidant effect. These nutrients, in combination with potassium, have also been shown to reduce the risk of high blood pressure. A 2007 study in the *Journal of Ethnopharmacology* reported that they also contain a natural diuretic compound that may reduce the risk for that condition.

## In a Nutshell

**Origin:** Egypt, Iran, northwest India
**Season:** Late summer to early autumn
**Why it's super:** High in vitamins A and C; good source of folate, vitamins B6 and K, niacin, thiamine, potassium, and magnesium; contains the antioxidant beta-carotene and various phenols
**Growing at home:** Easy to grow in the home garden

# Passionfruit

✪ *Passiflora edulis*

The passionfruit is native to South America, southeastern Asia, and Australia. In South America, Catholic missionaries gave the fruit its name, seeing in its unique structure certain symbols of the passion and crucifixion of Jesus. The fruit is eaten fresh by scooping the flesh out from the cavity, and the juice is added to other juices to improve aroma. Passionfruit is commercially grown in Brazil, the Caribbean, Australia, Africa, and some southern areas of the United States.

Passionfruit is an excellent source of vitamins A, B6, and C, fiber, protein, riboflavin, niacin, iron, magnesium, phosphorus, potassium, and copper, and a good source of folate. In addition, it contains a high level of the antioxidant beta-carotene and flavonoids.

BELOW Growers rely on the carpenter bee to pollinate passionfruit. It burrows into wood, so they place wooden beams near the flowers.

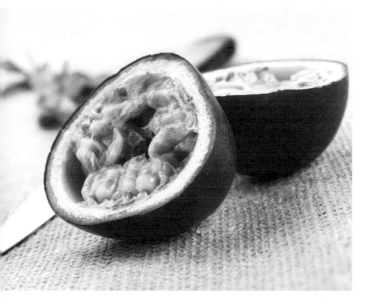

## In a Nutshell

**Origin:** South America, Southeast Asia, and Australia
**Season:** Autumn through winter
**Why it's super:** High in vitamins A, B6, and C, fiber, protein, riboflavin, niacin, iron, magnesium, phosphorus, potassium, and copper; good source of folate; contains the antioxidant beta-carotene and flavonoids
**Growing at home:** Easy to grow, but difficult to get the plant to fruit

## THE HEALTHY EVIDENCE

A 2009 study published in the journal *Experimental Biology and Medicine* reported on the effects of passionfruit extract on mice. The mice receiving the extract spent more time in the light, which suggested reduced anxiety, possibly due to a group of compounds, the C-glycosylflavonoids, in the fruit. Other studies have also shown that passionfruit reduces anxiety, though some of the data are conflicting. Additionally, researchers have identified the presence of numerous flavonoids that function as potent antioxidants.

## What's in a Serving?

**FRESH PASSIONFRUIT
(1 cup/236 g)**
**Calories:** 229 (958 kJ)
**Protein:** 5.2 g
**Total fat:** 1.7 g
**Saturated fat:** 0.1 g
**Carbohydrates:** 55.2 g
**Fiber:** 24.5 g

## Making the Most of Passionfruit

Eating the fruit fresh will retain the abundant supply of water-soluble vitamins (B6 and C). A traditional Australian recipe, pavlova, consists of a soft meringue shell filled with fruit and cream and topped with passionfruit. For a healthier version, replace the cream with low-fat yogurt.

# Grape

✪ *Vitis vinifera*

## What's in a Serving?

**FRESH GRAPES**

**(1 cup/92 g)**

**Calories:** 62 (258 kJ)

**Protein:** 0.6 g

**Total fat:** 0.3 g

**Saturated fat:** 0.1 g

**Carbohydrates:** 15.8 g

**Fiber:** 0.8 g

BELOW Although the *Vitis* genus includes dozens of species, commercially cultivated grapes of all colors normally belong to the *Vitis vinifera* species.

Grapes grow on the woody stems of the grapevine, in clusters of up to 300 individual fruits. There are thousands of cultivars and hybrids, and their colors range from light green, in the so-called white grape, to yellow, crimson, purple, and almost black. The plant is native to the Caucasus region, on the western side of the Black Sea and was cultivated in ancient Egypt—artworks

### In a Nutshell

**Origin:** The Caucasus region

**Season:** Autumn

**Why it's super:** High in vitamin K and manganese; good source of vitamins B6 and C, thiamine, and potassium; contains phytochemicals, including polyphenols and the compound resveratrol

**Growing at home:** Can be easily grown at home

from that time even depict horticultural techniques for producing larger-sized fruit.

### DIVERSE PRODUCTS

The Phoenicians took grapes to Greece shortly after 1000 BCE, where the Mediterranean climate proved favorable to the plant. The Romans then spread grapes throughout Europe and England. Greeks and Romans used grapes to make several food products, including wine and verjuice (juice from unripe grapes), which is still used in cooking. Although North America had indigenous grapes *(Vitis labrusca)*, Spanish missionaries introduced *Vitis vinifera* to California, where the climate and soil were ideal for wine-making. Worldwide today, nearly 71 percent of grapes are used to make wine and only 27 percent are used as fresh fruit, and 2 percent are dried to make raisins.

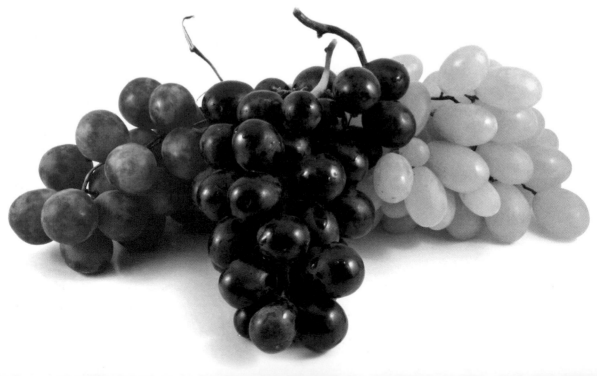

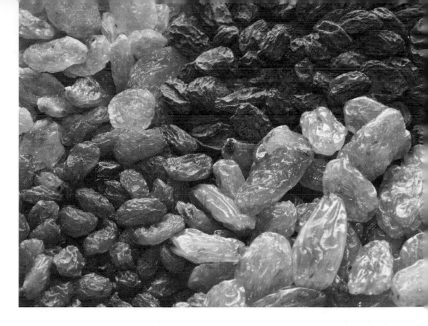

An excellent source of vitamin K and manganese, grapes are also a good source of vitamins B6 and C, thiamine, and potassium. They contain important phytochemicals, too, including polyphenols and the compound resveratrol. Both appear to reduce cardio-vascular disease risk by inhibiting platelet clumping and protecting LDL cholesterol from becoming oxidized, two processes that can cause heart attacks and strokes.

ABOVE The Thompson seedless grape cultivar accounts for up to 90 percent of raisin production in the United States.

## Making the Most of Grapes

To maximize the numerous benefits of grapes, use them in all their forms. Fresh grapes make not only an excellent snack, but also a nutritious addition to a wide variety of salads. To boost antioxidants and other phytochemical content, add raisins to baked goods and rice dishes. If wine is not your tipple, try a glass of cold grape juice.

## THE HEALTHY EVIDENCE

Numerous studies have reported on the benefits of grapes in the prevention of cardio-vascular disease, and a 2009 review of the evidence was published in the *Journal of Cardiovascular Pharmacology*. The authors noted that both wines and grapes appeared to lower the risk of heart disease through several mechanisms, with the key elements being resveratrol and a group of flavonoids known as proanthocyanidins. In addition, the authors pointed to evidence that wine may increase

*Wine makes daily living easier, less hurried, with fewer tensions and more tolerance.*

Benjamin Franklin, US statesman, scientist, and writer (1706–90)

## A Life-enchancing Compound

Resveratrol is a highly intriguing substance. Chemically, it is considered a phytoalexin, which other plants also produce to fight off bacteria or fungi. An early study, published in the journal *Nature* in 2003, reported that resveratrol extended the lifespan of a yeast; later studies showed the same effect in a species of worm and in fruit fly. Ongoing studies have focused on resveratrol's beneficial effects against diabetes, cancer, and cardiovascular disease.

life span by inducing longevity genes. They summarized their review by stating that the literature provides "evidence that grapes, wines, and resveratrol are equally important in reducing the risk of morbidity and mortality due to cardiovascular complications."

In a 2010 study published in the *British Journal of Nutrition*, researchers reported on their findings on the effects of grape juice in older people with memory decline but not dementia. Those who were given grape juice for 12 weeks experienced significant improvement in a measure of verbal learning and some enhancement of verbal and spatial recall. The authors concluded: "These pre-liminary findings suggest supplementation with … grape juice may enhance cognitive function for older adults with early memory decline."

## BERRIES

# Fig

✿ *Ficus carica*

The fig was one of the first plants to be cultivated by humans, even before wheat, barley, and legumes—the evidence dates back to 9400–9200 BCE in the Jordan Valley. Today, figs are grown throughout the Mediterranean region, Iran, and northern India, and other areas of the world with similar climates; figs may also be grown in climates with hot summers and are cultivated as far north as Hungary. Fresh figs do not transport or keep well, so they are often purchased dried.

Figs are an excellent source of vitamin K, fiber, calcium, magnesium, potassium, manganese, and copper, and a good source of vitamin B6, thiamine,

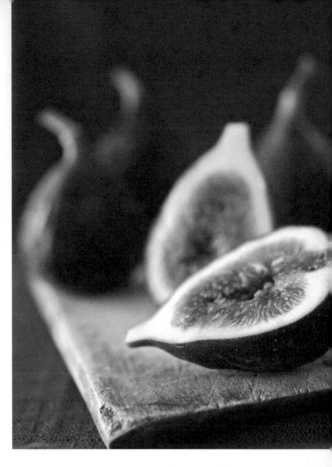

ABOVE The fig is the fruit mentioned most frequently in the Bible, and was said to have been grown in the Garden of Eden. The Romans adored figs, and gladiators ate them as a source of quick energy.

### Making the Most of Figs

Dried figs make an excellent and nutritious snack, as well as a good addition to baked goods, salads, meat entrees, and grain dishes. The majority of key nutrients and antioxidants are preserved in the dried product and will also be retained during the cooking process.

riboflavin, protein iron, and phosphorus. Figs also contain antioxidant phenols, including rutin, which has been studied for its health benefits.

### THE HEALTHY EVIDENCE

Figs contain numerous essential vitamins and minerals, and they also contain many phytochemicals of potential benefit to human health. A 2010 study published in the journal *Plant Foods for Human Nutrition* reported on an analysis of these phytochemicals, which found high antioxidant activity among the compounds. A similar study in 2009 reported high levels of phenols, such as rutin; several studies have shown that rutin may help prevent heart disease by inhibition of blood clotting and inflammation.

### In a Nutshell

**Origin:** Western Asia

**Season:** Summer through early autumn

**Why it's super:** High in vitamin K, fiber, calcium, magnesium, potassium, manganese, and copper; good source of vitamin B6, thiamine, riboflavin, protein, iron, phosphorus, and protein; contains antioxidant phenols, including rutin

**Growing at home:** Can be grown in the home garden

# Strawberry

✿ *Fragaria x ananassa*

No one knows for certain how the strawberry got its name. According to the California Strawberry Commission, "There is a legend that strawberries were named in the nineteenth-century by English children who picked the fruit, strung them on grass straws, and sold them as 'straws of berries.'" Whatever the case, the strawberry is now the most widely consumed berry in the world. The type that is most often available is a cross between a North American berry and a Central or South American berry, which was accidentally cross-bred in Normandy about 300 years ago by a French spy called Frézier. The resulting large, sweet berry soon became prized throughout Europe.

Strawberries are an excellent source of vitamin C, folate, fiber, and manganese. They are also a good source of vitamin K, potassium, and magnesium. In addition, they contain numerous antioxidant phytochemicals including ellagic acid and the flavonoids anthocyanin, catechin, quercetin, and kaempferol.

## THE HEALTHY EVIDENCE

A review published in the journal *Critical Reviews in Food Science and Nutrition* summarized some of the potential health benefits of strawberries deriving from the phytochemicals. The author pointed to studies demonstrating the ability of phytochemicals to prevent the oxidation of LDL cholesterol, improve the functioning of blood vessels, and reduce blood clotting and inflammation—effects that work together to lower the risk for heart disease.

### In a Nutshell

**Origin:** Uncertain
**Season:** Summer
**Why it's super:** High in vitamin C, folate, fiber, and manganese; good source of vitamin K, potassium, and magnesium; contains antioxidant phytochemicals
**Growing at home:** Can be grown in the home garden

### What's in a Serving?

**FRESH STRAWBERRIES**
**Sliced (1 cup/166 g)**
**Calories:** 53 (226 kJ)
**Protein:** 1.1 g
**Total fat:** 0.5 g
**Saturated fat:** 0 g
**Carbohydrates:** 12.8 g
**Fiber:** 3.3 g

## Making the Most of Strawberries

To take maximum advantage of strawberries' high levels of vitamin C and folate, enjoy them fresh. Strawberries make an excellent addition to whole-grain cereals, low-fat yogurt, and fruit salads and fresh green salads, instantly boosting their antioxidant and nutritional value.

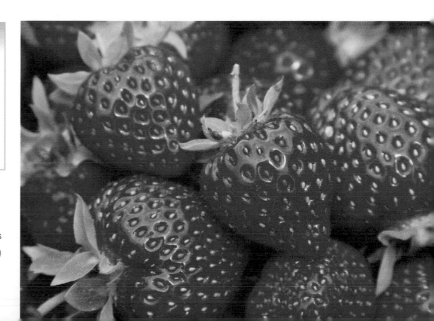

RIGHT Internationally, 73 countries produce strawberries on 529,000 acres (214,000 ha), with average crop yields of around 13,000 pounds (5,900 kg) per acre (0.4 ha). Top producers include the USA, Spain, and Turkey.

# Goji Berry or Wolfberry

✪ *Lycium barbarum*
✪ *Lycium chinense*

The terms "goji berry" and "wolfberry" are used interchangeably for two closely related species, *Lycium barbarum* and *Lycium chinense,* both woody perennial plants. Though they grow widely in China and have been used there for medicinal purposes for centuries, their origins are unclear. The plants are related to poisonous nightshade and to the tomato, which was named *Solanum lycopersicum,* meaning "wolf-peach," in 1753 by Carl Linnaeus, the famous Swedish taxonomist. This classification was the basis for the modern nomenclature of "wolfberry." The name "goji," most likely based on the Mandarin pronunciation of "wolfberry," was first popularized in 2004 during health-food marketing of the fruit.

Goji is available as dried berries, juice extracts, food additives, and dietary

## In a Nutshell

**Origin:** Southeastern Europe and Asia

**Season:** Mid-summer to late autumn

**Why it's super:** High in vitamins A and C and fiber, and a good source of calcium; contains the antioxidant beta-carotene and other antioxidant phytochemicals

**Growing at home:** Can be grown in the home garden

supplements. Dried goji berries are an excellent source of vitamins A and C and fiber and a good source of calcium. In addition, they contain the antioxidant beta-carotene and other antioxidant phytochemicals.

### THE HEALTHY EVIDENCE

A 2010 review article in the journal *Planta Medica* discussed the high level of anti-oxidants in the fruit and studies suggesting that it offered protection against athero-sclerosis and diabetes. It also noted possible interaction with warfarin, a blood-thinning medication, which may be of concern for certain individuals. In 2009, researchers published a study in the journal *Nutrition Research* on the effects the daily consumption of 4 fluid ounces (120 ml) of a goji-juice product over 30 days by a group of adults aged 55 to 72. They measured antioxidants and free radicals in the blood and found that the juice significantly reduced levels of free radicals.

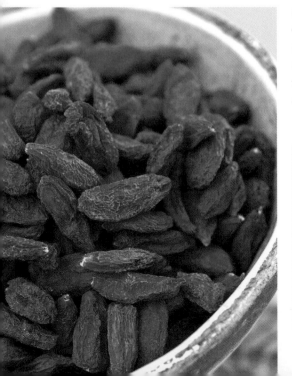

LEFT In the 1730s, Archibald Campbell, the third Duke of Argyll (nicknamed "the Treemonger") introduced the goji berry plant to Britain, where it became known as "Duke of Argyll's Tea Tree."

## What's in a Serving?

**DRIED GOJI BERRIES (¼ cup/28 g)**

**Calories:** 112 (469 kJ)

**Protein:** 1 g

**Total fat:** 1.6 g

**Saturated fat:** 0 g

**Carbohydrates:** 24 g

**Fiber:** 3 g

### Making the Most of Goji Berries

Both dried berries and juices will provide the nutrients and antioxidants, but the dried berries will also provide extra fiber. Add the dried berries to grain products, baked goods, and other dishes.

# Pomegranate

✿ *Punica granatum*

The pomegranate originated in Persia, modern Iran, where evidence of cultivation dates back 5,000 years. It is mentioned in the Greek myth of Persephone and in the Bible, which refers to the Israelites' desire for it during their desert trek. In the Middle Ages and beyond, it was regarded as a symbol of fertility—English king Henry VIII's first wife Catherine of Aragon ate the seeds in an effort to produce a son.

The fruit contains red seeds, or arils, which are separated from the peel and membrane. The juice is widely used, notably in pomegranate molasses, a traditional ingredient in Middle Eastern cuisine, which is made from the juice, sugar, and lemon juice. Pomegranate juice is an excellent source of vitamin K, folate, potassium, and manganese, and a good source of vitamins E and B6 and pantothenic acid. In addition, the juice is high in antioxidant tannins and flavonoids.

## THE HEALTHY EVIDENCE

In a 2009 review article published in the journal *Nutrition and Cancer*, the authors discussed the high level of antioxidant compounds in pomegranate juice. They summarized the results of studies showing that the juice extract inhibits the growth of breast, prostate, colon, and lung cancer cells. A clinical trial examined the effects of the extract on prostate cancer patients by measuring blood levels of PSA (prostate specific antigen), an indicator of the presence of prostate cancer cells. The extract significantly increased the time it took PSA levels to double, indicating that it was slowing the progress of the disease.

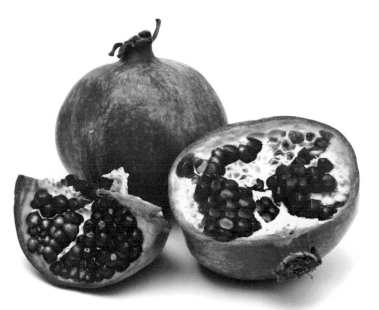

ABOVE The most popular cultivar of pomegranate is called the 'Wonderful', and is famed for its large and beautifully colored fruit.

## Making the Most of Pomegranates

The fruit is readily available; however, the juice provides a more concentrated source of antioxidants and nutrients, except for fiber. It can be used in cooking to make sauces, and in baked goods—combine with dark cocoa powder to mask the vivid color and add extra antioxidants.

## In a Nutshell

**Origin:** Persia (Iran)

**Season:** Late autumn

**Why it's super:** High in vitamin K, folate, potassium, and manganese; good source of vitamins E and B6 and pantothenic acid; contains antioxidant tannins and flavonoids

**Growing at home:** Can be grown in the home garden, but needs hot dry summers and may take three years to fruit

## What's in a Serving?

**POMEGRANATE JUICE (1 cup/235 ml)**

**Calories:** 134 (568 kJ)

**Protein:** 0.4 g

**Total fat:** 0.7 g

**Saturated fat:** 0.2 g

**Carbohydrates:** 32.7 g

**Fiber:** 0.2 g

# Blackberry

✪ *Rubus fruticosus*

## What's in a Serving?

**FRESH BLACKBERRIES
(1 cup/144 g)**
Calories: 62 (261 kJ)
Protein: 2 g
Total fat: 0.7 g
Saturated fat: 0 g
Carbohydrates: 13.8 g
Fiber: 7.6 g

The *Rubus* genus is native to all but the furthest reaches of the globe and grows well in cooler regions, and humans have collected the plants' sweet berries since prehistoric times. They grow on shrubs called brambles, most of which have thorny canes. Botanically, the fruits are not true berries, but rather aggregate fruits, forming from a single flower that has multiple separate carpels.

Interest in blackberries and other *Rubus* berries has grown significantly in recent years, following the discovery of their high

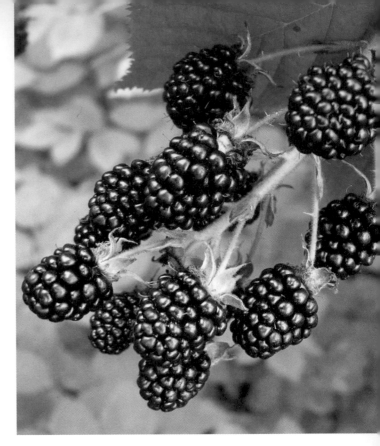

ABOVE Europeans have long used blackberries for food and medicines; they also grew the thorny plant as an effective barrier against intruders. The plant is invasive and must be pruned regularly to keep it under control.

### In a Nutshell

**Origin:** Ubiquitous
**Season:** Late summer
**Why it's super:** High in vitamins C and K, folate, fiber, manganese, and copper; good source of vitamins A and E, niacin, potassium, magnesium, zinc, and iron; contains antioxidant phenols and flavonoids
**Growing at home:** Easy to grow at home

### Making the Most of Blackberries

Although frozen blackberries usually have 20 percent less vitamin C, they retain the antioxidants and other nutrients of the fresh fruit and can be a convenient way to incorporate blackberries in your diet. Thaw frozen blackberries and add either sugar or sugar substitute and microwave for less than five minutes. Refrigerate and use as a topping for toast, cereal, or yogurt.

levels of antioxidants. Blackberries are an excellent source of vitamins C and K, folate, fiber, manganese, and copper, as well as a good source of vitamins A and E, niacin, potassium, magnesium, zinc, and iron. Blackberries are also high in antioxidant phenols and flavonoids, most notably the anthocyanins.

### THE HEALTHY EVIDENCE

A 2009 study published in the journal *Food and Chemical Toxicology* reported that the high level of anthocyanins and phenolic compounds in blackberry extracts worked together to exert powerful anticancer and antioxidant effects. The authors suggested that the potency of the extracts could possibly be the basis for the development of fruit-derived drug products.

# Raspberry

*Rubus idaeus*

Indigenous to Asia, Europe, and North America, raspberry is a hardy shrub that can withstand harsh temperatures. According to Pliny the Elder, the botanical name *idaeus* derives from Mount Ida in Asia Minor, where the fruits were gathered in ancient times. The Romans proliferated the plant throughout their empire and it was cultivated in Britain by the Middle Ages. Today raspberries are widely grown in North America, Europe, Russia, China, and Australia.

## What's in a Serving?

**FRESH RASPBERRIES
(1 cup/123 g)**
**Calories:** 64 (271 kJ)
**Protein:** 1.5 g
**Total fat:** 0.8 g
**Saturated fat:** 0 g
**Carbohydrates:** 14.7 g
**Fiber:** 8 g

## In a Nutshell

**Origin:** Asia, Europe, and North America
**Season:** Summer and autumn
**Why it's super:** High in vitamins C and K, fiber, and manganese; good source of vitamin E, folate, potassium, magnesium, copper, and iron; contains antioxidant phenols and flavonoids
**Growing at home:** Easy to grow at home

BELOW After the Romans took raspberries to Britain, the British steadily improved the plants over the centuries. They introduced them to North America in 1771.

One of the so-called bramble fruits, the raspberry grows on a thorny bush. Each berry is actually an aggregate fruit, a formation of numerous tiny fruits, with myriad tiny hairs between the individual fruits helping hold the berry together. Because of the fruit's fragility, only 10 percent of commercial raspberries are sold fresh; the rest of the international crop is processed, and much of it is frozen.

Raspberries are an excellent source of vitamins C and K, fiber, and manganese, and a good source of vitamin E, folate, potassium, magnesium, copper, and iron. Raspberries are high in antioxidant phenols and flavonoids, especially the anthocyanins.

### THE HEALTHY EVIDENCE

In 2007, the *Journal of Carcinogenesis* published a study of the relationship between raspberries and cancer. The authors noted a high level of antioxidant compounds in raspberries, such as polyphenols, anthocyanins, and ellagitannins, and found that raspberry extract inhibited several stages of colon cancer development. Another study, published in the *Journal of Biological Chemistry*, reported that a compound extracted from raspberries, cyanidin-3-rutinoside, inhibited leukemia cells.

## Making the Most of Raspberries

Use fresh raspberries as soon as possible to retain the vitamin C, and consider freezing any fresh berries that are not used immediately. Raspberries add antioxidants and nutrients to desserts, and make an excellent topping for whole-grain products, such as waffles and pancakes.

# Loganberry

✿ *Rubus x loganbaccus*

The loganberry was accidentally created in California in the late nineteenth century by American lawyer and horticulturist James Harvey Logan. While trying to breed a better commercial blackberry cultivar, he planted the blackberries next to European red raspberries; the plants flowered and fruited together, producing hybrids, among them a hardy plant with a larger berry that he dubbed the loganberry. The loganberry is not, however, popular with commercial growers, as the plant is thorny, the berries are often hidden by the leaves, and the fruit tends to mature at different times on the same plant.

Loganberries are an excellent source of vitamins C and K, folate, fiber, and manganese, and a good source of vitamins B6 and E, niacin, thiamine, iron, magnesium,

BELOW Suited to cooler climates, loganberries are widely grown in the northwestern United States, England, and Tasmania, Australia.

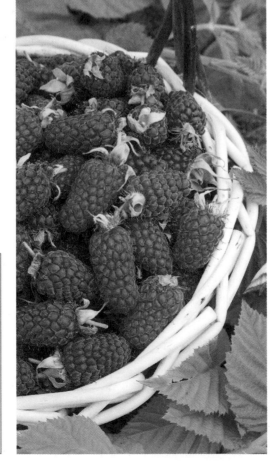

### In a Nutshell

**Origin:** California

**Season:** Late summer

**Why it's super:** High in vitamins C and K, folate, fiber, and manganese; good source of vitamins B6 and E, niacin, thiamine, iron, magnesium, potassium, and copper; contains antioxidant anthocyanins and polyphenols

**Growing at home:** Easy to grow in the home garden

potassium, and copper. The berries contain antioxidant anthocyanins and polyphenols.

## THE HEALTHY EVIDENCE

A 2007 study published in the *Journal of Medicinal Food* reported on the effect of loganberry extract on the antioxidant status of rats. The extract raised the antioxidant status of the rat's blood and reduced oxidative damage. A 2005 study published in the journal *Age* reported on the various phyto-chemicals in several varieties of berries, including loganberry, and found they were high in anthocyanins and polyphenols, which suggests they could help improve cognitive functioning in ageing.

### What's in a Serving?

**FROZEN LOGANBERRIES**
(1 cup/147 g)

**Calories:** 81 (338 kJ)

**Protein:** 2.2 g

**Total fat:** 0.5 g

**Saturated fat:** 0 g

**Carbohydrates:** 19.1 g

**Fiber:** 7.8 g

### Making the Most of Loganberries

Frozen loganberries are usually easier to find than fresh ones. Although the frozen fruit will have less vitamin C, it will normally retain most other nutrients. Thaw the frozen berries and combine them with whole-grain cereal and yogurt for a tasty, nutrient-packed breakfast or dessert.

# Elderberry

*Sambucus nigra*

Elderberry has an unusual flavor and is popular for use in jellies, jams, pies, drinks, and cordials. The plant is attractive and easy to grow. When eaten raw, the plant and its flowers are mildly poisonous, but cooking destroys the toxins. The stems of the elderberry are used as spiles to tap maple trees, and were used by Native Americans to make flutes and arrow shanks.

Elderberries are an excellent source of vitamins A, B6, and C, fiber, iron, and potassium, and a good source of thiamine, riboflavin, calcium, and phosphorus. They also contain antioxidant anthocyanins and flavonoids.

ABOVE Elderberry fruit grows in large clusters that hang down from the branches. In spring, the plant produces large, lacy white flowers.

## THE HEALTHY EVIDENCE

An earlier study that was recently published in a 2007 article in the *Journal of Alternative and Complementary Medicine* reported on the use of elderberry extract in treating influenza. The researchers concluded that, due to its efficacy, low cost, and absence of side-effects, "this preparation could offer a possibility for safe treatment for influenza A and B." The berry's content of anthocyanins was thought to enhance immune function. The high content of anthocyanins, flavonoids, and antioxidant nutrients in elderberry is also thought to make them effective in preventing chronic disease.

### In a Nutshell

**Origin:** Native to temperate-to-subtropical regions of both hemispheres

**Season:** Late summer

**Why it's super:** High in vitamins A, B6, and C, fiber, iron, and potassium; good source of thiamine, riboflavin, calcium, and phosphorus; contains antioxidant anthocyanins and flavonoids

**Growing at home:** Can be easily grown at home

### Making the Most of Elderberries

Since fresh elderberries contain a mild toxin, they require cooking, which causes some loss of vitamin C. Juice and frozen berries tend to be more widely available than the fresh fruit. Drink the juice or use the cooked fruit as a topping for cereals, baked goods, and yogurt.

# Blueberries

✿ *Vaccinium ashei* Rabbiteye Blueberry
✿ *Vaccinium corymbosum* Highbush Blueberry
✿ *Vaccinium lamarckii* Lowbush blueberry

RIGHT Blueberries probably grew and were gathered in the wild for millennia in North America and Eurasia before being domesticated in the twentieth century.

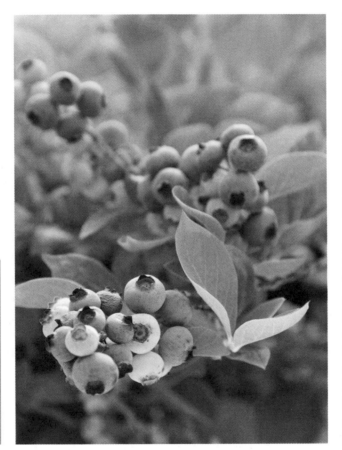

## In a Nutshell

**Origin:** Europe, North America, Asia
**Season:** Late spring through summer
**Why they're super:** High in vitamins C and K, fiber, and manganese; contain antioxidant flavonoids such as anthocyanins and kaempferol, and stilbenes
**Growing at home:** Can be grown in the home garden

## What's in a Serving?

**FRESH BLUEBERRIES**
**(1 cup/148 g)**
Calories: 84 (355 kJ)
Protein: 1.1 g
Total fat: 0.5 g
Saturated fat: 0 g
Carbohydrates: 21.5 g
Fiber: 3.6 g

Blueberries are among the few human foods that are naturally colored blue. The lowbush blueberry, also called wild blueberry, produces smaller, more intensely colored fruit than the highbush blueberry. The rabbiteye blueberry, grown principally in the southeastern United States, has large berries with more abundant seeds than the other species. Blueberry plants usually stand erect, but may grow prostrate as well. The leaves can be deciduous or evergreen; the flowers are usually bell-shaped and white, pale pink, or red, sometimes tinged with green.

## COMMERCIAL PRODUCTION

The blueberry is a relative newcomer to commercial production, having been harvested only from wild plants until the 1920s. The United States produces most of the world's supply, with Maine being the largest producer of the lowbush blueberry, and Michigan the largest producer of the highbush type. Blueberries can be used in juice, pies, jellies and jams, and pastries, or just eaten fresh.

Blueberries are an excellent source of vitamins C and K, fiber, and manganese and they contain high levels of various antioxidants including flavonoids such as anthocyanins and kaempferol, and stilbenes, as well as phytochemicals.

## THE HEALTHY EVIDENCE

Several phytochemical compounds found in blueberries may play a role in combating chronic disease. A 2010 study published in the *Journal of Agricultural and Food Chemistry*

*You ought to have seen what I saw on my way*
*To the village, through Mortenson's pasture to-day:*
*Blueberries as big as the end of your thumb …*

"Blueberries," Robert Frost, US poet (1874–1963)

compared the antioxidant content of several berry fruits and found that blueberries contain a "complex spectrum of anthocyanins" that is responsible for the fruit's high level of anti-oxidant activity. A large-scale study of nurses in the United States published in 2007 in the *International Journal of Cancer* reported that the highest level of intake of these compounds was associated with the lowest risk of ovarian cancer.

Another compound high in blueberries is kaempferol, a powerful antioxidant flavonoid, which studies show may reduce lung cancer risk in smokers, anxiety and depression, and inflammation. A 2010 study published in the journal *Inflammation* reported that flavonoids appear to work synergistically to counter the inflammatory response; blueberries contain several of the flavonoids identified in the study, which in combination will produce a greater effect than they would individually.

A 2010 study published in the journal *Carcinogenesis* reported on the high level of pterostilbene in blueberries and possible cancer-prevention effects. This compound

### Growing Blueberries

Although blueberries are not difficult to grow, they do require ground with high acidity, so your soil may need to be adjusted to obtain the best results. Since the plants have shallow roots, they require about 1–2 inches (2.5–5 cm) of water each week; adding mulch will help preserve moisture and discourage weed growth. Blueberry plants will generally begin to produce after three years, but it will normally take about six years for them to reach full production.

is part of a family of compounds known as stilbenes, and is related to the widely studied phytochemical, resveratrol, found in grapes. The researchers tested pterostilbene in human colon cancer cells and found that it significantly suppressed tumor development, cell growth, and inflammatory markers. The researchers concluded that their data "suggest the potential use of pterostilbene for colon cancer prevention."

BELOW Blueberries are quite perishable and have a shelf life of only two weeks, so freezing them is an excellent way to preserve their nutrients.

### Making the Most of Blueberries

Fresh blueberries provide maximum vitamin C along with the antioxidant phytochemicals. However, frozen blueberries are only slightly lower in vitamin C and retain the antioxidant benefits. Given their limited season, it is thus a good idea to freeze blueberries when they are available and then thaw them when required. Microwave the thawed berries for less than three minutes, then mash them and add the fruit and juice to rolled oats and yogurt for a nutrient-rich breakfast or dessert.

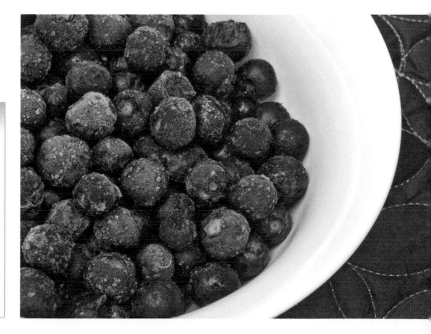

# Cranberries

✪ *Vaccinium macrocarpon* American Cranberry
✪ *Vaccinium oxycoccus* Northern Cranberry

Cranberries are native to North America, where they are common in cooler areas, usually growing on a low shrub or vine in acidic bogs. The American cranberry has larger leaves than the northern cranberry and a slight apple-like taste.

Cranberries were first cultivated on a farm in Massachusetts in the early nineteenth century and by the 1820s they were being shipped to Europe. Outside of North America, fresh cranberries can be difficult to find; most of the cranberries grown commercially are used in juices and other drinks, dried, or canned.

## What's in a Serving?

**FRESH CRANBERRIES**
**(½ cup/50 g)**
**Calories:** 23 (97 kJ)
**Protein:** 0.2 g
**Total fat:** 0.1 g
**Saturated fat:** 0 g
**Carbohydrates:** 6.1 g
**Fiber:** 2.3 g

**CRANBERRY JUICE**
**(1 cup/235 ml)**
**Calories:** 116 (491 kJ)
**Protein:** 0.1 g
**Total fat:** 0.3 g
**Saturated fat:** 0 g
**Carbohydrates:** 30.8 g
**Fiber:** 0.3 g

## In a Nutshell

**Origin:** North America
**Season:** Late autumn to early winter
**Why they're super:** High in vitamin C and a good source of fiber and manganese; contain antioxidant anthocyanins and phenols
**Growing at home:** Difficult to grow at home

Cranberries are an excellent source of vitamin C, and a good source of fiber and manganese. The berries contain numerous antioxidants, such as anthocyanins and other flavonoids, and phenols.

### THE HEALTHY EVIDENCE

Many people are aware of cranberry juice's ability to protect against urinary-tract infections; fewer know that it also protects against another infection, *Helicobacter pylori*, which causes ulcers and stomach cancer. Indeed, the fruit is a powerhouse of nutrients and disease-fighting antioxidants. A 2010 study published in the journal *Food and Chemical Toxicology* reported on the protective effects of cranberries against a chemotherapy drug that damages the heart. A study published in *Nutrition and Cancer* reported that cranberry extract inhibited growth of cancer cells in the brain, colon, and prostate.

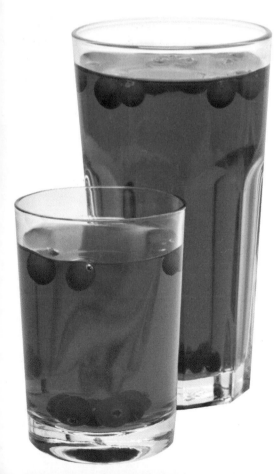

LEFT Almost 95 percent of the cranberry crop is processed into juices and sauces. Juice blends have become particularly popular in recent years.

## Making the Most of Cranberries

Fresh cranberries are too tart to eat on their own—combine them with other sweet berries for a good mix of flavors and antioxidants. Cranberries freeze well, so purchase the bagged fruit when available, and place the entire bag into the freezer. When ready to use, rinse well and thaw at room temperature.

# Bilberry

✿ *Vaccinium myrtillus*

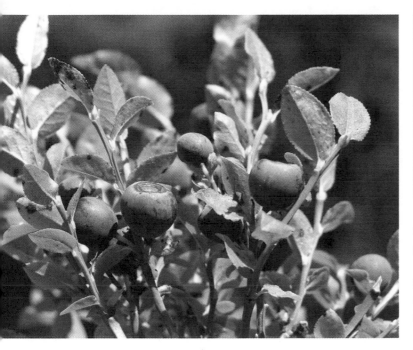

## Making the Most of Bilberries

Bilberries are not widely available except in juice and extract forms, although they sometimes can be bought frozen. When purchasing juice, select a product that is at least 70 percent bilberry juice. The juice will only be missing the fiber found in the fresh berries, but it will contain all the antioxidants and vitamin C. Use the juice to make smoothies and also to make fruit sauces.

LEFT The bilberry shrub thrives in damp, acid, and sandy or rocky soils, growing throughout the cooler regions of Europe, Asia, and North America.

Native to temperate and subarctic regions, where it grows in soil poor in nutrients and of high acidity, the bilberry is related to, resembles, and is often mistaken for the blueberry. It is also known as the whortleberry, European blueberry, hurts, whinberry, winberry or wimberry, myrtle blueberry, and fraughan. For a variety of reasons, bilberries are seldom cultivated or grown commercially; as a result, when they are found in shops they are frequently very expensive.

Bilberries are an excellent source of vitamin C and fiber. They also contain high levels of antioxidant anthocyanins and other flavonoids, and phenols.

### THE HEALTHY EVIDENCE

A 2010 study published in the *Journal of Nutrition* reported that bilberry extract improved blood glucose and insulin levels. The researchers suggested that "the use of bilberry fruits has important implications for the prevention and treatment of type 2 [diabetes]." In a 2010 study published in the *Journal of Medicinal Foods*, the researchers found that bilberry extract significantly inhibited breast cancer cell growth; they concluded that "bilberry extract as ingested by humans, not just the purified anthocyanins it contains, inhibits proliferation of and induces apoptosis in breast cancer cells at its lowest effective concentrations."

## What's in a Serving?

**BILBERRY JUICE**
**72 percent bilberry**
**(½ cup/118 ml)**
**Calories:** 157.5
**Protein:** 0 g
**Total fat:** 0 g
**Saturated fat:** 0 g
**Carbohydrates:** 19 g
**Fiber:** 0 g

### In a Nutshell

**Origin:** Europe, northern Asia, far northern regions of North America
**Season:** Late summer
**Why it's super:** Juice is high in vitamin C and contains antioxidant anthocyanins and other flavonoids and phenols
**Growing at home:** Extremely difficult to grow

# Nuts and Oils

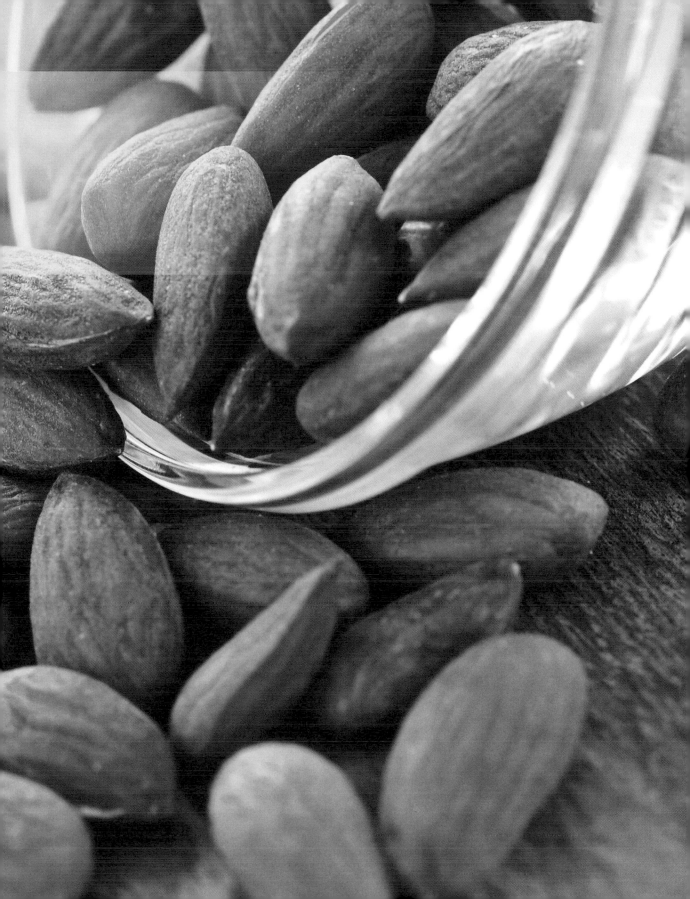

# Cashew

✿ *Anacardium occidentale*

RIGHT The cashew is enclosed in a shell containing anacardic acid, a skin irritant, which is chemically related to poison ivy toxin.

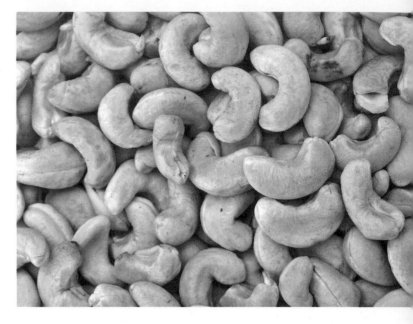

Cashews grow on a small evergreen tree that is native to the tropical regions of America, and most likely originated in Brazil. The nut's name derives from the Native American word *acaju*, which means "to pucker the mouth" and which was misheard by Portuguese sailors as *caju*. The scientific name of the plant refers to a potent skin irritant in the shells, anacardic acid.

The fruit of the tree is pear-shaped and known as the cashew apple. It is an accessory fruit that gives rise to the true fruit, or drupe, that grows at the end of the cashew apple; the familiar cashew nut is the seed inside. The cashew apple ripens to a yellow and red color with juicy flesh, which is edible.

Cashews are an excellent source of vitamin K, copper, magnesium, and phosphorus, and a good source of folate, protein, potassium, selenium, manganese, zinc, and iron. They contain beta-sitosterol, which may lower blood cholesterol, and antioxidant proanthocyanidins, and squalene, another antioxidant.

## What's in a Serving?

**DRY ROASTED CASHEWS**
**(1 ounce/28.4 g)**
**Calories:** 163 (681 kJ)
**Protein:** 4.3 g
**Total fat:** 13.1 g
**Saturated fat:** 2.6 g
**Carbohydrates:** 9.3 g
**Fiber:** 0.9 g

## Making the Most of Cashews

Cashews are a good addition to stir-fries, where they increase antioxidants and protein. Another way to use the nuts is to make cashew butter: Place the cashews in a food processor, add 3 tablespoons of canola oil to 2 cups (274 g) of nuts, and process until smooth.

## In a Nutshell

**Origin:** Brazil

**Season:** Several weeks only during the dry season (winter); available year-round

**Why it's super:** High in vitamin K, copper, magnesium, and phosphorus; good source of folate, protein, potassium, selenium, manganese, zinc, and iron; contains beta-sitosterol, proanthocyanidins, and squalene

**Growing at home:** Possible, but requires a tropical climate

## THE HEALTHY EVIDENCE

A 2010 study published in the journal *Food and Chemical Toxicology* reported on the effects of squalene on human breast cancer cells and normal breast cells. Squalene protected against oxidative DNA damage in normal breast cells, suggesting it may help prevent breast cancer.

In 2006, researchers published an article in the *American Journal of Hypertension* on an eight-week study of a diet rich in cashews. The diet improved an important component of blood pressure regulation.

# Brazil Nut

### ✿ *Bertholletia excelsa*

Brazil nuts grow on enormous slow-growing trees, known as evergreen titans—which can reach up to 150 feet (45 m) in height—in the rain forests of South America. In 1633, Dutch explorers took the nuts back to the Netherlands and within the next 200 years they were exported throughout Europe. It takes 12–15 years for the titan to bear fruit. Because of the height of the tree and weight of the fruit, which ranges from 3¼–4½ pounds (1.5–2 kg), falling fruits are a significant danger to people.

Brazil nuts have recently been in the nutrition spotlight for their high content of the essential mineral selenium. They are also an excellent source of vitamin E, fiber, copper, manganese, magnesium, zinc, and phosphorus, and a good source of protein. They contain beta-sitosterol, which may lower blood cholesterol, and squalene, an antioxidant.

## THE HEALTHY EVIDENCE

In 2010, Australian researchers published an article in the *American Journal of Clinical Nutrition* on Brazil nuts and selenium status in adult males, and found that just one Brazil nut a day is sufficient in raising blood levels of this important essential mineral. Selenium serves as a cofactor, or helper compound, to key antioxidant enzymes, and plays a similar role in the functioning of the thyroid gland. Studies, notably in animals and human cell lines, suggest that selenium helps protect against cancer; however, clinical trials are needed to provide definitive evidence.

---

### In a Nutshell

**Origin:** Amazon region of South America

**Season:** Five to six months during the rainy season (summer); available year-round

**Why it's super:** High in vitamin E, fiber, selenium, copper, manganese, magnesium, zinc, and phosphorus; good source of protein; contains beta-sitosterol and squalene

**Growing at home:** Difficult to grow as it requires a particular type of tropical rain forest

---

### What's in a Serving?

**DRY ROASTED BRAZIL NUTS**
**(1 ounce/28.4 g)**
**Calories:** 186 (778 kJ)
**Protein:** 4.1 g
**Total fat:** 18.8 g
**Saturated fat:** 4.3 g
**Carbohydrates:** 3.5 g
**Fiber:** 2.1 g

---

### Making the Most of Brazil Nuts

Brazil nuts can be used in place of any nut—even coconut—in recipes. Traditionally they are used in desserts, but they can also be added to grain side dishes to boost the fiber and protein content. Note that Brazil nuts contain a high level of fat—even more than other nuts. This makes them especially susceptible to rancidity, so make sure you store them in the refrigerator.

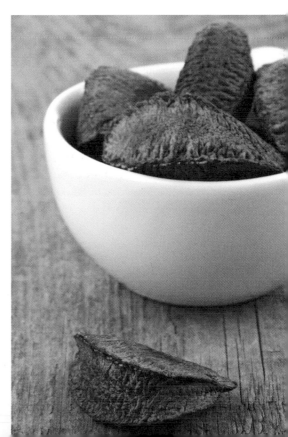

RIGHT Brazil nuts are among the most important crops of the Amazon region. They are harvested almost entirely from wild trees.

# Pecan

✿ *Carya illinoinensis*

Pecans are native to many parts of North and Central America, including the state of Illinois, which gave the plant its scientific name, and they have been a staple food in the southern United States for the past two centuries, figuring prominently in numerous traditional foods and beverages of that region. Prior to that, the nuts were also a staple for Native Americans, who referred to them as *pacane*, a name subsequently adopted and adapted by French settlers in Louisiana. Thomas Jefferson planted several hundred pecan trees at his estate in Monticello and sent some to George Washington to plant at Mount Vernon. The pecan tree is the state tree of Texas.

Pecans are an excellent source of fiber, manganese, and copper, and a good source of protein, thiamine, magnesium, phosphorus, and zinc. They contain beta-sitosterol, which may help lower blood cholesterol, as well as squalene, an antioxidant.

### THE HEALTHY EVIDENCE

A 2006 study published in the journal *Nutrition Research* reported that eating 1 ounce (28.4 g) of pecans daily lowered the blood level of oxidized LDL cholesterol, a promoter of cardiovascular disease. Other studies have shown that an important phytochemical found at high levels in pecans, beta-sitosterol, lowers blood cholesterol levels. An analysis published in the *Journal of Agricultural and Food Chemistry* found that pecans ranked in the highest category of nuts for antioxidant capacity, which can potentially protect against both cancer and heart disease.

## In a Nutshell

**Origin:** North America

**Season:** Early autumn; available year-round

**Why it's super:** High in fiber, manganese, and copper; good source of protein, thiamine, magnesium, phosphorus, and zinc; contains beta-sitosterol and squalene

**Growing at home:** Easy to grow in a temperate climate; grows up to 100 feet (30 m).

## What's in a Serving?

**DRY ROASTED PECANS
(1 ounce/28.4 g)**

**Calories:** 201 (842 kJ)

**Protein:** 2.7 g

**Total fat:** 21.1 g

**Saturated fat:** 1.8 g

**Carbohydrates:** 3.8 g

**Fiber:** 2.7 g

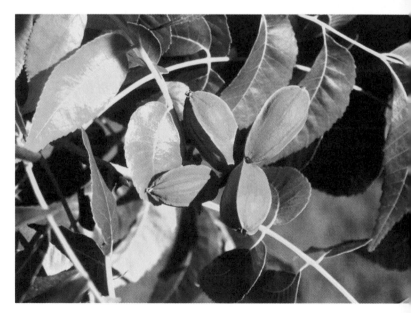

ABOVE Native Americans used pecans to produce an intoxicating drink known as *powcohicora*, the source of the word "hickory."

## Making the Most of Pecans

Pecans make an excellent substitute for walnuts in recipes, because of their similarly high fat content. Combining them with vegetables and a whole grain provides a complete protein and therefore a nutritious main dish. Pecans also boost nutrients in baked goods, from cookies to fruit breads.

# Hazelnuts

✿ *Corylus avellana* Hazelnut
✿ *Corylus maxima* Filbert

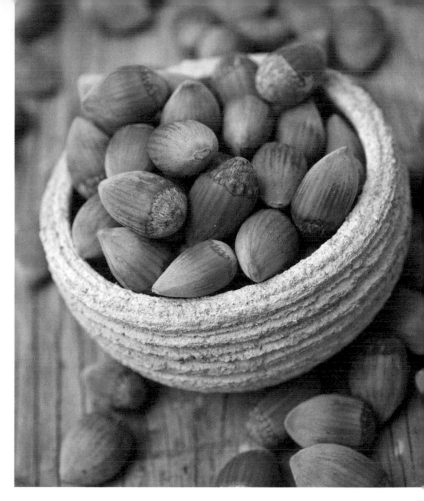

The name "hazelnut" is used commercially to refer to any of the nuts of the genus *Corylus*. The two most widely available species are the hazelnut, also known as a cobnut, and the filbert; the former is rounder than the latter, which has a more elongated shape. In terms of their nutritional content, the two nuts are, however, identical and they can be used interchangeably in cooking. Oil is sometimes extracted from these nuts and used in baked goods and salad dressings. It is, however, expensive, not readily available, and high in saturated fats.

Hazelnuts are an excellent source of vitamin E, fiber, manganese, copper, and magnesium, and a good source of phosphorus, iron, potassium, and zinc. They also contain beta-sitosterol, which may help lower blood cholesterol, and several antioxidants, including squalene and phenols.

## THE HEALTHY EVIDENCE

Turkish researchers published an article in 2010 on their study of hazelnuts and LDL cholesterol oxidation. They gave members of a control group 1 g of nuts per kilogram of body weight for four weeks—for the average person this would be about 2–3 ounces (57–85 g)

ABOVE The Black Sea coast region of Turkey provides around three-quarters of the world's hazelnut crop. Other major centers of cultivation include Italy, Spain, China, Iran, and the northeastern United States.

### Making the Most of Hazelnuts

Chopped hazelnuts add protein and antioxidants to fruit salads and fresh green salads. They also make an excellent addition to any baked goods, such as quick breads, muffins, and biscuits. Hazelnuts also contribute texture and protein to cooked vegetables.

### What's in a Serving?

**DRY ROASTED HAZELNUTS**
(1 ounce/28.4 g)
**Calories:** 183 (766 kJ)
**Protein:** 4.3 g
**Total fat:** 17.7 g
**Saturated fat:** 1.3 g
**Carbohydrates:** 5 g
**Fiber:** 2.7 g

### In a Nutshell

**Origin:** Europe and western Asia
**Season:** Mid-autumn; available year-round
**Why they're super:** High in vitamin E, fiber, manganese, copper, and magnesium; good source of phosphorus, iron, potassium, and zinc; contain beta-sitosterol, squalene, and phenols
**Growing at home:** Easy to grow at home

per day. They found that hazelnuts reduced LDL oxidation and also increased the ratio of large-sized LDL particles to small-sized particles—this is significant in relation to heart disease, because small LDL particles are more likely to penetrate the blood vessel wall, causing injury.

# Pumpkin Seed

✿ *Cucurbita maxima*

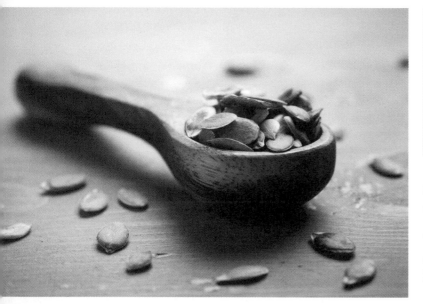

### In a Nutshell

**Origin:** South America
**Season:** Late autumn; available year-round
**Why it's super:** High in fiber, magnesium, and zinc; good source of protein, manganese, potassium, copper, and iron; contains phytosterols
**Growing at home:** Easy to grow at home

LEFT Native Americans valued pumpkin seeds as a dietary staple and, like many other peoples, used the seed as an ingredient in medicines.

During the annual pumpkin-carving season prior to Halloween, most people regularly toss away large amounts of pumpkin seeds, which is a pity, as they are a highly nutritious food in their own right. For centuries they were widely used in folk medicine. Among the conditions they have been purported to treat are irritable bowel syndrome and prostate problems; Germans even used the seed oil to combat tapeworms.

### What's in a Serving?

**DRY ROASTED PUMPKIN SEEDS
(1 ounce/28.4 g)**
**Calories:** 126 (529 kJ)
**Protein:** 5.3 g
**Total fat:** 5.5 g
**Saturated fat:** 1 g
**Carbohydrates:** 15.2 g
**Fiber:** 5.2 g

### Making the Most of Pumpkin Seeds

Using the whole pumpkin seed, rather than just the kernel, provides three times the fiber and reduces the calorie level. Pumpkin seeds are easy to collect and prepare at home from fresh pumpkins. Scoop out the seeds and spread them on a baking sheet. Spray with nonfat cooking spray and seasoning, if desired. Bake until the seeds are slightly brown.

Today the oil is still widely used, both as a salad oil and as a cooking oil in Central European cuisine.

Whole pumpkin seeds are an excellent source of fiber, magnesium, and zinc, and a good source of protein, manganese, potassium, copper, and iron. They contain numerous phytochemicals; of particular interest are the phytosterols, which may lower cholesterol levels and be helpful to the prostate gland.

### THE HEALTHY EVIDENCE

A 2006 study published in the *Journal of Medicinal Foods* reported on the use of pumpkin seed oil in the treatment of a condition known as benign prostatic hyperplasia (BPH), or enlarged prostate. This is a common condition in middle-aged and elderly men. In the study, the researchers injected rats with testosterone to cause the prostate enlargement. Doses of pumpkin seed oil significantly inhibited enlargement, and the authors concluded that the oil "therefore may be beneficial in the management of benign prostatic hyperplasia."

# Sunflower Seed

✿ *Helianthus annuus*

Sunflowers originated in Central America, where they were cultivated as early as 2600 BCE, and were taken to Europe in the 1500s by Spanish explorers. The plant's name most likely refers to the phenomenon of heliotropism, whereby certain plants move in response to the motion of the sun. However, sunflowers only do this in the bud stage, so the name could also be a reference to the flower's resemblance to the sun, and, indeed, for some indigenous American cultures, the plant symbolized their solar deity.

The head of the sunflower is made up of numerous florets. The florets within the circular head are disc florets, which mature into the seeds. The seeds are used to make many products, especially oil, which first became popular in Europe in the 1700s.

Sunflower seeds are an excellent source of vitamins B6 and E, folate, fiber, protein, pantothenic acid, selenium, manganese, phosphorus, and copper, and a good source of zinc, potassium, magnesium, and iron. Sunflower seeds also contain phytosterols.

## What's in a Serving?

**DRY ROASTED SUNFLOWER SEEDS**
**(1 ounce/28.4 g)**
**Calories:** 165 (690 kJ)
**Protein:** 5.5 g
**Total fat:** 14.1 g
**Saturated fat:** 1.5 g
**Carbohydrates:** 6.8 g
**Fiber:** 3.1 g

## THE HEALTHY EVIDENCE

Sunflower seeds contain numerous compounds that promote good health, including essential nutrients and phytochemicals. A 2005 study published in the *Journal of Agricultural and Food Chemistry* reported that, of 27 nut and seed products commonly eaten, sunflower seeds and pistachios had the highest levels of phytosterols, which can lower blood cholesterol.

### Making the Most of Sunflower Seeds

The small size of sunflower seeds means they can easily be added to a wide variety of recipes without the need for chopping. Try them in baked goods and vegetable dishes, where they add texture, fiber, and nutrients. Sunflower seeds are also an excellent addition to fruit salads and fresh leaf salads.

### In a Nutshell

**Origin:** Central America
**Season:** Late autumn; available year-round
**Why it's super:** High in vitamins B6 and E, folate, fiber, protein, pantothenic acid, selenium, manganese, phosphorus, and copper; good source of zinc, potassium, magnesium, and iron; contains phytosterols
**Growing at home:** Easy to grow at home

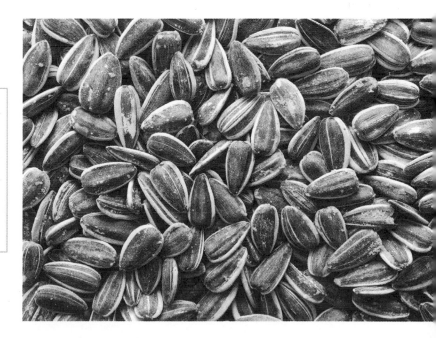

RIGHT The Aztecs enjoyed eating sunflower seeds, and their priestesses wore sunflower-shaped crowns. In the early 1700s, Peter the Great took the plant to Russia, which became the largest seed producer in Europe.

# Walnuts

☸ *Juglans cinerea* Butternut Walnut
☸ *Juglans nigra* Black Walnut
☸ *Juglans regia* Walnut, Persian Walnut

The genus name for walnuts comes from the Roman phrase *Jupiter glans*, meaning "Jupiter's acorn," an indication of the high esteem in which the Romans held the nut—it was, as it were, fit for a god. The word "walnut" comes from an Old English term, *walhnutu*, which in turn derives from the Welsh *wealh* for "foreign" and *hnutu* for "nut"—a reference to the fact that the nut had been introduced from France and Italy. The walnut may have originally reached Europe from Persia; the black and butternut walnuts originated in North America, though they are now cultivated elsewhere, too. These three are the most widely available walnuts, but there are 21 species in the genus.

Wood from walnut trees is highly prized as a hardwood, especially for furniture-making, and it commands a hefty price. As well as the nut, which has been adapted for numerous culinary uses, walnut oil has also been widely used for centuries; recently, its health benefits, substantiated by scientific evidence, have made it particularly popular.

Walnuts are an excellent source of manganese, copper, and magnesium, and a good source of vitamin B6, folate, fiber, protein, thiamine, zinc, potassium, and iron. Walnuts also contain alpha-linolenic acid, antioxidants, and phytosterols, and especially beta-sitosterol, which may lower blood cholesterol.

## In a Nutshell

**Origin:** Asia, North America

**Season:** Early to mid-autumn; available year-round

**Why they're super:** High in manganese, copper, and magnesium; good source of vitamin B6, folate, fiber, protein, thiamine, zinc, potassium, and iron; contain antioxidants, alpha-linolenic acid, and beta-sitosterol

**Growing at home:** Easy to grow at home, although the plant may take up to five years to produce nuts

## What's in a Serving?

**FRESH WALNUTS
(1 ounce/28.4 g)**
**Calories:** 175 (733 kJ)
**Protein:** 6.8 g
**Total fat:** 16.7 g
**Saturated fat:** 1 g
**Carbohydrates:** 2.8 g
**Fiber:** 1.9 g

BELOW Spanish missionaries took walnuts to California, now the source of a fifth of the world crop.

### THE HEALTHY EVIDENCE

Walnuts contain high levels of many compounds that help prevent cardiovascular disease. A study published in the journal *Circulation* reported on a four-week-long human clinical trial during which subjects regularly ate walnuts. It found that walnuts improved blood cholesterol levels, blood-vessel functioning, and other factors related to cardiovascular disease.

## Making the Most of Walnuts

Walnuts are highly susceptible to oxidation and become rancid quickly, so store them in the freezer to optimize shelf life. Add chopped walnuts to cooked grains, such as brown rice, for extra flavor and nutrients. Walnuts also combine well with blue cheese, dried cranberries, and any leafy green to make a nutrient-rich salad that can also be a main course.

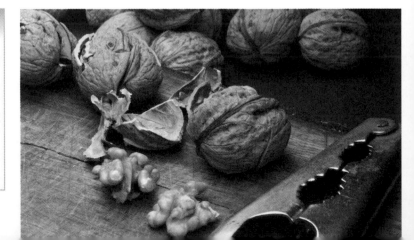

# Flax Seed or Linseed

✿ *Linum usitatissimum*

## What's in a Serving?

**GROUND FLAX SEEDS**
**(¼ cup/28 g)**
**Calories:** 150 (626 kJ)
**Protein:** 5.1 g
**Total fat:** 11.8 g
**Saturated fat:** 1 g
**Carbohydrates:** 8.1 g
**Fiber:** 7.6 g

The flax plant is native to the area extending from the eastern shore of the Mediterranean Sea to India. The ancient Egyptians and Ethiopians cultivated the plant for many uses, particularly the production of linen cloth. In Georgia in the Caucasus, archaeologists have found dyed flax fibers dating to 34,000 BCE.

The flax plant is an annual that grows to a height of just over 3 feet (1 m) and produces a small round fruit that contains the brown glossy seeds. Oil from the seeds, known as both flax seed and linseed oil, has been used for varnishing and in painting for hundreds of years.

Flax seeds are an excellent source of fiber, protein, thiamine, magnesium, phosphorus, and copper, and a good source of vitamin B6, folate, calcium, potassium, iron, zinc, and selenium. Flax seeds also contain alpha-linolenic acid and lignans, both of which may help prevent cancer and heart disease.

### THE HEALTHY EVIDENCE

A 2008 study published in the journal *Cancer Epidemiology, Biomarkers and Prevention* reported on a study of flax seed consumption by men. They found that flax caused changes indicative of protection against prostate cancer, concluding that "flax seed is safe and associated with biological alterations that may be protective for prostate cancer."

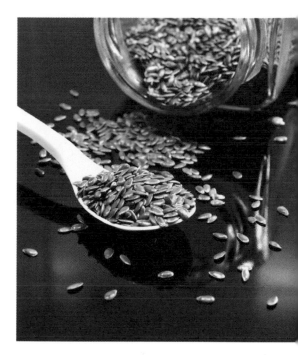

ABOVE As a result of its significant content of fiber, as well as the presence of a gummy compound known as mucilage, flax has been widely used throughout history as a form of laxative.

### In a Nutshell

**Origin:** Eastern Mediterranean to India
**Season:** Early to late autumn; available year-round
**Why it's super:** High in fiber, protein, thiamine, magnesium, phosphorus, and copper; good source of vitamin B6, folate, calcium, potassium, iron, zinc, and selenium; contains alpha-linolenic acid and lignans
**Growing at home:** Easy to grow at home

### Making the Most of Flax Seeds

For the best absorption of nutrients, flax seed should be consumed in ground or milled form. Use ground flax seed as a fat substitute in any baked goods recipe: 3 tablespoons of flax replaces 1 tablespoon of solid or liquid fat. Ground flax can also be added to smoothies, using 3 tablespoons of flax to 2 cups (470 ml) of liquid and up to 3 cups (450 g) of fruit.

# Macadamia

✪ *Macadamia integrifolia*

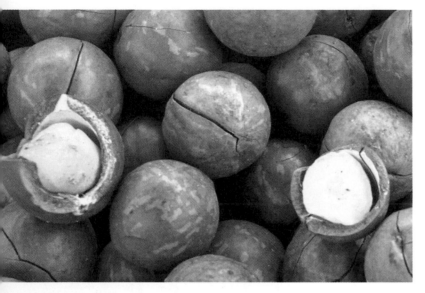

LEFT Macadamia nuts are the only commercially important food crop that is native to Australia. All of the country's major crops are imported species.

## Making the Most of Macadamia Nuts

Since they are one of the most expensive nuts and one of the most delicious, most people prefer to eat them out of hand. However, their flavor combines well with tropical fruits, such as mango, papaya, and coconut, to create a nutrient-rich fruit salad. Chopped macadamia nuts make an excellent addition to baked goods, particularly those containing dark chocolate.

## What's in a Serving?

**DRY ROASTED MACADAMIA NUTS
(1 ounce/28.4 g)**

**Calories:** 204 (852 kJ)
**Protein:** 2.2 g
**Total fat:** 21.6 g
**Saturated fat:** 3.4 g
**Carbohydrates:** 3.8 g
**Fiber:** 2.3 g

The macadamia nut is native to Australia and was named in 1857 for Dr. John Macadam, a Scottish-born Australian chemist and politician. Other names for the tasty round nut include the bush nut, Maroochi nut, Queen of Nuts, and bauple nut, as well as Aboriginal names including *gyndl*, *jindilli*, and *boombera*. In the 1880s, the nut was introduced to Hawaii, with which many Americans associate the nut, although Australia is the major international exporter.

### In a Nutshell

**Origin:** Australia
**Season:** Late autumn to spring; available year-round
**Why it's super:** High in thiamine and manganese; good source of fiber, magnesium, phosphorus, copper, and selenium; contains a high proportion of monounsaturated fat
**Growing at home:** Requires subtropical climate

The macadamia tree is an evergreen that grows from a range of 6–33 feet (2–10 m) in height. While people highly prize this typically expensive nut, it is toxic to dogs.

Macadamia nuts are an excellent source of thiamine and manganese, as well as a good source of fiber, magnesium, phosphorus, copper, and selenium. Furthermore, they contain a high proportion of fat as monounsaturated fat, which is thought to be beneficial in the prevention and treatment of cardiovascular disease.

### THE HEALTHY EVIDENCE

A 2008 study published in the *Journal of Nutrition* reported on the effects of macadamia nuts on men and women with high blood-cholesterol levels. The subjects were given 1½ ounces (42.5 g) of the nuts daily for five weeks, after which researchers rechecked their cholesterol levels. The results demonstrated that "macadamia nuts can be included in a heart-healthy dietary pattern that reduces lipid/lipoprotein cardiovascular disease risk factors."

# Pistachio

✪ *Pistachia vera*

Pistachio nuts are native to many areas of the Mediterranean and Middle East, including Turkey, Greece, Pakistan, Syria, and Afghanistan. They have been enjoyed since antiquity—nuts discovered in Jordan have been carbon-dated to 6760 BCE. The pistachio was brought back to Rome by the Roman consul in Syria. Pliny wrote in his treatise on natural history that "*pistacia* is well known among us." In Iran, an important commercial producer of the nuts, there is a pistachio tree that is reputed to be more than 700 years old.

## What's in a Serving?

**DRY ROASTED PISTACHIOS**
**(1 ounce/28.4 g)**
**Calories:** 162 (678 kJ)
**Protein:** 6.1 g
**Total fat:** 13 g
**Saturated fat:** 1.6 g
**Carbohydrates:** 7.8 g
**Fiber:** 2.9 g

## Making the Most of Pistachios

Pistachios go well with a wide range of foods and being small can be easily added to dishes. Add them whole to salads or chop them into a dessert. They'll not only add a crunchy texture, but also a host of nutrients and antioxidants.

Vendors of pistachios often dye the shells red. Originally this was done to conceal stains left by those picking the nuts. Although machines do the work today, the practice continues because that is the way most consumers recognize the nuts.

Pistachios are an excellent source of vitamin B6, fiber, protein, thiamine, copper, manganese, and phosphorus. They are also a good source of vitamin K, potassium, magnesium, and iron, and contain anti-oxidants and phytosterols.

### THE HEALTHY EVIDENCE

A 2008 study published in the *American Journal of Clinical Nutrition* reported on the effects of two levels of daily pistachio intake, 1 ounce (28.4 g) and 2 ounces (56.7 g), on cardiovascular disease markers. They found that pistachios significantly lowered cholesterol levels and raised the level of a protective lipoprotein at both intake levels; however, the higher level of intake had an even more pronounced effect.

## In a Nutshell

**Origin:** The Mediterranean and Middle East
**Season:** Early autumn; available year-round
**Why it's super:** High in vitamin B6, fiber, protein, thiamine, copper, manganese, and phosphorus; good source of vitamin K, potassium, magnesium, and iron; contains antioxidants and phytosterols
**Growing at home:** Can be grown at home but requires a dry sunny climate; fruits in four to six years

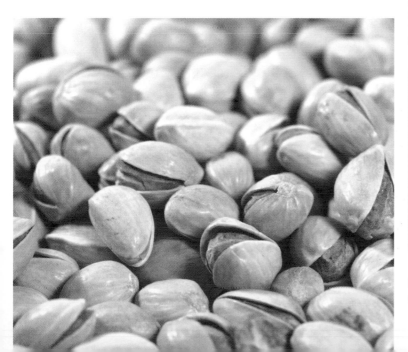

LEFT King Nebuchadnezzar had pistachio trees planted in the Hanqing Gardens of Babylon, one of the Seven Wonders of the Ancient World.

# Olive Oil

✿ *Olea europaea*

### What's in a Serving?

**FRESH OLIVE OIL**
**(1 tablespoon /13.5 g)**
**Calories:** 119 (499 kJ)
**Protein:** 0 g
**Total fat:** 13.5 g
**Saturated fat:** 1.9 g
**Carbohydrates:** 0 g
**Fiber:** 0 g

For thousands of years, olive trees have been cultivated in temperate climates not only for their fruit, but also for the oil that is pressed from the fruit. Olive oil's ancient history includes use in all three major world religions. It was incorporated in religious rites in Judaism, under the laws of which it was consecrated for use in the Temple. In the Koran, the olive tree is mentioned as being blessed; Muhammad wrote: "Consume olive oil and anoint it upon your bodies since it is of the blessed tree." And even today Christians bless the oil and use it as the Oil of Catechumens (for baptisms), the Oil of the Sick, and the Holy Chrism (confirmation).

### A VERSATILE REMEDY

Olive oil is the main cooking oil in countries surrounding the Mediterranean Sea, and Spain, Italy, Greece, and Portugal are the largest producers. In addition to its culinary uses, olive oil has long been used as a natural remedy for constipation, because of its mild laxative effect, and as an ear-wax softener. It is also used as both a skin and hair moisturizer and for shaving.

Olive oil is a good source of vitamins E and K, and also contains antioxidant polyphenols, phytosterols, and monounsaturated fat. Indeed, it is the richest source of monounsaturated fatty acids among common vegetable oils, being 77 percent monounsaturated and only 14 percent saturated. This is one of the many reasons why it helps prevent cardiovascular disease.

### THE HEALTHY EVIDENCE

A Swiss researcher published a review article on the antioxidants and health benefits of olive oil in the *International Journal of Vitamin*

BELOW About 90 percent of the world's olives are made into olive oil. Olive trees require a long period of hot, dry weather in order to ripen fully. When ripe, the fruit turns almost black.

*Except the vine, there is no plant which bears a fruit of as great importance as the olive.*

Pliny the Elder, Roman statesman, historian, and scientist (CE 23–79)

### Making the Most of Olive Oil

To maximize olive oil's benefits, select extra virgin oil. Store the container in a cool dark area, as it is susceptible to oxidation. Use it as your main fat for cooking (such as sautéing and roasting) and in salads. Olive oil also works well in recipes that call for vegetable oil, such as fruited quick breads.

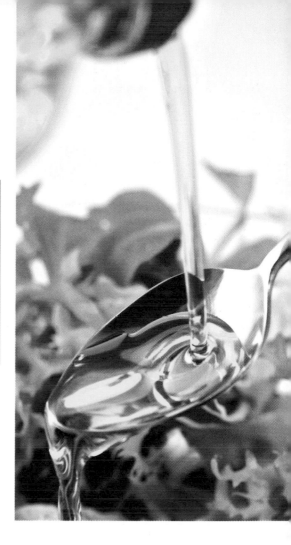

*Research* in 2009. He discussed the multitude of data providing evidence for the oil's prevention of cardiovascular disease, and cited the major antioxidant, hydroxytyrosol, as the source of this effect. Hydroxytyrosol is well absorbed by humans, and it has the highest antioxidant potency compared to other polyphenols in the oil. Studies suggest that it reduces LDL oxidation and improves other markers of oxidative damage in the blood.

RIGHT The diverse tastes of different kinds of olive oil are influenced by the soil in which the trees grow, as well as the timing of the harvest.

A 2010 human study published in the *FASEB Journal* reported on the effects of olive oil on several markers of cardiovascular disease. The researchers found that the oil reduced LDL oxidation, inflammation, and oxidative damage in subjects consuming a diet containing olive oil. They attributed the results to virgin olive oil's rich concentration of polyphenols.

The high concentration of antioxidants and phytosterols would also suggest olive oil might help protect against cancers, particularly breast cancer. A 2008 study published in the *International Journal of Molecular Medicine* reported on the effects of olive oil on the development of breast cancer. Spanish researchers focused on an enzyme involved

### In a Nutshell

**Origin:** The Mediterranean and Middle East
**Season:** Autumn and winter; available year-round
**Why it's super:** Good source of vitamins E and K; contains antioxidant polyphenols, monounsaturated fat, and phytosterols
**Growing at home:** Olive trees require a temperate climate and are moderately difficult to grow

in a key step of carcinogenesis, fatty acid synthase. They found that phenols from extra virgin olive oil suppressed the enzyme in breast cancer cells, and concluded that their data showed "a previously unrecognized mechanism for extra virgin olive oil's cancer-preventive effects."

# Almond

✿ *Prunus dulcis*

Almonds originated in the ancient Middle East and spread throughout the Mediterranean region. The Romans introduced them to England during the first century CE. The tree is quite similar to a peach tree, which along with plums and apricots are members of the rose family. The fruit resembles a small peach, and the pit inside is the almond. The almond is used to make oil, and almond butter, which is similar to peanut butter. Almonds can be ground into meal or flour and used for specialty desserts such as the Italian cookies called Amaretti. Almond meal is also used to make gluten-free products, such as cookies and snack foods, for people with Celiac disease.

Almonds are an excellent source of vitamin E, fiber, protein, riboflavin, manganese, magnesium, copper, and phosphorus. They are also a good source of niacin, calcium, potassium, iron, and zinc, and contain antioxidants and phytosterols.

## THE HEALTHY EVIDENCE

A 2008 study published in the journal *Metabolism* reported on the effects of almonds on blood-glucose regulation in people with

### What's in a Serving?

**DRY ROASTED ALMONDS**

**(1 ounce/28.4 g)**

**Calories:** 169 (708 kJ)

**Protein:** 6.3 g

**Total fat:** 15 g

**Saturated fat:** 1.2 g

**Carbohydrates:** 5.5 g

**Fiber:** 3.3 g

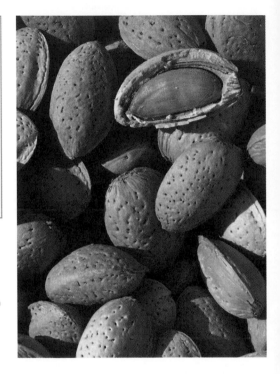

RIGHT California leads the world in almond production, and the almond tree is the most widely planted tree in the state.

### In a Nutshell

**Origin:** Middle East and Mediterranean

**Season:** Late summer to early autumn; available year-round

**Why it's super:** High in vitamin E, fiber, protein, riboflavin, manganese, magnesium, copper, and phosphorus; good source of niacin, calcium, potassium, iron, and zinc; contain antioxidants and phytosterols

**Growing at home:** Can be grown at home

### Making the Most of Almonds

Almonds are versatile and easy to include in a variety of foods. They can be used chopped or whole in stir-fries and salads, and chopped in baked goods. Ground almonds, or almond meal, can also be used to replace at least a quarter of the flour in most recipes.

high blood cholesterol. Almonds significantly reduced a blood marker of insulin secretion. The authors concluded that reducing this marker "helps to explain the association of nut consumption with reduced CHD [coronary heart disease] risk." The same group published another study in the *Journal of Nutrition* showing that antioxidants in almonds reduced blood markers of oxidative stress.

# Sesame Seed

✿ *Sesamum orientale*

The sesame plant originated in Africa or India. An annual with yellow or, occasionally, blue flowers, it grows to a height of about 3 feet (1 m), and produces pods holding the seeds. The familiar command, "Open sesame," a phrase used in the *Arabian Nights*, derives from the sesame seed pod, which pops open when mature.

Sesame seeds were widely used in ancient times. The Romans and Greeks ate them out of hand or made them into a paste flavored with cumin. Sesame oil is also a staple in Asian cuisine, imparting a distinctive flavor to many dishes. In the Middle East and Asia, sesame seeds are ground into a paste known as tahini.

Sesame seeds are an excellent source of fiber, copper, manganese, calcium, magnesium, iron, and zinc, and a good source of vitamin B6, protein, and thiamine. Sesame seeds also contain various antioxidants and phytosterols.

## THE HEALTHY EVIDENCE

A 2006 study published in the *Journal of Nutrition* reported on the effects of sesame seed consumption on postmenopausal women. A daily intake of 1¾ ounces (50 g) lowered LDL oxidation and cholesterol levels in such women. The researchers attributed some of the benefit to a compound known as sesamin, a lignin or form of phytosterol, in sesame seeds. Another study, published in 2009 in the *Journal of Nutritional Science and Vitaminology* found that sesamin reduced blood pressure in people with mild hypertension.

| What's in a Serving? | |
| --- | --- |
| **DRIED SESAME SEEDS (2 tablespoons/18 g)** | |
| **Calories:** 103 (431 kJ) | |
| **Protein:** 3.2 g | |
| **Total fat:** 8.9 g | |
| **Saturated fat:** 1.3 g | |
| **Carbohydrates:** 4.2 g | |
| **Fiber:** 2.1 g | |

BELOW An ancient Assyrian legend states that the gods drank wine made from sesame seeds the night before they created the world.

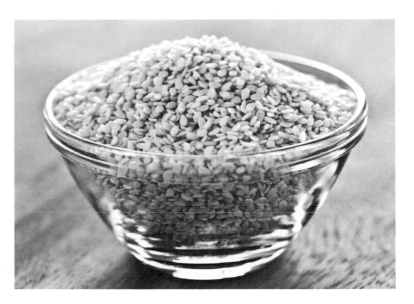

### In a Nutshell

**Origin:** Africa or India

**Season:** Mid-summer; available year-round

**Why it's super:** I ligh in fiber, copper, manganese, calcium, magnesium, iron, and zinc; good source of vitamin B6, protein, and thiamine; contains antioxidants and phytosterols

**Growing at home:** Can be grown at home

### Making the Most of Sesame Seeds

Sesame seeds instantly boost the nutrients and antioxidants of any recipe they are added to. They are particularly good in vegetable stir-fries, and make a nutrient-rich addition to baked goods. Another effective way to include more sesame seeds in your diet is to add them to soups and chili, or include them in a salad dressing.

# Herbs and Spices

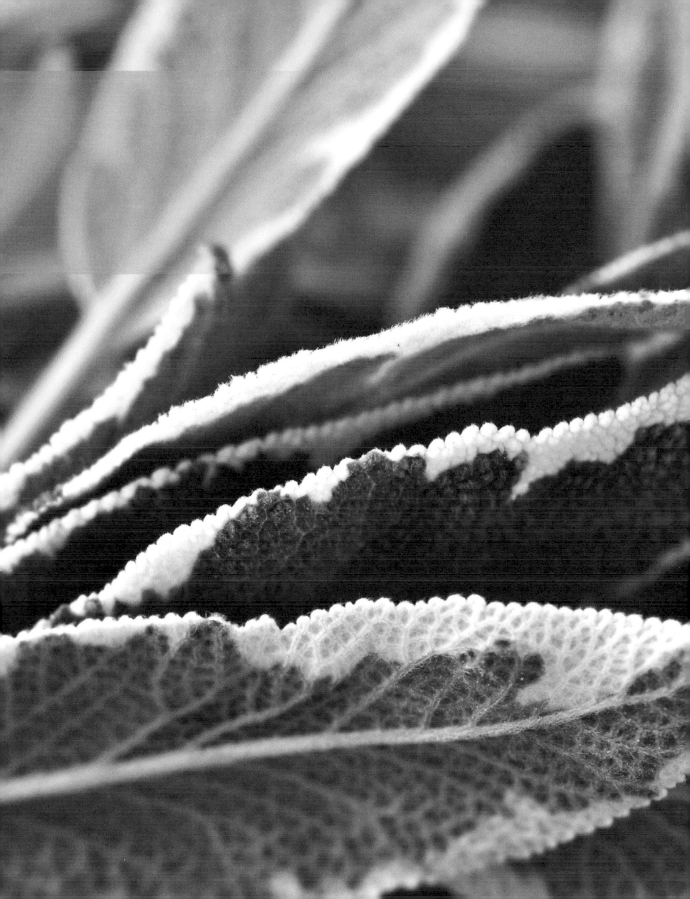

# Garlic

✪ *Allium sativum* Garlic
✪ *Allium scordoprasum* Giant Garlic, Sand Leek
✪ *Allium ursinum* Bear's Garlic, Ramson

## What's in a Serving?

**FRESH GARLIC**
**(4 cloves/12 g)**
**Calories:** 18 (75 kJ)
**Protein:** 0.8 g
**Total fat:** 0.1 g
**Saturated fat:** 0 g
**Carbohydrates:** 4 g
**Fiber:** 0.3 g

There is perhaps no other plant food that has been the subject of as much disdain and as much adulation as the garlic bulb. Garlic is native to the Mediterranean and Syria, although Central Asia is where it now grows most abundantly in its wild form. Writings from Babylonia, China, and India indicate that garlic was well known in ancient times. Giant garlic, however, was not discovered until the 1500s. Another variety, bear's garlic, is native to Western Europe; it gets its name from a folktale asserting that the brown bear eats large quantities of the plant after its long hibernation.

Garlic has always been considered a medicinal plant. The ancient Greeks and Romans believed that it conferred protection and strength, and in the Middle Ages it was widely used as a medicine in Europe and Asia. Many superstitions surround it, perhaps due to its odiferous nature. The best known is that it can be used to ward off vampires; centuries prior to that belief, midwives in ancient Greece would string cloves around newborns' necks to protect them from evil spirits.

Garlic is an excellent source of manganese as well as a good source of vitamins B6 and C. It contains several important phytochemicals, including thiosulfinate allicin, and S-allylcysteine, which act as antioxidants and have other functions that help fight disease.

### In a Nutshell

**Origin:** The Mediterranean, Syria, Central Asia
**Season:** Throughout the year in mild climates; late autumn in northern climates
**Why it's super:** High in manganese; good source of vitamins B6 and C; contains numerous phytochemicals
**Growing at home:** Relatively easy to grow in the home garden

### THE HEALTHY EVIDENCE

For a long time it was claimed that garlic would lower blood cholesterol, but this idea was dismissed after the results of a large 2007 clinical trial were published in the *Archives of Internal Medicine.* The American Heart Association reviewed the evidence and confirmed that the study "found absolutely no effects of raw garlic or garlic supplements on LDL, HDL, or triglycerides."

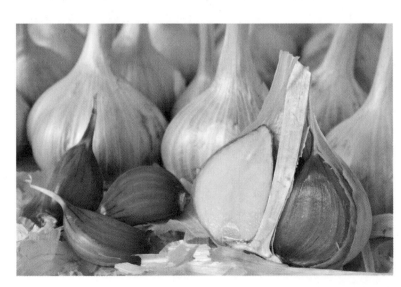

RIGHT In medieval times, people used to eat garlic as a vegetable. However, it gradually came to be regarded as more appropriate for use as a seasoning.

However, garlic may have other benefits, particularly with regard to other aspects of cardiovascular disease. A 2010 study published in the *Journal of Cardiovascular Medicine* reported on the use of various agents, one of which was garlic, on markers for heart disease. Some of the markers that were reduced included inflammation and platelet aggregation (which can cause clotting and, consequently, heart attacks).

Garlic has also been shown in some scientific studies to improve aspects of cancer development. A 2009 study published in the journal *Public Health Nutrition* reported on garlic intake and rates of cancer of the endometrium (the lining of the uterus). The researchers found that consumption of alliums, particularly garlic, was associated with a reduced risk of the cancer.

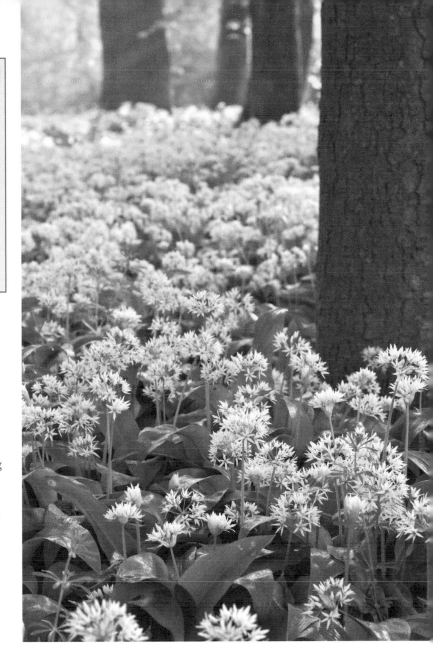

ABOVE Bear's garlic is native to Europe and is still harvested exclusively from the wild. Its leaves and its white flowers have a strong garlic scent. The leaves can be crushed and used to make a type of pesto.

*It is not really an exaggeration to say that peace and happiness begin, geographically, where garlic is used in cooking.*

Marcel Boulestin, French chef (1878–1943)

# Cinnamon Cassia

✪ *Cinnamomum aromaticum*

What is called "cinnamon" in North America and other Western countries is usually cinnamon cassia, which comes from an evergreen tree native to China, Bangladesh, India, and Vietnam. It is closely related to true cinnamon, *Cinnamomum verum*, also known as Ceylon cinnamon.

Cinnamon has been an important spice for thousands of years, and was once even more valuable than gold. It is most often ground into powder and used as a flavoring for desserts, curries, and in baking, but it is also used in religious rites and medicinally.

Cinnamon is an excellent source of fiber and manganese, and a good source of calcium. It contains antioxidant anthocyanidins and chalcone polymers, which lower blood glucose.

## What's in a Serving?

**GROUND CINNAMON
(1 tablespoon/7.8 g)**
**Calories:** 19 (81 kJ)
**Protein:** 0.3 g
**Total fat:** 0.1 g
**Saturated fat:** 0 g
**Carbohydrates:** 6.3 g
**Fiber:** 4.1 g

## In a Nutshell

**Origin:** Southern China, Bangladesh, India, and Vietnam
**Season:** Available year-round
**Why it's super:** High in fiber and manganese; good source of calcium; contains antioxidant anthocyanidins and chalcone polymers
**Growing at home:** Moderately difficult to grow: must be protected from hard frost and cold weather

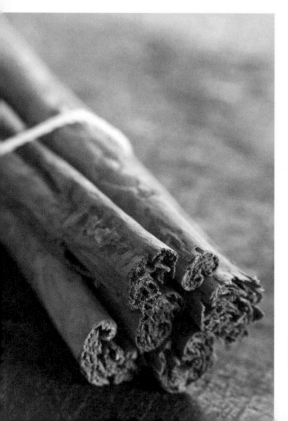

LEFT In 2004, researchers showed that chewing cinnamon-flavored gum or even just breathing the scent of cinnamon enhanced performance on mental tasks.

## THE HEALTHY EVIDENCE

A 2009 study published in the *Journal of American Board of Family Medicine* reported on a clinical trial to assess cinnamon's effectiveness in countering diabetes. In patients with diabetes, taking a 1 gram cinnamon capsule daily for 90 days significantly lowered an important blood marker of blood glucose control, HbA1C. The researchers concluded that "cinnamon could be useful" to regulate blood glucose.

Another 2009 study published in the *Journal of the American College of Nutrition* reported on the effect of cinnamon extract on overweight people with impaired glucose regulation, which is widely acknowledged as a high risk factor for diabetes. Cinnamon lowered the level of oxidized compounds in the blood; consequently, the authors stated that "cinnamon compounds could reduce risk factors associated with diabetes and cardiovascular disease."

## Making the Most of Cinnamon

An intake of at least 1 tablespoon a day of cinnamon can be beneficial to health. Mix cinnamon to vanilla yogurt—1 teaspoon of the spice for every 1 cup (245 g) of yogurt works well or add it to hot beverages, such as coffee, tea, or cocoa.

# Turmeric

✺ *Curcuma longa*

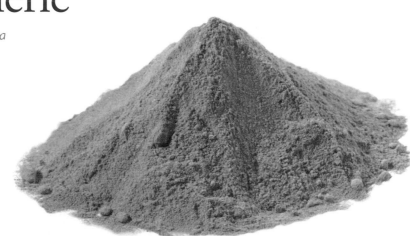

ABOVE Turmeric's peppery and slightly bitter flavor has hints of ginger and oranges. It is often used to add color to mustard products.

The spice known as turmeric comes from the root of the herbaceous perennial plant of the same name, which originated in India or nearby Southeast Asia. For 4,000 years turmeric has had a wide range of medicinal, religious, and culinary applications, especially in South Asian countries. The spice is most often used in its powdered form and is valued for its dark yellow color and unusual flavor. It is sometimes used in India as a substitute for the much more expensive spice, saffron, and was once known as "Indian saffron."

Medicinally, turmeric has long been used as an antiseptic and as an antibacterial. It is also touted for its efficacy in relieving gastro-intestinal discomfort due to irritable bowel syndrome, as well as other digestive disorders.

Turmeric is an excellent source of manganese, and iron, as well as a good source of vitamin B6, fiber, and potassium. Additionally, it contains the polyphenol curcumin, which is an antioxidant.

## Making the Most of Turmeric

The potent flavor of turmeric works well with bland foods, such as whole-grain side dishes. It also can be incorporated in vegetable stir-fries, and makes a good addition to soups and sauces, helping to boost antioxidant levels. Try making your own spice combination using turmeric and other high antioxidant spices such as cumin and coriander, and keep it handy for quick use in diverse dishes.

## What's in a Serving?

**GROUND TURMERIC (1 tablespoon/6.8 g)**

**Calories:** 24 (101 kJ)
**Protein:** 0.5 g
**Total fat:** 0.7 g
**Saturated fat:** 0.2 g
**Carbohydrates:** 4.4 g
**Fiber:** 1.4 g

### THE HEALTHY EVIDENCE

A 2010 study published in the journal *Cancer Research* reported on the anticancer effects of turmeric. The researchers isolated two compounds, known as FLLL31 and FLLL32, from curcumin, the main bioactive compound of turmeric, and applied these to pancreatic and breast cancer cells. The curcumin compound effectively inhibited several processes that lead to the cancer. The researchers concluded, "Our findings high-light the potential of these new compounds and their efficacy in targeting pancreatic and breast cancers."

## In a Nutshell

**Origin:** India or Southeast Asia
**Season:** Available year-round
**Why it's super:** High in manganese and iron; good source of vitamin B6, fiber, and potassium; contains the polyphenol curcumin
**Growing at home:** Moderately difficult to grow; grows best in hot, humid climates

# Basil

✿ *Ocimum americanum* Spice Basil      ✿ *Ocimum citriodorum* Lemon Basil
✿ *Ocimum basilicum* Basil, Sweet Basil      ✿ *Ocimum sanctum* Sacred Basil, Holy Basil

Basil or sweet basil *(Ocimum basilicum)* is a popular culinary herb strongly associated with tomato sauces and pesto. Sacred basil, also called holy basil and *tulsi*, is native to Malaysia and India; in Asia, it is not only used as a flavoring but also as a medicine and for religious purposes—it plays an important role in the rituals of some Hindu sects. Spice basil, also known as hoary basil, hairy basil, and American basil, is an annual whose flavor has hints of camphor, cinnamon, citrus, and lavender. Lemon basil is a more recently created hybrid of basil and spice basil; it contains a chemical, citrol, that gives it a lemony smell and taste. The color of basil varies from pale green to dark purple.

Basil is an excellent source of vitamins A and K, and a good source of vitamin C and manganese. Its essential oils contain antioxidant compounds and carotenoids.

## THE HEALTHY EVIDENCE

A 2006 study in the *Journal of Agricultural and Food Chemistry* analyzed the phytochemicals in basil. They found that basil contains essential oils, which function as antioxidants and antimicrobial agents, and that these inhibited specific bacteria and fungi.

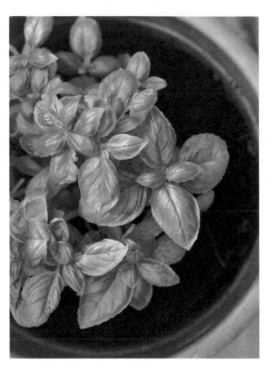

LEFT The leaves of the basil plant resemble those of its close relative, peppermint. As well as green, they can be dark red or even purple.

---

### What's in a Serving?

**FRESH BASIL
(1 cup/24 g)**
**Calories:** 6 (23 kJ)
**Protein:** 0.8 g
**Total fat:** 0.2 g
**Saturated fat:** 0 g
**Carbohydrates:** 0.6 g
**Fiber:** 0.4 g

---

### In a Nutshell

**Origin:** Old World tropics
**Season:** Year-round in warm climates
**Why it's super:** High in vitamins A and K; good source of vitamin C and manganese; contains antioxidant essential oils and carotenoids
**Growing at home:** Easy to grow

---

### Making the Most of Basil

Many people add only small amounts of basil to dishes, but to maximize your intake of nutrients and antioxidants try using larger quantities of the fresh leaves—for example, 3 cups (72 g) in a standard recipe for spaghetti sauce (ten servings). Even larger amounts can be sautéed with onions and olive oil and used as a base for any vegetable dish.

In 2008, researchers at the Swiss Federal Institute of Technology published a report on a compound in basil, (E)-beta-caryophyllene (BCP). They suggested that this powerful anti-inflammatory agent could be effective in treating diseases in which inflammation plays a key role, such as arthritis and inflammatory bowel disease.

# Marjoram and Oregano

✪ *Origanum majorana* Sweet Marjoram
✪ *Origanum onites* Pot Marjoram
✪ *Origanum vulgare* Oregano

Sweet marjoram, pot marjoram, and oregano are the best known of the 36 species belonging to the genus *Origanum*. By far the most widespread and best known is oregano, now inextricably linked with Italian foods such as pasta sauces and pizza. Native to Europe, it was, however, originally used more widely as a medicinal herb. Spanish explorers in what is now Oregon may have mistakenly conferred its name after spying an aromatic herb resembling oregano on the coastline.

Marjoram is closely associated with England and cottage gardens, but it was not introduced to England until 1573, when it was brought from Portugal. As its name implies, sweet marjoram has a sweet scent (it is sometimes incorporated in perfumes) and a sweet flavor, milder than oregano. Pot marjoram, which originated in the Mediterranean region, has a stronger flavor, more akin to oregano; it is widely used in Turkish cuisine.

Marjoram and oregano are an excellent source of vitamin K, and a good source of fiber, calcium, iron, and manganese. They also contain antioxidants such as phenols, flavonoids, and carvacrol.

## Making the Most of Oregano and Marjoram

The best way to maximize the benefits of these herbs is to use them in both fresh and dried forms. Incorporate them in tomato sauces and pizza toppings, or try them fresh in salads. Dried oregano and marjoram can also be used to add antioxidants and flavor to vegetables and roasted meats.

## In a Nutshell

**Origin:** Oregano: the Mediterranean to central Europe; sweet marjoram: North Africa and southwest Asia; pot marjoram: the Mediterranean

**Season:** Summer to autumn

**Why they're super:** High in vitamin K; good source of fiber, calcium, iron, and manganese; contain antioxidant phenols, flavonoids, and carvacrol

**Growing at home:** Easy to grow

## What's in a Serving?

**DRIED MARJORAM/ OREGANO**

**(2 teaspoons/3.6 g)**

**Calories:** 10 (40 kJ)
**Protein:** 0.4 g
**Total fat:** 0.2 g
**Saturated fat:** 0 g
**Carbohydrates:** 2.4 g
**Fiber:** 1.6 g

BELOW Oregano is widely used in both Mediterranean and Mexican cuisines for its scent and flavor.

### THE HEALTHY EVIDENCE

A 2005 study published in the *Journal of Agricultural and Food Chemistry* reported on the antioxidants contained in oregano. The plant's essential oils were tested for their ability to inhibit specific pathogenic bacteria, *Listeria monocytogenes*, and were found to be highly effective in suppressing its growth. In addition, the compounds exhibited antioxidant functions.

A 2010 study published in the journal *Arthritis and Rheumatism* reported that a compound found in both marjoram and oregano, carvacrol, "had an unprecedented capacity" to affect an important immune system marker; the researchers concluded that this may help prevent inflammation and protect against arthritis.

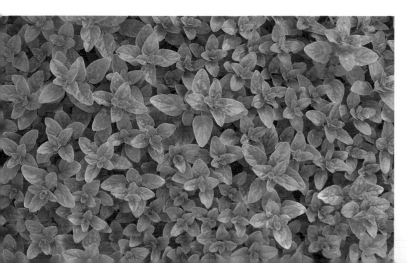

# Rosemary

✿ *Rosmarinus officinalis*

A member of the mint family, rosemary is a perennial plant that blooms in the summer in cooler climates and all year in warm climates. Its name comes from the Latin *rosmarinus*, meaning "dew of the sea," a reference to the fact that it is often found growing near the ocean. The plant's flowers may be white, pink, purple, or blue. It is frequently used in cooking, either fresh or dried, especially in Mediterranean cuisine. Highly aromatic, it has a somewhat bitter,

## What's in a Serving?

**DRIED ROSEMARY**
**(2 teaspoons/2.4 g)**
**Calories:** 8 (33 kJ)
**Protein:** 0.1 g
**Total fat:** 0.4 g
**Saturated fat:** 0.2 g
**Carbohydrates:** 1.5 g
**Fiber:** 1 g

## In a Nutshell

**Origin:** Mediterranean region of North Africa and southern Europe
**Season:** Available year-round
**Why it's super:** Good source of fiber and iron; contains the antioxidants carnosic acid, rosmarinic acid, camphor, caffeic acid, ursolic acid, betulinic acid, rosmaridiphenol, and rosmanol
**Growing at home:** Easy to grow

astringent taste that works well in stews, soups, casseroles, salads, and other dishes.

Rosemary is a good source of iron and fiber and contains antioxidants such as carnosic acid, rosmarinic acid, camphor, caffeic acid, ursolic acid, betulinic acid, rosmaridiphenol, and rosmanol.

## THE HEALTHY EVIDENCE

A pair of 2007 studies published in the *Journal of Neurochemistry* and *Nature Reviews Neuroscience* reported on the health benefits of rosemary. Researchers at the Burnham Institute for Medical Research, who carried out both studies, found that rosemary contains numerous compounds that protect brain cells from the ravages of free radicals. They focused on one compound in particular, carnosic acid (CA). Its action, similar to a drug in that it exerts its effects only when needed, is referred to as a "pathological-activated therapeutic" or PAT. This PAT action of CA makes it especially effective at protecting the brain from disorders such as Alzheimer's and Lou Gehrig's disease, and, potentially, slowing the ageing process.

LEFT Rosemary's upright sprigs are reminiscent of the needles of the pine, a distant relative, and its pine-like aroma complements meat dishes nicely.

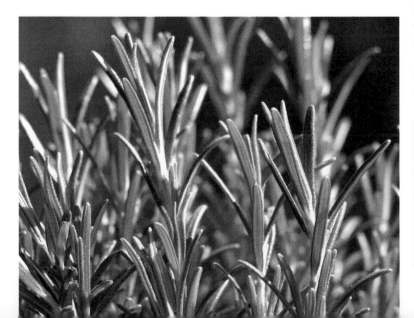

## Making the Most of Rosemary

Ground rosemary is easier to incorporate into foods than whole fresh rosemary. Brush the top of breads with olive oil and sprinkle liberally prior to broiling. Fresh rosemary can, however, be placed in a cheesecloth pouch and used as an infusion for soups and sauces, thereby boosting antioxidants.

# Parsley

✿ *Petroselinum crispum*

Although it has been cultivated for centuries, parsley remains an afterthought for many in the West, frequently being relegated to the role of a garnish. In contrast, Middle Eastern cuisine has made good use of this nutrient-rich herb, notably in the traditional salad known as tabbouleh, where it is the main ingredient.

The genus name, *Petroselinum*, is derived from the Greek words for "rock" and "celery," a reference to the herb's tendency to grow on rocky cliffs. There are numerous cultivars of parsley, but the most common are curly parsley and Italian or flat leaf parsley. The latter variety is more aromatic and less bitter than curly parsley.

Fresh parsley is an excellent source of vitamins A, C, and K, folate, fiber, and iron, and a good source of potassium, calcium, magnesium, and manganese. It also contains antioxidant flavonoids, and the carotenoids beta-carotene, lutein, and zeaxanthin.

## THE HEALTHY EVIDENCE

In a 2007 study published in the journal *International Journal of Oncology*, researchers at Case Western Reserve University reviewed

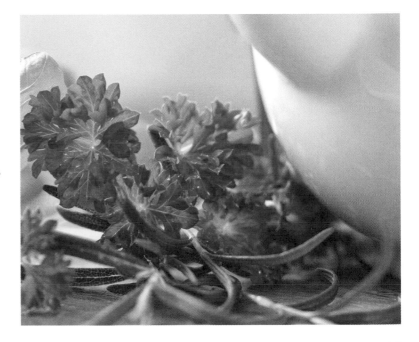

ABOVE In ancient Greece, parsley was planted on graves, and if someone was said "to be in need of parsley" it meant they were close to death.

## Making the Most of Parsley

Eating parsley fresh will provide maximum levels of nutrients. Try using it as a salad green in combination with mild-flavored greens. Adding legumes or cheese, and a side serving of whole-grain bread, will make it a nutrient-rich meal.

## What's in a Serving?

**FRESH PARSLEY
(1 cup/60 g)**
**Calories:** 22 (91 kJ)
**Protein:** 1.8 g
**Total fat:** 0.5 g
**Saturated fat:** 0.1 g
**Carbohydrates:** 3.8 g
**Fiber:** 2 g

## In a Nutshell

**Origin:** Southeastern Europe and western Asia
**Season:** Summer; available year-round
**Why it's super:** High in vitamins A, C, and K, folate, fiber, and iron; good source of potassium, calcium, magnesium, and manganese; contains antioxidant carotenoids, including beta-carotene, lutein, and zeaxanthin, as well as flavonoids
**Growing at home:** Easily grown in the home garden

international epidemiologic data on cancer and dietary intake. They found that apigenin, a flavonoid in parsley, has been "shown to possess remarkable anti-inflammatory, antioxidant and anticarcinogenic properties." The anti-inflammatory and antioxidant effects would also suggest that parsley can also help prevent cardiovascular disease.

# Sage
✪ *Salvia officinalis*

## What's in a Serving?

**DRIED SAGE**
**(2 teaspoons/1.4 g)**
**Calories:** 4 (18 kJ)
**Protein:** 0.2 g
**Total fat:** 0.2 g
**Saturated fat:** 0 g
**Carbohydrates:** 0.9 g
**Fiber:** 0.6 g

The genus name of this herb comes from the Latin word for "save," and over the centuries sage has been used to treat a wide range of diseases. To the Romans, it was a sacred herb and its harvesting included rituals; the Greeks used it to treat snakebites. The scientific name of the plant refers to the fact that in ancient times it was often the official sage of the apothecary.

Other notable varieties of sage include pineapple sage *(Salvia elegans)* and clary sage *(Salvia sclarea)*. The scientific name of pineapple sage refers to its elegant appearance; that of clary sage derives from its use in treating eye disorders, *sclarea* meaning "to clarify."

Sage has a slight peppery taste, and its use in recipes is varied. In the West, it is mainly used as a seasoning for poultry stuffing and sauces. Germans season sausage with sage, as do the British in English Lincolnshire sausage.

Sage is a good source of vitamin K, and it contains numerous phytochemicals including phenols and flavonoids.

## THE HEALTHY EVIDENCE

A 2010 study published in the *Journal of Medicinal Food* reported on extracts of several herbs and their potential health effects. Sage showed a high level of antioxidant activity against oxidative stress in liver cells. In 2008, Pakistani researchers demonstrated that sage was an effective antimicrobial agent against specific bacteria, including common pathogens such as salmonella, shigella, and staphylococcus. That sage extract can enhance memory has been demonstrated in a number of studies, including one 2008 Australian study that noted this effect in people over the age of 65.

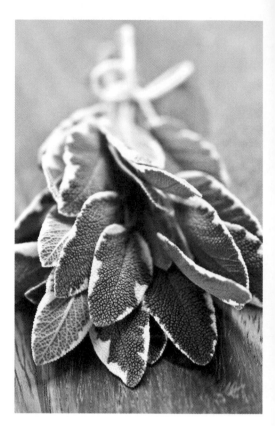

ABOVE The leaves of the sage plant have a texture almost akin to reptile skin. The plant also produces attractive white to dusky mauve flowers. Together these features make it an appealing ornamental plant.

## In a Nutshell

**Origin:** Southeastern Europe and Asia Minor
**Season:** Summer; available year-round
**Why it's super:** Good source of vitamin K; contains phenols and flavonoids
**Growing at home:** Easy to grow in the home garden

## Making the Most of Sage

Most people only make stuffing, the most common use for sage, during the holidays. One way to add more sage to your diet, and thereby increase antioxidant intake, is to use it in grain side dishes such as wild and brown rice, and barley and lentils. Sage will also enliven sauces and stews.

# Thyme

- *Thymus* x *citriodora* Lemon Thyme
- *Thymus serpyllum* Wild Thyme
- *Thymus vulgaris* Thyme, Garden Thyme

Thyme, or garden thyme, has been a popular culinary and medicinal herb for many thousands of years. Ancient Greeks used it in baths, and ancient Egyptians used it in embalming. Like most of the herbs it has many culinary uses: as a flavoring for meats, in stews, and in soups. Thyme retains its flavor after drying better than most herbs. Wild thyme is not generally commercially available and is usually picked wild or grown in gardens; it may be used as a substitute for garden thyme. Lemon thyme has a faint lemon scent and a mild lemony flavor.

Thyme is an excellent source of vitamin K and iron, as well as a good source of manganese. The leaves and essential oils contain antioxidant phenols and flavonoids, and the compound thymol, which is an effective antibacterial agent and a key ingredient in antiseptic mouthwash.

## THE HEALTHY EVIDENCE

A 2010 study published in the journal *Phytomedicine* reported on the effects of thyme extract on the growth of Methicillin-resistant *Staphylococcus aureus* (MRSA), a highly dangerous bacteria that is of major concern in hospitals and community facilities worldwide, as it is difficult to treat and sometimes fatal. The results indicated that the thymol compound from thyme could potentially be used to treat MRSA.

---

### What's in a Serving?

**DRIED THYME**
**(2 teaspoons/2.8 g)**
**Calories:** 8 (32 kJ)
**Protein:** 0.3 g
**Total fat:** 0.2 g
**Saturated fat:** 0.1 g
**Carbohydrates:** 1.8 g
**Fiber:** 1 g

---

### Making the Most of Thyme

Thyme does not have an overpowering flavor and combines well with other herbs. This makes it easy to add to many different recipes to enhance the nutrients and antioxidants in foods. It is especially good in soups, stews, and sauces, as this way all of the herb will be consumed with the liquid.

---

### In a Nutshell

**Origin:** Western Mediterranean
**Season:** Available year-round
**Why it's super:** High in vitamin K and iron; good source of manganese; contains antioxidant phenols and flavonoids, and thymol
**Growing at home:** Easy to grow

---

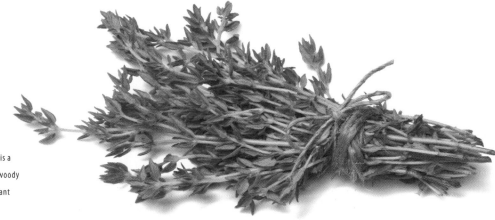

RIGHT Easy to grow, thyme is a perennial plant with stiff, woody stems. In summer, its fragrant pink flowers attract bees.

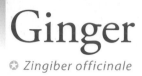

# Ginger

✤ *Zingiber officinale*

Ginger has a long history of medicinal and culinary use, dating back to at least the fifth century BCE. However, since ginger does not grow wild, its place of origin is unclear. The plants in India show the most biological variability, which suggests that the species may have originated there.

The part of the plant that is used is called the rhizome, the fleshy stalk. It looks like a root—and, indeed, is often referred to as "ginger root"—with thin brown skin and pale flesh inside. Younger rhizomes have a milder taste; the later harvest is more pungent. Ginger can also be purchased in powdered

### A Versatile Age-old Remedy

Throughout history, ginger has been used in most cultures to treat an amazing array of illnesses, including indigestion, upset stomach, diarrhea, nausea, arthritis, colic, heart conditions, the common cold, flu-like symptoms, headaches, and even painful menstrual periods. And ginger is still considered highly beneficial. According to researchers at the University of Maryland Medical Center, "Today, health care professionals commonly recommend ginger to help prevent or treat nausea and vomiting associated with motion sickness, pregnancy, and cancer chemotherapy, and as support in inflammatory conditions such as arthritis."

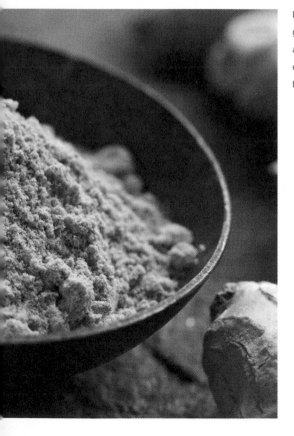

LEFT The ancient Romans imported ginger from China 2,000 years ago. The costs of this made it an expensive food; nevertheless, it became extremely popular.

form. The spice is used in many dishes, in many different cuisines, and is particularly popular in Asian, Indian, Middle Eastern, and Western cooking.

Ginger contains several compounds that act as antioxidants and anti-inflammatory agents, including shogaols, gingerols, and 6-dehydrogingerdione (DGE).

### THE HEALTHY EVIDENCE

The potential health benefits of ginger include protection against cancer, cardiovascular disease, and a host of other ailments and conditions. A 2010 review published in the journal *Biofactors* discussed one of the main bioactive ingredients of ginger, 6-gingerol,

### Making the Most of Ginger

Fresh ginger root is easy to use and stores well in the freezer, if tightly wrapped. To use, cut thin slices and add to vegetable stir-fries. Another quick way to add ginger to your diet is to boil some of the root and make ginger honey tea—just add honey and lemon to taste. Dried ginger can also be sprinkled liberally onto fresh fruit or stirred into vanilla yogurt.

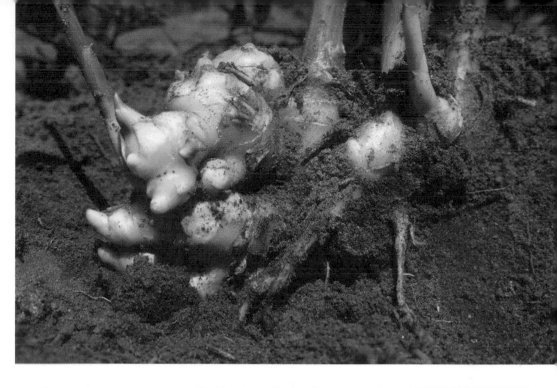

which functions as an antioxidant and anti-inflammatory agent, and can inhibit tumors. Based on their review, the authors suggested that the compound "presents a promising future alternative to therapeutic agents that are expensive [and] toxic."

A 2010 study published in the journal *Molecular Nutrition and Food Research* reported on another potent compound in ginger, 6-dehydrogingerdione (DGE). Researchers at the Graduate Institute of Medicine in Taiwan used DGE in breast cancer cells and found that it suppressed cell growth by inducing cancer cells to undergo apoptosis, or cell suicide. In 2009, a review published in the *Journal of Gynecologic Oncology* noted ginger's effectiveness in preventing nausea after chemotherapy in ovarian cancer patients as one of nine "major clinical advances in gynecology for 2009."

In 2009, researchers at Rutgers University in New Jersey reported on another group of compounds, called shogaols, in ginger that may account for some of its numerous health benefits. These compounds were even more effective than gingerols at inhibiting the growth of human lung cancer cells and colon cancer cells. The shogaols also demonstrated a stronger anti-inflammatory effect.

A 2008 study published in the *Saudi Medical Journal* reported on a human clinical trial using ginger in subjects with elevated blood lipids, such as cholesterol and tri-glycerides. Researchers gave the treatment group of subjects capsules containing 3 g of ginger daily for 45 days. The group experienced a significant reduction in levels of serum triglyceride, cholesterol, low density lipoprotein (LDL), and very low-density lipoprotein (VLDL), all of which, when elevated, increase the risk of heart disease. In addition, subjects taking ginger had an increase in high-density lipoprotein (HDL), which protects against heart disease.

## What's in a Serving?

**FRESH GINGER ROOT**
**(¼ cup/24 g)**
**Calories:** 19 (80 kJ)
**Protein:** 0.4 g
**Total fat:** 0.2 g
**Saturated fat:** 0.1 g
**Carbohydrates:** 4.3 g
**Fiber:** 0.5 g

## In a Nutshell

**Origin:** Unknown
**Season:** Autumn; available year-round
**Why it's super:** Contains antioxidant and anti-inflammatory compounds including shogaols, gingerols, and 6-dehydrogingerdione (DGE)
**Growing at home:** Easy to grow at home

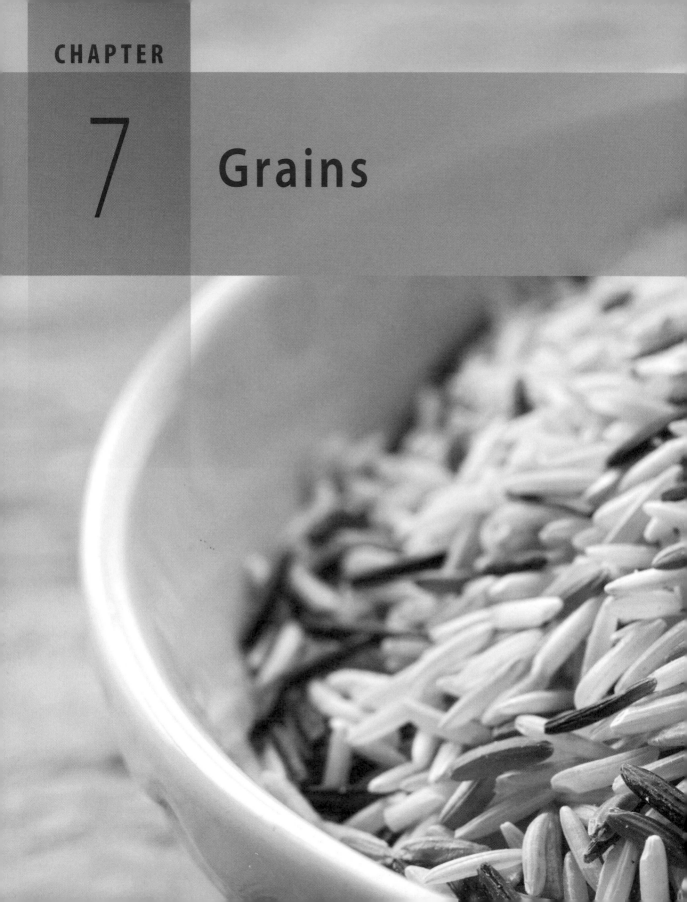

CHAPTER

7

Grains

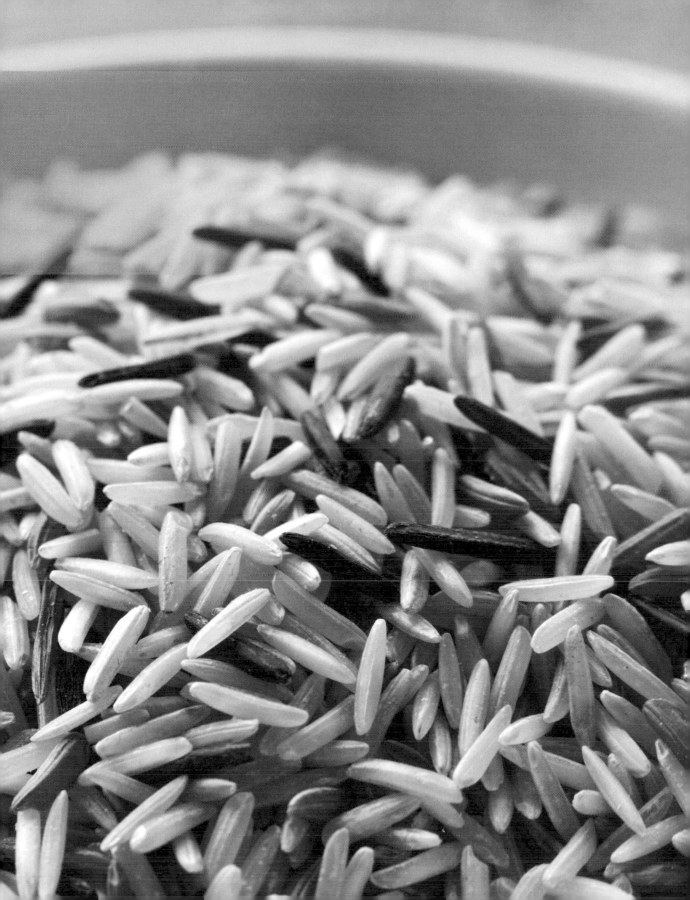

# Oats

✪ *Avena sativa*

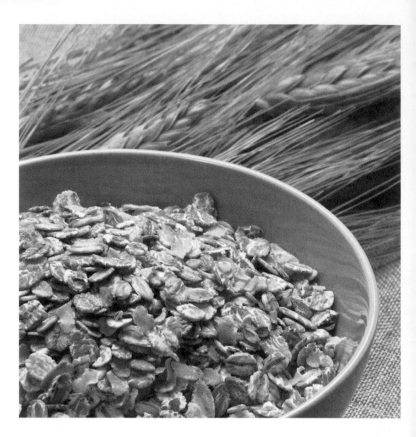

Oats were not cultivated as early as other grains, and the wild plant often grew as a weed among crops. Ancient Europeans were the first to cultivate the plant, and Pliny the Elder wrote in the first century CE of its use as food for animals and humans. Since then many cultures have enjoyed oat porridge, in which the grain is boiled in water or milk to a thick consistency, and found a variety of other uses for these grains.

Oats can be purchased as "steel-cut," "rolled," or "instant." Steel-cut oats are the least processed, having simply been cut into two or three pieces, whereas rolled oats have been flattened and steamed or toasted lightly. Rolled oats are a major ingredient in muesli, along with fruits and nuts. Instant oatmeal has usually been precooked and dried—this reduces subsequent cooking time, but it also increases the glycemic load. Furthermore, this type of oats has often had sugar and flavorings added.

Oats are an excellent source of fiber, protein, thiamine, manganese, selenium, phosphorus, magnesium, zinc, copper, and iron, and a good source of pantothenic acid and potassium. They also contain beta-glucans, soluble fiber, and polyphenols known as avenanthramides, which are antioxidants.

## Making the Most of Oats

Make sure to purchase either steel-cut or rolled oats. An easy way to incorporate more oats in your diet is to use them to replace other more refined grains. For example, you could replace up to half the breadcrumbs in a meatloaf and up to one-third of the flour in baked goods with oats.

## In a Nutshell

**Origin:** Europe
**Season:** Early autumn
**Why they're super:** High in fiber, protein, thiamine, manganese, selenium, phosphorus, magnesium, zinc, copper, and iron; good source of pantothenic acid and potassium; contain beta-glucans and antioxidant polyphenols
**Growing at home:** Can be grown in the home garden

ABOVE Rolled oats were first popularized in the United States in 1881 by Ferdinand Schumacher and Henry Crowell, who packaged it under the brand "Quaker Oats."

## THE HEALTHY EVIDENCE

A 2009 review published in *Nutrition Reviews* discussed the health benefit of oats. The author cited studies showing that oats reduce total plasma cholesterol and LDL-cholesterol levels, both risk factors for heart disease. This benefit is usually attributed to the beta-glucans, but he also pointed to the avenanthramides, which exhibit antioxidant, anti-inflammatory, and anticancer effects.

## What's in a Serving?

**DRY ROLLED OATS**
**(½ cup/41 g)**
**Calories:** 153 (642 kJ)
**Protein:** 5.3 g
**Total fat:** 2.6 g
**Saturated fat:** 0.5 g
**Carbohydrates:** 27.4 g
**Fiber:** 4.1 g

# Bran

- *Avena sativa* Oat Bran
- *Hordeum vulgare* Barley Bran

Bran refers to the outer layer of a grain kernel, which encases the endosperm and the germ, and, when considered with these components, constitutes the whole grain. The bran from many grains is sold as a health food, including rice, oat, wheat, corn, and barley. Oat and barley bran have become particularly popular as a result of studies reporting their health benefits. Most notably, oat bran made headlines in the late 1980s after a study showed that it reduced blood cholesterol in people with elevated levels. Barley bran has also been shown to contain disease-fighting compounds.

Oat and barley bran are excellent sources of fiber, protein, thiamine, manganese, selenium, phosphorus, magnesium, and iron. They are also good sources of folate, pantothenic acid, riboflavin, potassium, zinc, and copper. Studies have shown that they both contain beta-glucan (soluble fiber) and antioxidants.

## Making the Most of Bran

Bran can be used to make a hot cereal, and it provides very high fiber and nutrients. Another way to add more to your diet is in baked goods and grain side dishes. In baked goods, you may need to increase the leavening agent when adding bran.

### THE HEALTHY EVIDENCE

A 2008 article published in the *European Journal of Nutrition* provided a comprehensive review of the health-promoting properties of oat bran. The author cited studies showing that bran may help treat diabetes and cardiovascular disease. An article in the *Journal of Agricultural and Food Chemistry* in 2001 described the antioxidant and antibacterial compounds in barley bran.

BELOW Physicians were particularly keen on espousing the use of bran during the 1980s, and a dosing cup of dry bran was a common fixture on in-patients' hospital trays during that period.

## What's in a Serving?

**DRY OAT BRAN**
(½ cup/47 g)
**Calories:** 116 (484 kJ)
**Protein:** 8.1 g
**Total fat:** 3.3 g
**Saturated fat:** 0.5 g
**Carbohydrates:** 31.1 g
**Fiber:** 7.2 g

**DRY BARLEY BRAN**
(½ cup/47 g)
**Calories:** 134 (564 kJ)
**Protein:** 5.6 g
**Total fat:** 1.9 g
**Saturated fat:** 0.2 g
**Carbohydrates:** 23.5 g
**Fiber:** 8.7 g

## In a Nutshell

**Origin:** Oats: Europe; barley: Middle East

**Season:** Early autumn

**Why it's super:** High in fiber, protein, thiamine, manganese, selenium, phosphorus, magnesium, and iron; good source of folate, pantothenic acid, riboflavin, potassium, zinc, and copper; contains beta-glucan (soluble fiber) and antioxidants

**Growing at home:** The grains can be grown in a garden, but milling to produce bran is difficult

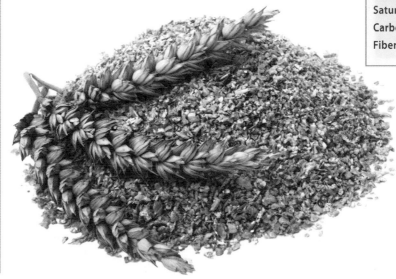

# Quinoa

✪ *Chenopodium quinoa*

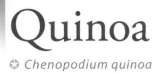

Although it has become more widely known only recently, quinoa (pronounced either *keen-wa* or *kin-wa*) has an ancient history in its native region of the Andes Mountains of South America. To the Incas, quinoa was a sacred crop, referred to as *chisaya mama* or "mother of all grains," though it is not a member of the grass (Poaceae) family and therefore not a true cereal. Quinoa remains a staple food in much of South America, and has gained popularity in Western countries because of its high protein and nutrient content.

Fresh quinoa must be soaked for a few hours to remove bitter compounds known

## What's in a Serving?

**COOKED QUINOA**
**(1 cup/185 g)**
**Calories:** 222 (931 kJ)
**Protein:** 8.1 g
**Total fat:** 3.6 g
**Saturated fat:** 0 g
**Carbohydrates:** 39.4 g
**Fiber:** 5.2 g

## Making the Most of Quinoa

Quinoa makes a nutrient-rich substitute for virutally any grain dish. Use it as an excellent base for polenta instead of cornmeal—topping it with tomato sauce will boost its antioxidant power. Another excellent use of quinoa is as a hot breakfast cereal; it works particularly well with a generous topping of cinnamon. Quinoa is gluten-free, so it is an ideal food for people with celiac disease.

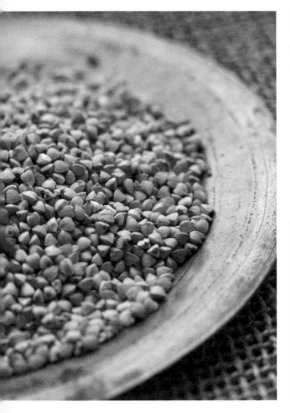

LEFT Quinoa seeds are only about ⅓–1¼ inches (1–3 cm) in length, but plump up to roughly four times that size after cooking.

as saponins; the water then has to be extracted and the quinoa rinsed before cooking. With prepackaged quinoa, however, the saponins have usually already been removed.

Quinoa is an outstanding source of vitamin B6, folate, fiber, protein, thiamine, riboflavin, manganese, magnesium, phosphorus, copper, iron, and zinc, and a good source of vitamin E, potassium, and selenium. Quinoa contains antioxidant polyphenols and flavonoids.

### THE HEALTHY EVIDENCE

A 2010 study published in the journal *Plant Foods for Human Nutrition* demonstrated that quinoa was effective in protecting against oxidative damage in rats. A 2009 review in *Advances in Food and Nutrition Research* noted that quinoa contains a high level of nutrients and antioxidant phytochemicals, such as polyphenols and flavonoids, which could combat disease.

## In a Nutshell

**Origin:** The Andes
**Season:** Summer
**Why it's super:** High in vitamin B6, folate, fiber, protein, thiamine, riboflavin, manganese, magnesium, phosphorus, copper, iron, and zinc; good source of vitamin E, potassium, and selenium; contains antioxidant polyphenols and flavonoids
**Growing at home:** Easy to grow in the home garden

# Millet

- ☻ *Eleusine coracana* Finger Millet
- ☻ *Panicum miliaceum* Proso Millet
- ☻ *Pennisetum glaucum* Pearl Millet
- ☻ *Setaria italica* Foxtail Millet

Millet represents a group of small-seeded cereal crops, many of which are grown worldwide for both human food and animal fodder. Of the numerous millet species, the most important are pearl, finger, proso, and foxtail millet. Proso millet is also known as common millet, broom corn millet, hog millet, or white millet.

Archaeological evidence suggests that in ancient times cultivation of millet was more widespread than that of rice in Asia and Africa. Millet has been cultivated in Asia for at least 10,000 years, and it reached Europe by 5000 BCE. Millet porridge, made with whole millet, is a traditional dish in both Russia and China. Millet grits can be made from the whole grain, but are cut for faster cooking.

Millet is an excellent source of protein, thiamine, niacin, manganese, magnesium, phosphorus, zinc, and copper, and in addition is a good source of vitamin B6, folate, fiber, riboflavin, and iron. Millet also contains numerous polyphenols.

## THE HEALTHY EVIDENCE

A 2008 study published in the journal *Bioscience, Biotechnology and Biochemistry* reported on the effects of millet on markers

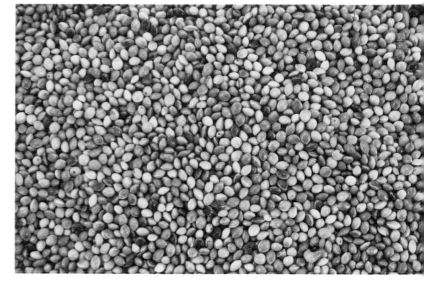

ABOVE In ancient China, proso millet was considered a sacred grain, and it became the staple food in the north, where rice was not cultivated. Today, proso is the most widely traded form of millet in the world.

for diabetes. In obese diabetic mice, a concentrate of proso millet raised HDL cholesterol level, the protective particle, and reduced the levels of other blood compounds that increase the risk for diabetes. The authors noted that their data might suggest a potential therapeutic role for millet in type 2 diabetes.

### What's in a Serving?

**COOKED MILLET
(1 cup/174 g)**

**Calories:** 207 (867 kJ)
**Protein:** 6.1 g
**Total fat:** 1.7 g
**Saturated fat:** 0.3 g
**Carbohydrates:** 41.2 g
**Fiber:** 2.3 g

## Making the Most of Millet

The traditional Russian millet porridge is a nutrient-rich breakfast, and with minor tweaking is also heart-healthy. Use 3 cups (700 ml) of water to 1 cup (200 g) of millet grits, bring to a boil, and simmer for 15 minutes. Add honey, nuts, and dried fruit to boost nutrients, and enjoy as a breakfast or even as dessert.

## In a Nutshell

**Origin:** Africa and Asia
**Season:** Summer
**Why they're super:** High in protein, thiamine, niacin, manganese, magnesium, phosphorus, zinc, and copper; good source of vitamin B6, folate, fiber, riboflavin, and iron; contains antioxidant polyphenols
**Growing at home:** Can be grown at home

# Buckwheat

✿ *Fagopyrum esculentum*

Though its name would suggest it is a grain, and it is used as such, buckwheat is not in fact a cereal or grass. Rather, it belongs to a separate group of crops known as pseudocereals (which also includes quinoa), and its "grain" is actually the dried fruit, or kernel, of the plant. Buckwheat, or common buckwheat, is the most widely cultivated species; two others, tartary buckwheat (*Fagopyrum tartaricum*) and perennial buckwheat (*Fagopyrum cymosum*), are also grown, but neither is widespread and perennial buckwheat is seldom raised for its seeds.

Buckwheat has many uses, most famously perhaps in buckwheat pancakes, which are made from buckwheat flour and known as *blini* in Russia, *galettes* in France, *ployes* in the Acadia region of Canada, and *bouketes* in Belgium. The hulled "grains," or groats, are also used in porridge, and mixed with broth to make kasha, a kind of porridge used in Poland and Russia to make knishes and blintzes.

Buckwheat is an excellent source of fiber, niacin, manganese, magnesium, phosphorus, and copper, and a good source of vitamin B6, thiamine, riboflavin, pantothenic acid, zinc, iron, and selenium. It contains antioxidant phenols and D-chiro-inositol (DCI), a compound with insulin-like bioactivity.

## In a Nutshell

**Origin:** China and eastern Russia

**Season:** Early autumn

**Why it's super:** High in fiber, niacin, manganese, magnesium, phosphorus, and copper; good source of vitamin B6, thiamine, riboflavin, pantothenic acid, zinc, iron, and selenium; contains antioxidant phenols and D-chiro-inositol

**Growing at home:** Easy to grow at home

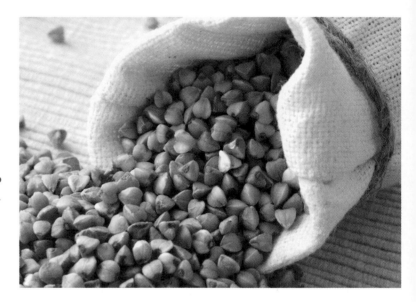

ABOVE After its introduction to Europe in the fourteenth century, common buckwheat became popular because it flourished when other grains did not.

## THE HEALTHY EVIDENCE

A 2009 study in the *Journal of Agricultural and Food Chemistry* reported that buckwheat extract lowered blood cholesterol in rats with high cholesterol, and exhibited antioxidant activity in the blood. A 2008 study from the same journal reported on DCI in buckwheat extract, and its ability to lower blood glucose and improve glucose tolerance in mice.

## Making the Most of Buckwheat

Cooked buckwheat groats make a quick and nutrient-rich breakfast cereal. To boost the antioxidants, add dried cranberries and walnuts. Cooked groats also make a nutritious side dish to accompany any entrée, adding fiber and a bevy of nutrients to the meal.

## What's in a Serving?

**TOASTED BUCKWHEAT (¼ cup/41 g)**

**Calories:** 142 (594 kJ)

**Protein:** 4.8 g

**Total fat:** 1.1 g

**Saturated fat:** 0.2 g

**Carbohydrates:** 30.7 g

**Fiber:** 4.2 g

# Barley

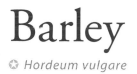
*Hordeum vulgare*

## What's in a Serving?

**COOKED BARLEY**
**(1 cup/157 g)**
**Calories:** 193 (809 kJ)
**Protein:** 3.6 g
**Total fat:** 0.7 g
**Saturated fat:** 0.2 g
**Carbohydrates:** 44.3 g
**Fiber:** 6 g

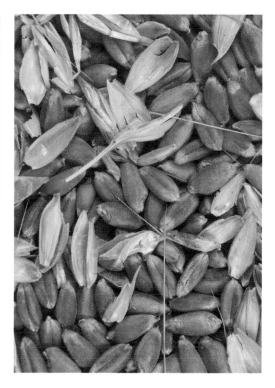

RIGHT Barley was the first cereal to be cultivated in the Middle East and Europe, and the most important grain in ancient times.

### In a Nutshell

**Origin:** Mediterranean and Central Asia
**Season:** Summer
**Why it's super:** High in fiber, niacin, manganese, selenium, and iron; good source of vitamin B6, folate, thiamine, riboflavin, magnesium, phosphorus, zinc, and copper; contains beta-glucan (soluble fiber) and antioxidants
**Growing at home:** Easy to grow at home

Barley is widely used as animal food and in the production of beer and whiskey, but it is also an important human food, regularly incorporated in the stews, soups, and breads of many cultures. The most widely available form of barley is known as "pearl" or "pot" barley, which has had its tough outer hull removed and then been polished. It can be boiled and used like rice as a side dish, or used as an ingredient in salads or other dishes to provide a chewy texture as well as a healthy dose of fiber. Barley is also available as flakes, which can be cooked like rolled oats for a breakfast cereal, and used in breads, cookies, and muffins. Barley grass is also used to make a nutritious drink (see p. 219).

Barley is an excellent source of fiber, niacin, manganese, selenium, and iron, and a good source of vitamin B6, folate, thiamine, riboflavin, magnesium, phosphorus, zinc, and copper. It also contains beta-glucan (BG, a soluble fiber) and antioxidants.

### THE HEALTHY EVIDENCE

A 2009 study published in the journal *Molecular Nutrition and Food Research* reported on the effect of barley's BG in mice fed a high-fat diet. The BG reduced weight gain, fat accumulation, and insulin resistance. The authors concluded that, "Consumption of barley BG could be an effective strategy for preventing obesity, insulin resistance, and the metabolic syndrome."

## Making the Most of Barley

For a nutrient-packed entrée, sauté ½ cup (100 g) pearl barley, ¼ cup (40 g) chopped onion, ¼ cup (25 g) chopped celery, and ¼ cup (32 g) carrot in 2 tablespoons of olive oil until the barley is browned. Add 2 cups (470 ml) of chicken broth and 1 teaspoon of thyme. Bring to boil, reduce heat, cover, and simmer for 45 minutes. Cut an acorn squash in half, scoop out the seeds, and place in a microwave dish in ¼ inch (0.7 cm) of water for ten minutes on high. Place the barley mixture into the squash halves on a baking sheet and then bake for ten minutes at 350°F (180°C).

# Brown Rice

✿ *Oryza sativa*

Brown rice is rice that has not been milled, leaving the bran intact and preserving the whole grain. Although rice, which is native to tropical regions of India, China, and Indochina, is a staple throughout the world, brown rice has traditionally been considered a food for the poor or a substitute during food shortages. But better understanding of its

## What's in a Serving?

**COOKED BROWN RICE**
**(1 cup/195 g)**
**Calories:** 216 (905 kJ)
**Protein:** 5 g
**Total fat:** 1.8 g
**Saturated fat:** 0.4 g
**Carbohydrates:** 44.8 g
**Fiber:** 3.5 g

nutritional advantages over white rice has increased its use and made it more expensive than white rice. One disadvantage with brown rice, however, is that it becomes rancid more quickly than milled rice.

Brown rice is an outstanding source of vitamin B6, fiber, niacin, thiamine, manganese, selenium, magnesium, phosphorus, and copper, as well as a good source of protein, zinc, and iron. Research shows it contains beta-glucan and pectin, which are forms of soluble fiber, and antioxidant tocotrienols, as well as beta-sitosterol, a plant sterol that has been shown to reduce cholesterol levels.

## In a Nutshell

**Origin:** Tropical India, China, and Indochina
**Season:** Year-round
**Why it's super:** High in vitamin B6, fiber, niacin, thiamine, manganese, selenium, magnesium, phosphorus, and copper; good source of protein, zinc, and iron; contains beta-glucan, pectin, antioxidant tocotrienols, and beta-sitosterol
**Growing at home:** Difficult to grow, as it requires simulating a flooded rice paddy

BELOW Although brown rice does not contain a complete protein, its protein quality is higher than that of most other grains.

### THE HEALTHY EVIDENCE

A 2007 study published in the *British Journal of Nutrition* reported on the effects of rice bran on cancer. In mice, rice bran reduced intestinal adenomas—benign tumors that are similar to colonic polyps, which have been linked to colon cancer. The authors concluded: "Rice bran might be beneficially evaluated as a putative chemopreventive intervention in humans with intestinal polyps." A 2010 study in *Nutrition Journal* reported that germinated brown rice reduced cancerous colon tumors in rats, in which cancer had been induced.

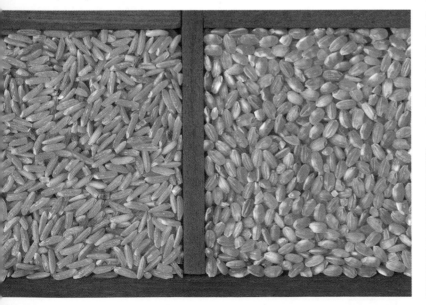

## Making the Most of Brown Rice

Soaking brown rice for 20 hours in warm water prior to cooking stimulates germination, which in turn activates certain enzymes. These enzymes provide a more complete amino acid profile. For those with celiac disease, brown rice flour can be an excellent alternative to products containing gluten.

# Whole Wheat Berries

✿ *Triticum* species

Wheat berries are the entire wheat kernel (except for the hull): the bran, germ, and endosperm. They have a crunchy consistency and are higher in fiber and nutrients than some types of processed wheat. As their nutritional benefits have become better known, wheat berries have become more widely available. They are often used as a healthful whole-grain side dish or as a hot breakfast cereal and are sometimes added to fresh vegetable salads.

Wheat berries are sometimes simply cut or crushed, to make what is known as cracked wheat. Many whole-grain breads contain either wheat berries or cracked wheat to increase the fiber content and add a crunchy texture.

Wheat berries are an excellent source of fiber, thiamine, niacin, manganese, magnesium, and phosphorus, and a good source of vitamin B6, folate, protein, zinc, potassium, iron, and copper. Wheat berries contain numerous polyphenols.

**THE HEALTHY EVIDENCE**

A 2010 study published in the *Journal of Agricultural and Food Chemistry* reported

## Making the Most of Whole Wheat Berries

Try this wheat and bean salad for a one-dish meal of nutrient-dense ingredients: combine 1 cup each of cooked wheat berries and navy beans (182 g), ½ cup each of chopped celery (100 g), onion (160 g), and tomato (180 g). Toss with an olive oil and balsamic vinaigrette dressing.

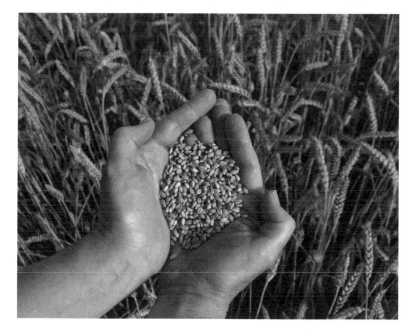

ABOVE Wheat berries can add a distinctive texture and taste, as well as highly beneficial whole-grain nutrients, to a wide range of recipes.

on the effects of a wheat component, aleurone, on human colon cells. Wheat aleurone is a layer of tissue in the endosperm, which accounts for 30 percent of the kernel's protein. An extract of the aleurone reduced cell growth and increased apoptosis (cell suicide), suggesting that it could modulate cell growth to help prevent cancer.

## In a Nutshell

**Origin:** Fertile Crescent region of the Middle East

**Season:** Summer

**Why they're super:** High in fiber, thiamine, niacin, manganese, magnesium, phosphorus; good source of vitamin B6, folate, protein, zinc, potassium, iron, and copper; contain numerous polyphenols

**Growing at home:** All types of wheat can be grown at home; some will grow even in poor soil

## What's in a Serving?

**COOKED WHEAT BERRIES**

**(1 cup/195 g)**

**Calories:** 278 (1164 kJ)

**Protein:** 8.8 g

**Total fat:** 1.4 g

**Saturated fat:** 0.2 g

**Carbohydrates:** 62.4 g

**Fiber:** 10.2 g

# Bulgur

✪ *Triticum* species

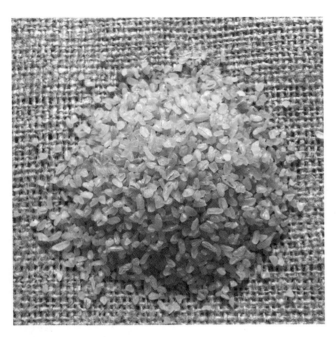

LEFT Because it has usually already been parboiled and partially cracked, bulgur can be made into a type of "instant" cereal by simply adding liquid.

Bulgur is a common ingredient in Middle Eastern dishes, most notably tabouleh, a parsley and tomato salad, and is also used as a main ingredient in pilaf, soups, stuffing, and breads. In India, bulgur, or *daliya*, as it is known there, is eaten as a cereal with milk and sugar.

Bulgur is an excellent source of fiber, protein, manganese, magnesium, and iron, and a good source of vitamin B6, folate, pantothenic acid, thiamine, niacin, zinc, copper, and phosphorus. It also contains antioxidant polyphenols.

Bulgur, or burghul, is made from several species of whole wheat, but usually durum wheat *(Triticum durum)*. The wheat is parboiled and dried, and then some of the bran (typically about 5 percent) is removed. (This is different from cracked wheat, which is crushed but not parboiled.) Bulgur can be purchased in forms of varying coarseness, typically in four grinds: #1 (fine), #2 (medium), #3 (coarse), and #4 (extra coarse).

## Making the Most of Bulgur

An easy way to incorporate more bulgur in your diet is to add it to recipes, especially those in which a binding ingredient is needed, such as meatloafs. It will boost vitamins, minerals, and fiber content. You can also make a healthy breakfast treat by cooking bulgur in skim milk and adding fresh fruits and almonds.

## THE HEALTHY EVIDENCE

Bulgur contains an exceptionally high level of fiber relative to its caloric value, and fiber can help combat a range of diseases. A 2005 study published in the *American Heart Journal* reported on the effects of cereal and whole-grain intake in postmenopausal women. It found that a higher intake was associated with reduced progression of atherosclerosis in women with existing coronary artery disease.

### What's in a Serving?

**COOKED BULGUR**
**(1 cup/182 g)**
**Calories:** 151 (632 kJ)
**Protein:** 5.6 g
**Total fat:** 0.4 g
**Saturated fat:** 0.1 g
**Carbohydrates:** 33.8 g
**Fiber:** 8.2 g

# Wheat Germ

✪ *Triticum* species

Wheat germ is the reproductive portion of the seed from wheat, the part that germinates the new plant. It is contained in the endosperm, which is encased by the bran covering. It is usually discarded in the milling process when the grain is refined, but it is a rich nutrient source in itself. As people have become aware of this, they have increasingly added it to casseroles, baked goods, cereals, yogurt, and many other foods to boost fiber, protein, and other nutrients.

One drawback of wheat germ is that it is high in unsaturated fat and therefore susceptible to becoming rancid. To prevent this, keep it in a tightly sealed container and it will remain fresh for several months.

Wheat germ is an outstanding source of vitamins B6 and E, folate, fiber, protein, thiamine, riboflavin, niacin, pantothenic acid, manganese, phosphorus, zinc, selenium, magnesium, iron, potassium, and copper. It is also a good source of vitamins C and K, and calcium, and contains antioxidants and alpha-linolenic acid.

## THE HEALTHY EVIDENCE

A 2006 study published in the journal *Arteriosclerosis, Thrombosis, and Vascular*

---

### What's in a Serving?

**ROASTED WHEAT GERM**

**(½ cup/57 g)**

**Calories:** 216 (903 kJ)

**Protein:** 16.4

**Total fat:** 6.1 g

**Saturated fat:** 1 g

**Carbohydrates:** 28 g

**Fiber:** 8.5 g

RIGHT A half-cup of wheat germ provides almost half the Daily Value of vitamin E, and is one of the best sources of this nutrient.

---

### Making the Most of Wheat Germ

An excellent use for wheat germ is as a cereal by itself, with milk and dried fruits, or in combination with other cereals. Combine ⅓ cup (40 g) of wheat germ, ⅔ cup (155 ml) of nonfat milk, 1 tablespoon of dried cranberries, and 1 tablespoon of chopped walnuts. Place in the microwave for a minute, stirring once after 30 seconds or so.

*Biology* reported on the effects of wheat-germ oil on markers of cardiovascular disease. The researchers gave wheat-germ oil to patients with elevated blood cholesterol. They found that the oil reduced oxidative stress and platelets—clotting cells that play a role in the development of atherosclerosis and heart attack. They concluded: "Wheat germ oil is an important source of n-3 fatty acids, which may exert an anti-atherosclerotic effect."

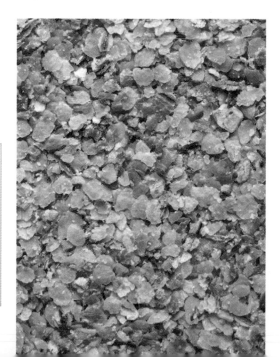

---

### In a Nutshell

**Origin:** Fertile Crescent region of the Middle East

**Season:** Available year-round

**Why it's super:** High in vitamins B6 and E, folate, fiber, protein, thiamine, riboflavin, niacin, pantothenic acid, manganese, phosphorus, zinc, selenium, magnesium, iron, potassium, and copper; good source of vitamins C and K, and calcium; contains antioxidants and alpha-linolenic acid

**Growing at home:** Not applicable

# Whole-wheat Pasta

✪ *Triticum* species

In Italy, the home of pasta, whole-wheat pasta was traditionally only to be endured during periods of hardship. However, a multitude of recent research has shown the health benefits of consuming whole grains, and whole-wheat pasta is now in demand around the world.

In Italy, food labeling laws direct that dry pasta must be made from durum sticks wheat flour or durum wheat semolina, but in other countries, pasta is made from a variety of flour types, especially wheat flour, and most whole-wheat pastas contain a mixture of whole-grain and regular-grain ingredients. In the United States, the Food and Drug Administration permits grain products containing 51 percent or more whole-grain

## What's in a Serving?

**COOKED WHOLE-WHEAT PASTA**
**(1 cup/57 g)**
**Calories:** 210 (879 kJ)
**Protein:** 7 g
**Total fat:** 1 g
**Saturated fat:** 0 g
**Carbohydrates:** 41 g
**Fiber:** 2 g

## In a Nutshell

**Origin:** Fertile Crescent region of the Middle East
**Season:** Available year-round
**Why it's super:** High in fiber, protein, thiamine, manganese, and copper; good source of vitamin B6, folate, niacin, biotin, and iron; contains antioxidants and alpha-linolenic acid
**Growing at home:** Not applicable

ingredients to make a health claim about a reduction in cancer and heart-disease risk.

Whole-wheat pasta is an excellent source of fiber, protein, thiamine, manganese, and copper, and a good source of vitamin B6, folate, niacin, biotin, and iron. It also contains antioxidants and alpha-linolenic acid.

### THE HEALTHY EVIDENCE

A 2008 study in *Nutrition, Metabolism, and Cardiovascular Disease* reported on the health benefits of whole-grain foods. The authors pooled seven large studies and found that two and a half daily servings compared to one-fifth of a daily serving was associated with a 21 percent lower risk for cardiovascular disease. They concluded, "There is a consistent, inverse association between dietary whole grains and cardiovascular disease."

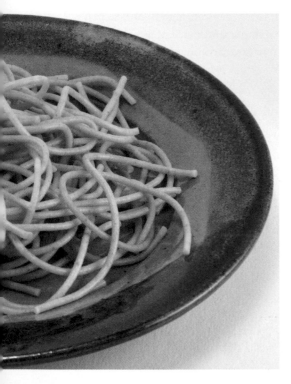

LEFT A specialty item until quite recently, whole-wheat pasta is now readily available in a wide variety of shapes.

## Making the Most of Whole-wheat Pasta

The wide variety of whole-wheat pasta shapes now available makes it easy to include this versatile product in your diet. For example, whole-wheat spaghetti can be used instead of rice to accompany a vegetable stir-fry, and whole-wheat lasagne can be layered with mashed chili beans, diced tomatoes, shredded romaine lettuce, and taco spices to make a whole-grain taco casserole.

# Whole-wheat Bread

✪ *Triticum* species

Inspired by the whole-grain health movement, manufacturers now market a vast array of whole-wheat or whole-grain breads. These offer the benefits of many different grains, while providing an excellent source of B vitamins, fiber, and antioxidants from the whole wheat. However, the labeling of such products can be confusing, as it often uses diverse terms such as "multigrain," "stone-ground," "100 percent whole wheat," "seven-grain," and "cracked wheat." In the United States, the Food and Drug Administration defines "whole grain" as a product containing grains in their entirety, whether it is whole, ground, or cracked. When selecting bread, look first for the words "whole wheat" or "whole grain," or "100 percent whole grain." "Multigrain" is acceptable as a secondary designation, but by itself does not ensure that all the grain components are included.

Whole-wheat bread is normally an excellent source of folate, fiber, protein, thiamine, niacin, manganese, phosphorus, selenium, and magnesium. In addition, it is a good source of vitamin B6, iron, zinc, and copper, and it also contains antioxidants and alpha-linolenic acid.

## What's in a Serving?

**FRESH WHOLE-WHEAT BREAD**
**(2 slices/52 g)**
**Calories:** 138 (576 kJ)
**Protein:** 7 g
**Total fat:** 2.2 g
**Saturated fat:** 0.5 g
**Carbohydrates:** 22.5 g
**Fiber:** 3.8 g

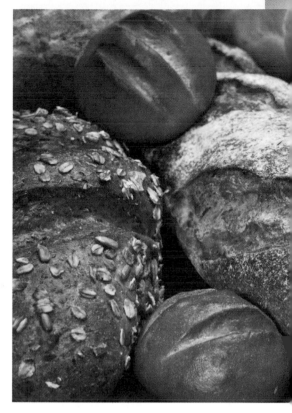

RIGHT The benefits of the fiber in whole-wheat bread were only fully appreciated in the 1960s.

## Making the Most of Whole-wheat Bread

An easy way to increase your consumption of whole-wheat breads is to use them in all bread-based recipes. For example, use whole-wheat bread for your favorite bread pudding recipe; and make sure you use whole-wheat bread in casseroles and stuffing recipes that call for bread cubes or breadcrumbs.

## In a Nutshell

**Origin:** Fertile Crescent region of the Middle East
**Season:** Available year-round
**Why It's super:** High in folate, fiber, protein, thiamine, niacin, manganese, phosphorus, selenium, and magnesium; good source of vitamin B6, iron, zinc, and copper; contains antioxidants and alpha-linolenic acid
**Growing at home:** Not applicable

### THE HEALTHY EVIDENCE

A 2006 study published in the *European Journal of Clinical Nutrition* reported on the effect of replacing a low-fiber refined bread product with high-fiber whole-grain bread. The researchers checked blood levels of glucose, insulin, HDL-cholesterol, and triglyceride in women with impaired glucose tolerance, a high risk for developing type 2 diabetes. They found that the simple substitution improved their insulin response to a subsequent glucose challenge. They concluded: "Increased intake of whole grain helps prevent against development of type 2 diabetes."

# Spelt

⭑ *Triticum spelta*

A species of wheat that was an important staple grain in much of Europe up to the fifteenth century, spelt is now popular among nutrition-conscious consumers for its numerous health benefits, and among environmentalists, as it requires low levels of fertilizers. Spelt appears to have originated in Europe and evidence of its early cultivation there has been gathered from Neolithic sites. It was not introduced to the United States until the 1890s, and never became a major crop there. Spelt is harvested in an immature state, when it is still green, and is sometimes referred to as whole green spelt.

An excellent source of fiber, protein, thiamine, niacin, manganese, magnesium, phosphorus, zinc, copper, and iron, spelt is also a good source of vitamin B6, folate, selenium, and potassium, and contains numerous antioxidant polyphenols.

## THE HEALTHY EVIDENCE

A 2008 study published in the *Journal of Agricultural and Food Chemistry* reported on the effects of wheat antioxidants in rats. Wheat antioxidants, like those found in spelt, significantly lowered an enzyme involved in cholesterol synthesis, and increased an enzyme

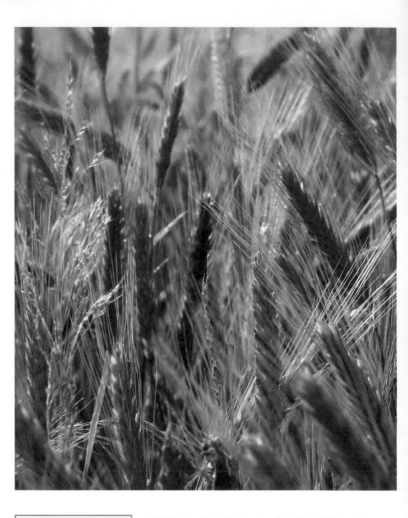

ABOVE Spelt was thought to have been first cultivated in Bronze Age Europe; new evidence suggests it was also grown then in what is now Iran.

that metabolizes cholesterol. The authors concluded that their data "indicated the potential of wheat antioxidants in reducing the risk of atherosclerosis."

### What's in a Serving?

**COOKED SPELT**

**(1 cup/194 g)**

**Calories:** 246 (1028 kJ)

**Protein:** 10.7 g

**Total fat:** 1.7 g

**Saturated fat:** 0.3 g

**Carbohydrates:** 51.3 g

**Fiber:** 7.6 g

### In a Nutshell

**Origin:** Europe

**Season:** Summer

**Why it's super:** High in fiber, protein, thiamine, niacin, manganese, magnesium, phosphorus, zinc, copper, and iron; good source of vitamin B6, folate, selenium, and potassium; contains antioxidant polyphenols

**Growing at home:** Can be grown in the home garden

### Making the Most of Spelt

For a nutritious grain side dish, try a spelt pilaf. Add 1 cup of spelt (174 g) to 3 cups (700 ml) of boiling water or vegetable stock, then cover and simmer for an hour and a half. After most of the liquid has been absorbed, add 2 tablespoons of olive oil, fresh herbs, chopped mushrooms, and diced carrots. Allow to simmer until the carrots have softened.

# Wild Rice

- *Zizania aquatica* Wild Rice
- *Zizania latifolia* Manchurian Wild Rice
- *Zizania palustris* Northern Wild Rice
- *Zizania texana* Texas Wild Rice

Wild rice has been eaten since prehistoric times and was a staple grain of many Native American peoples; it was early British explorers in North America who gave it the name of wild or Indian rice. There are four different species of wild rice, all belonging to the genus *Zizania*. Three, *Z. palustris, Z. aquatica,* and *Z. texana*, are native to North America, and one, *Z. latifolia*, is native to Asia. Texas wild rice is in danger of extinction as a result of habitat reduction and pollution. The same has occurred with Manchurian wild rice in China. It was accidentally introduced to New Zealand, where it is now considered an invasive species.

Wild rice can be purchased at specialty shops or online, although the price can be up to ten times that of white rice. It is used mostly in grain side dishes, but it can also be added to soups and salads.

Wild rice is an outstanding source of vitamin B6, folate, fiber, protein, niacin, manganese, magnesium, phosphorus, zinc, and copper, and a good source of potassium and iron. It contains both insoluble and soluble fibers, such as beta-glucans, and plant sterols.

## Making the Most of Wild Rice

Wild rice is widely used in grain side dishes, but it can be a nutrient-rich ingredient in a variety of salads. Add 1 cup (164 g) of cooked wild rice to a three-bean salad for a complete protein combination, as well as extra soluble fiber and plant sterols. Wild rice also adds protein and fiber to a salad of fresh greens.

## THE HEALTHY EVIDENCE

A 2009 review published in *Current Opinion in Clinical Nutrition and Metabolic Care* discussed phytochemicals, like those found in wild rice, and their importance in human health. The authors cited studies showing that plant sterols "appear to play an important role in the regulation of serum cholesterol and to exhibit anticancer properties."

One such study published in 2009 in the *Journal of Nutrition* reported on the effects of plant sterols in adults with both normal blood cholesterol levels and adults with elevated levels of cholesterol. The results demonstrated that a daily dose of 3 grams of plant sterols lowered LDL cholesterol in both groups.

### What's in a Serving?
**COOKED WILD RICE
(1 cup/164 g)**
**Calories:** 166 (694 kJ)
**Protein:** 6.5 g
**Total fat:** 0.6 g
**Saturated fat:** 0.1 g
**Carbohydrates:** 35 g
**Fiber:** 3 g

BELOW Joseph Bowron suggested using wild rice as a field crop in 1852, but it was seldom grown in the United States until the 1960s.

### In a Nutshell

**Origin:** North America and Asia

**Season:** Late summer and early autumn

**Why it's super:** High in vitamin B6, folate, fiber, protein, niacin, manganese, magnesium, phosphorus, zinc, and copper; good source of potassium and iron; contains soluble fibers, beta-glucan, and plant sterols

**Growing at home:** Difficult: requires a steady supply of moving water and temperatures above 70°F (21°C) for at least 40 days

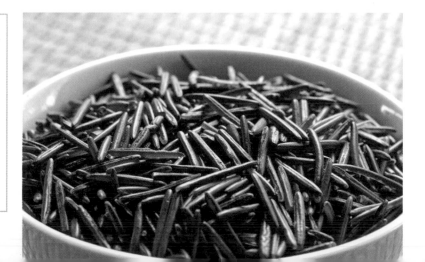

# Corn or Maize

✪ *Zea mays*

## What's in a Serving?

**BOILED CORN**
**(1 cup/149 g)**
**Calories:** 143 (299 kJ)
**Protein:** 5 g
**Total fat:** 2.2 g
**Saturated fat:** 0.3 g
**Carbohydrates:** 31.2 g
**Fiber:** 3.6 g

Corn, as it is known in the United States, Australia, New Zealand, and Canada, or maize, as it is known to the British, is a cereal crop that thrives in a wide variety of conditions and is consequently grown in many parts of the world. It was discovered by European explorers being cultivated by the Mayans and Aztecs, and was taken to Europe in the late fifteenth and early sixteenth centuries and then disseminated further through trade.

## Making the Most of Corn

Corn makes a high-nutrient and antioxidant addition to many foods. For example, adding corn to soups, stews, and chili is an excellent way to get more corn in the diet. Another way to benefit from corn's antioxidants and nutrients is to add this colorful vegetable to fresh salads. Corn also adds fiber to hamburger patties and meatloaf.

### ON AND OFF THE COB

The cultivar of *Zea mays* that is most widely consumed by humans is the yellow or white form, usually known as "sweet corn," or "corn on the cob." Another type of corn, *Zea mays averta*, which is not edible on the cob, is used to make the popular snack known as popcorn. When the corn is exposed to a dry heat, the inside breaks through the outer hull, creating a white, fluffy, crunchy kernel.

Coarse-ground corn kernels, known as grits, are a popular breakfast food, especially in the southern United States. Medium-ground corn, or cornmeal, is used in polenta, corn bread, and other baked goods. Fine-ground corn is used as flour for baking. Corn is also wet-milled and soaked in an alkali solution to make masa dough, which is used for tortillas and fried corn chips, and steamed in corn husks to make tamales.

Corn is an outstanding source of vitamin C, folate, fiber, protein, pantothenic acid, thiamine, niacin, magnesium, phosphorus, potassium, and manganese. It is also a good source of vitamins A and B6, riboflavin, and zinc, and contains the antioxidant carotenoids lutein, zeaxanthin, and beta-cryptoxanthin, as well as phenols.

BELOW Corn, or maize, is related to millet and sorghum, and all are varieties of grasses.

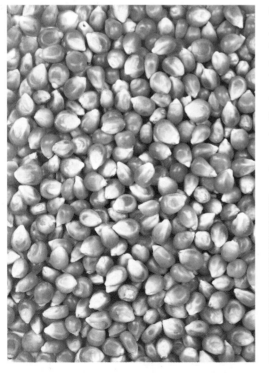

## In a Nutshell

**Origin:** Central and South America
**Season:** Autumn
**Why it's super:** High in vitamin C, folate, fiber, protein, pantothenic acid, thiamine, niacin, magnesium, phosphorus, potassium, and manganese; good source of vitamins A and B6, riboflavin, and zinc; contains the antioxidant carotenoids lutein, zeaxanthin, beta-cryptoxanthin, and phenols
**Growing at home:** Can easily be grown in the home garden

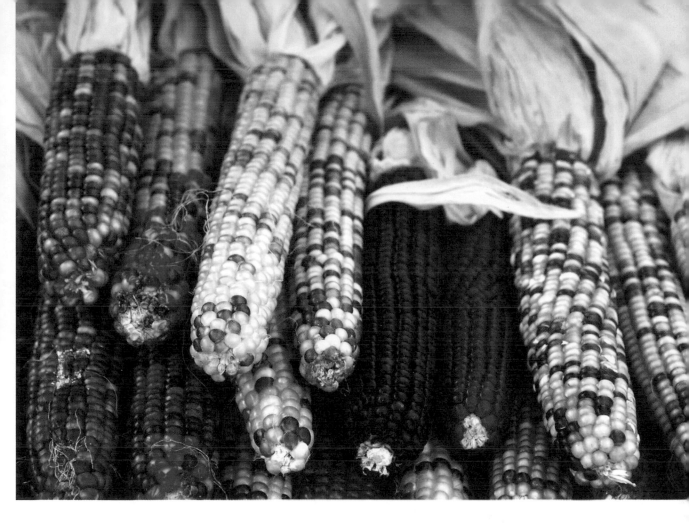

## THE HEALTHY EVIDENCE

A 2009 study published in the *Journal of Hypertension* reported on the effects of carotenoids on blood pressure—high blood pressure is a major contributing factor to heart attacks and strokes. The authors noted that several population studies have shown that higher blood levels of carotenoids are associated with a lower risk for cardiovascular disease, and they hypothesized and confirmed a similar effect for high blood pressure.

A 2009 study published in the *American Journal of Clinical Nutrition* reported on the relationship between dietary intake of carotenoids and breast cancer risk in postmenopausal women. The researchers reported that their results add "to the evidence of an inverse association of specific carotenoids with breast cancer."

*Plough deep,*
*while Sluggards sleep;*
*And you shall have Corn,*
*to sell and to keep.*

Benjamin Franklin, US statesman (1706–90)

ABOVE Some types of corn produce kernels in a range of colors. This has made their cobs a popular form of autumn decoration.

### Missing in the Maize

When maize was first cultivated outside of the Americas, it was enthusiastically received because of its productivity. But it was soon discovered that those who consumed it as a staple food developed a potentially deadly vitamin deficiency called pellagra, caused by a lack of niacin or vitamin B3. Native Americans did not seem to be affected in the same way, however. Eventually, it was discovered that they had learned that soaking the maize in lime, an alkali, caused the corn to release its niacin. As soon as others followed suit, pellagra ceased to be a problem.

# Meat, Seafood, and Dairy Foods

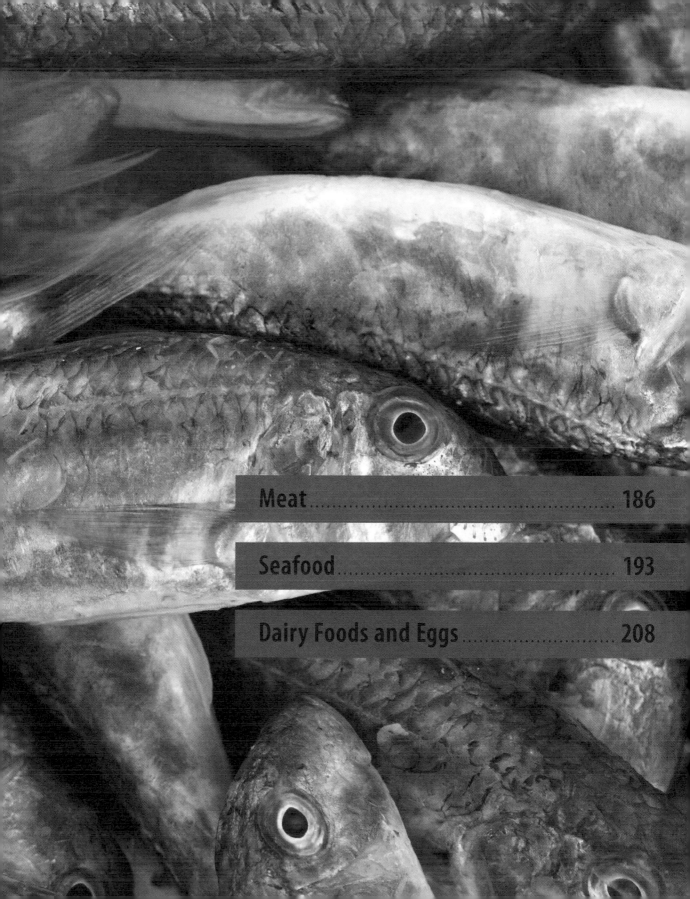

## MEAT

# Lean Red Meats

In Western societies at least, the most widely consumed lean red meats are beef and lamb. Sheep were first domesticated between 9,000 and 11,000 years ago, and were one of the earliest staple foods that provided a protein source for humans after the transition from hunting and gathering to agrarian societies. The exact ancestry of the domestic sheep is not known for certain, although it is likely to be descended from the wild mouflon of Asia and Europe. Lamb is meat that comes from a sheep that is less than one year old; the meat from an older animal is called mutton.

First domesticated 8,000 years ago, cattle are descended from the auroch, which was a much larger and fiercer beast than the modern cow. The last-known aurochs died in Poland in the early seventeenth century. Most commercially available beef comes from heifers, cows that have not yet produced young, or steers, bulls that have been castrated. The meat from steers is somewhat leaner than heifer meat.

A lean cut of beef or lamb is an outstanding source of vitamins B6 and B12, protein, niacin, selenium, zinc, and phosphorus, and a good source of pantothenic acid, thiamine, riboflavin, potassium, iron, and magnesium.

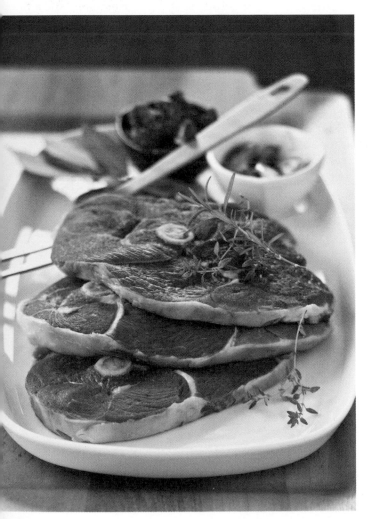

LEFT Lamb is usually brought to market between six and eight months old, and "spring lamb" refers to lamb that was slaughtered in spring or summer.

---

### What's in a Serving?

**BROILED LEAN RED MEAT**

**(3 ounces/85 g)**

**Calories:** 152 (638 kJ)

**Protein:** 23.9 g

**Total fat:** 5.6 g

**Saturated fat:** 2.1 g

**Carbohydrates:** 0 g

**Fiber:** 0 g

---

### In a Nutshell

**Origin:** Europe and Asia

**Season:** Available year-round

**Why they're super:** High in vitamins B6 and B12, protein, niacin, selenium, zinc, phosphorus; good source of pantothenic acid, thiamine, riboflavin, potassium, iron, and magnesium

**Growing at home:** Not applicable

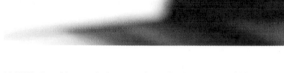

## Making the Most of Lean Red Meat

Broiling, roasting, and grilling are excellent ways to cook expensive lean-meat cuts, such as beef tenderloin. However, lean cuts that are tougher work best with long cooking times and moist heat, as with stewing or using an electric cooking pot. For a nutrient-rich meal, use an electric pot to cook lean stewing beef, carrots, green peas, and herbs, such as thyme and rosemary. Serve with a high-fiber grain, such as brown or wild rice.

ABOVE The United States is the largest producer of beef, yielding one-fifth of world production, followed by Brazil and the European Union.

## THE HEALTHY EVIDENCE

A 2009 study published in the *Journal of the American Dietetic Association* reported on the effect of lean red meat intake on body muscle. Researchers at the Graduate Center for Gerontology at the University of Kentucky, Lexington, conducted a study to determine if high-quality protein from lean beef could be effective in protecting the elderly from sarcopenia. This is the loss of muscle mass, strength, and function that occurs in ageing. The process generally begins after the age of 40 and accelerates after 75. While it is more common in people who are physically inactive, it also occurs in those who maintain physical activity into their senior years. This means that other factors are important in its development, and one of these is a reduction in protein synthesis. Previous studies have shown that older adults have lower rates of muscle protein synthesis than younger adults, which results in loss of body mass.

The researchers tested the effects of varying amounts of lean beef on muscle protein synthesis, in both elderly subjects and young adults. In both groups, a daily 4-ounce (113-g) serving of lean beef increased muscle protein synthesis by about 50 percent. The researchers noted that, "There is little debate that the ingestion of high-quality protein is of paramount importance in the maintenance of muscle mass and function in elderly people."

*Beef is the soul of cooking.*

Marie-Antoine Carême, French chef (1784–1833)

## Choice Cuts

The cuts of beef that are considered extra lean are eye of round roast, top round steak, mock tender steak, bottom round roast, and top sirloin steak. Lean cuts include round steak, chuck shoulder roast, arm pot roast, shoulder steak, strip steak, tenderloin steak, and T-bone steak. Lean lamb cuts are sirloin and shank cuts from the leg, loin chops, arm chops, and foreshanks. An easy way to add high-quality protein to your diet is to purchase extra-lean ground beef, which has only ½ ounce (4 g) of fat in a 3-ounce (85-g) serving.

# Game

The word "game" originally referred to any mammal killed during a hunt and included deer, hares, wild pigs, and many other species. These days, it most often refers to venison (from the Latin *venari*, meaning "to hunt"), the meat of deer, though in Australia it would also include kangaroo meat. Both deer and kangaroos browse on grasslands used for cattle, sheep, and cultivation, and are therefore hunted to keep their numbers down and protect farmland, as well as for their meat and, in some communities, for sport.

Lean cuts of venison and kangaroo are outstanding sources of vitamins B6 and B12, protein, niacin, thiamine, riboflavin, selenium, zinc, potassium, copper, phosphorus, and iron. They are also good sources of pantothenic acid and magnesium.

## THE HEALTHY EVIDENCE

In a 2010 study published in the *British Journal of Nutrition*, researchers at the University of Sydney, Australia, assessed blood levels of inflammatory markers—associated with chronic diseases including cardiovascular disease—in subjects consuming either kangaroo meat or a hybrid form of beef, wagyu, also known as Kobe. They found that wagyu significantly increased

inflammatory markers compared to kangaroo meat. A 2010 study published in the *Journal of Microbiology and Biotechnology* reported on the discovery of a compound in venison protein, antioxidative peptide (APVPH I). The researchers found that APVPH I inhibited the production of oxidized compounds, which are believed to be involved in the development of chronic diseases such as cancer and cardiovascular disease.

---

### What's in a Serving?

**BROILED VENISON TOP ROUND**
**(3 ounces/85 g)**
Calories: 129 (540 kJ)
Protein: 26.8 g
Total fat: 1.6 g
Saturated fat: 0.9 g
Carbohydrates: 0 g
Fiber: 0 g

**BROILED KANGAROO LOIN FILLET**
**(3 ounces/85 g)**
Calories: 115 (481 kJ)
Protein: 26.1 g
Total fat: 1.2 g
Saturated fat: 0.3 g
Carbohydrates: 0 g
Fiber: 0 g

---

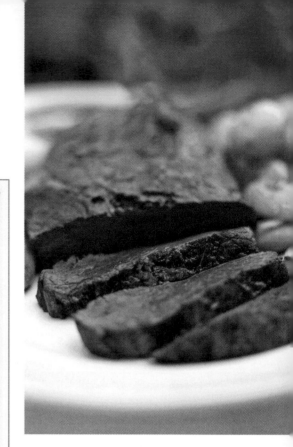

ABOVE Venison farming is an important industry in parts of Europe and in New Zealand, but the meat is not so widely available in the United States.

---

### In a Nutshell

**Origin:** Venison: Europe, Asia, North America; kangaroo: Australia
**Season:** Available year-round
**Why it's super:** High in vitamins B6 and B12, protein, niacin, thiamine, riboflavin, selenium, zinc, potassium, copper, phosphorus, and iron; good sources of pantothenic acid and magnesium
**Growing at home:** Not applicable

---

### Making the Most of Game

Tender cuts of venison, such as the back strap, are excellent if broiled or grilled. Tougher cuts, such as shoulder cuts, work best with slower, moister cooking methods such as stewing. One way to tenderize tougher cuts is to include an acidic ingredient, such as tomato, which helps break down the muscle fibers.

# Liver

## What's in a Serving?

**BRAISED LIVER
(3 ounces/85 g)**

**Calories:** 162 (681 kJ)

**Protein:** 24.7 g

**Total fat:** 4.5 g

**Saturated fat:** 1.4 g

**Carbohydrates:** 4.4 g

**Fiber:** 0 g

Liver has long been a part of the human diet and nearly every cuisine has a special liver recipe, and it's no wonder since, ounce for ounce, liver may contain more nutrients than any other food. Liver from most domestic animals is widely consumed. Chicken and other poultry liver is baked, made into sausage, used in gravy, and puréed and seasoned to make pâté. Calf liver is often more popular than beef liver, because it's more tender. Fried lamb's liver, or lamb's fry, is a popular dish in Australia.

The high level of vitamin A in liver makes it a potentially lethal food—a number of early polar explorers became sick or died after eating polar bear and dog liver. However, to consume a toxic dose, you would have to eat ⅔ pound (286 g) a day for several months.

Liver is an exceptional source of vitamins A and B12, folate, pantothenic acid, protein, niacin, thiamine, riboflavin, copper, selenium, iron, phosphorus, manganese, and zinc, and a good source of potassium.

### Making the Most of Liver

Since chicken liver is lower in vitamin A than beef liver, you can consume it more frequently. Liver pâté is thought to be susceptible to contamination with the *Listeria monocytogenes* bacteria. To prevent this, make sure you store the pâté at below 39°F (4°C).

### THE HEALTHY EVIDENCE

Liver has been shown to be an outstanding source of nutrients, indeed one of the most nutritious of all foods. But at one point, it was believed that its high content of vitamin A could cause birth defects. This was disproved by a study published in the journal *Teratology*, which found no congenital malformations among infants exposed daily to 50,000 IU (International Units) of vitamin A. Another study, published in the *International Journal of Vitamin and Nutrition Research*, found that a daily dose of 30,000 IU resulted in blood levels that had no link with birth defects.

RIGHT When it comes to choosing liver, favor calf or lamb's liver, as it is less likely that toxins will have accumulated in young animals.

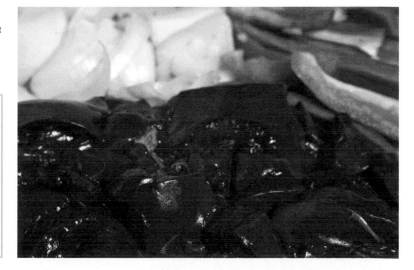

### In a Nutshell

**Origin:** Worldwide

**Season:** Available year-round

**Why it's super:** High in vitamins A and B12, folate, pantothenic acid, protein, niacin, thiamine, riboflavin, copper, selenium, iron, phosphorus, manganese, zinc; good source of potassium

**Growing at home:** Not applicable

# Lean White Meats

Lean white meats are widely available and highly nutritious. Pork accounts for about 38 percent of meat production worldwide. The leanest cuts are the tenderloin, loin chops, or leg. Veal, the meat of a calf, is considered white meat (as is the meat of all young animals), even though cattle normally yield red meat. The best veal cuts are round cuts, such as top round veal.

Pork is an excellent source of vitamins B6 and B12, protein, thiamine, niacin, riboflavin, selenium, phosphorus, potassium, and zinc, and a good source of pantothenic acid, iron, and magnesium. Veal is high in vitamins B6 and B12, protein,

## Making the Most of Pork and Veal

From the nutritional and gastronomic points of view, pork and veal roasts work well with rosemary and garlic, which both contain significant levels of antioxidants. Carefully make small cuts into the raw roast and insert as many garlic cloves as desired. Rub the meat with olive oil, and then either sprinkle it with ground rosemary or insert snips of fresh rosemary into small cuts.

## What's in a Serving?

| | ROASTED PORK LOIN (3 ounces/85 g) | ROASTED VEAL TOP ROUND (3 ounces/85 g) |
|---|---|---|
| Calories: | 147 (615 kJ) | 128 (534 kJ) |
| Protein: | 23.2 g | 23.9 g |
| Total fat: | 5.3 g | 2.9 g |
| Saturated fat: | 1.6 g | 1 g |
| Carbohydrates: | 0 g | 0 g |
| Fiber: | 0 g | 0 g |

BELOW Most veal comes from animals aged up to 18 weeks, but about 15 percent is from calves up to 3 weeks old, which are called bob calves.

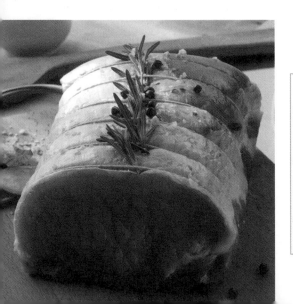

niacin, riboflavin, zinc, phosphorus, selenium, and potassium, and a good source of pantothenic acid, magnesium, and copper.

### THE HEALTHY EVIDENCE

Pork is a nutrient-rich food containing high-quality protein. Its only drawback is a tendency for the meat to become infected with a type of roundworm, *Trichinella spiralis*, which can cause an illness called trichinosis. Research cited by the USDA has shown, however, that the risk can be avoided if the meat is cooked in a conventional oven rather than a microwave (which distributes heat unevenly); the meat is cooked to a minimum internal temperature of 160°F (70°C); and you increase cooking time to allow for variation in internal temperature and thermometer errors.

## In a Nutshell

**Origin:** Asia and Europe

**Season:** Available year-round

**Why they're super:** Pork: high in vitamins B6 and B12, protein, thiamine, niacin, riboflavin, selenium, phosphorus, potassium, and zinc, and a good source of pantothenic acid, iron, and magnesium. Veal: high in vitamins B6 and B12, protein, niacin, riboflavin, zinc, phosphorus, selenium, and potassium; good source of pantothenic acid, magnesium, and copper.

**Growing at home:** Not applicable

# Skinless Chicken

The fact that there are more domestic chickens in the world than any other kind of bird is an indication of the popularity of chicken as a food source. The domestic chicken is descended from the red junglefowl, *Gallus gallus,* and is still classified as part of the same species. Recent research suggests *Gallus gallus* was first domesticated in Vietnam about 10,000 years ago; the practice then spread through India, western Asia, and Asia Minor, reaching Greece in the fifth century BCE. Since then, chicken meat has featured prominently in the cuisines of most cultures, no doubt because it is one of the least expensive sources of high-quality protein available.

The skin of the chicken contains most of the fat, so removing it will reduce calories while leaving the high protein and other nutrients in the flesh. Skinless breast is an excellent source of vitamin B6, protein, niacin, selenium, and phosphorus, and a good source of vitamin B12, pantothenic acid, riboflavin, iron, potassium, zinc, and magnesium. Dark meat is similar but has higher levels of all the minerals.

> **In a Nutshell**
>
> **Origin:** Asia and Europe
> **Season:** Available year-round
> **Why it's super:** High in vitamin B6, protein, niacin, selenium, and phosphorus; good source of vitamin B12, pantothenic acid, riboflavin, iron, potassium, zinc, and magnesium; dark meat contains higher levels of minerals
> **Growing at home:** Not applicable

RIGHT Chicken was much favored by the ancient Egyptians, who developed incubators to hatch large numbers of eggs at a time.

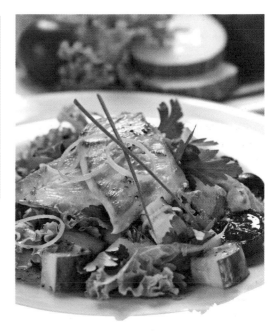

> **Making the Most of Skinless Chicken**
>
> Eating different kinds of chicken meat will provide the widest range of the abundant proteins and nutrients. Chicken breast is highest in protein and lowest in fat; however, dark meat from the thigh or leg is higher in vitamins and essential minerals.

### What's in a Serving?

| ROASTED CHICKEN BREAST (3 ounces/85 g) | ROASTED DARK MEAT (3 ounces/85 g) |
|---|---|
| **Calories:** 142 (593 kJ) | **Calories:** 178 (743 kJ) |
| **Protein:** 26.7 g | **Protein:** 22 g |
| **Total fat:** 3 g | **Total fat:** 9.3 g |
| **Saturated fat:** 0.9 g | **Saturated fat:** 2.6 g |
| **Carbohydrates:** 0 g | **Carbohydrates:** 0 g |
| **Fiber:** 0 g | **Fiber:** 0 g |

## THE HEALTHY EVIDENCE

Dietary protein has been shown to be especially important for the health of particular groups of people, including growing children, adolescents, pregnant women, and the elderly. Chicken not only contains high levels of protein, but is also widely available and relatively inexpensive. It also contains the correct balance of all the essential amino acids, along with plentiful vitamins and minerals, and low calories.

# Skinless Turkey

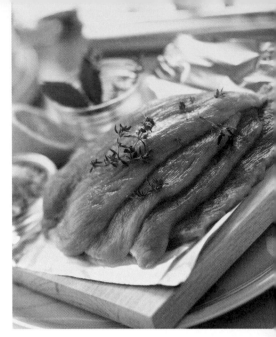

Native to North America, the turkey was imported to Europe by the first explorers to reach the New World. The bird was domesticated in the early 1500s and became extremely popular in England, Italy, and France. By the time the Pilgrims migrated from England to America, they knew all about raising turkeys and enjoying their meat. In 1621, the first Thanksgiving dinner took place in what would become the United States of America; in 1863, President Abraham Lincoln proclaimed the festival a national holiday, by which time turkey was the staple dish of the occasion. Despite its popularity as a food, the turkey was rejected as the national bird of the United States by the Founding Fathers, despite numbering among its supporters Benjamin Franklin, who disapproved of the final choice, the bald eagle, due to its "bad moral character."

Like chicken, turkey is best consumed without the skin, which contains high levels of fat. Skinless white turkey meat is an excellent source of vitamin B6, protein, niacin, phosphorus, selenium, and zinc, as well as a good source of vitamin B12, pantothenic acid, riboflavin, iron, potassium, and magnesium.

RIGHT Consumption of turkey meat has doubled over the past 25 years, partly due to the much wider range of turkey products on offer.

## What's in a Serving?

**ROAST TURKEY BREAST**
**(3 ounces/85 g)**
**Calories:** 114 (481 kJ)
**Protein:** 25.5 g
**Total fat:** 2.9 g
**Saturated fat:** 0.8 g
**Carbohydrates:** 0 g
**Fiber:** 0 g

**ROAST DARK MEAT**
**(3 ounces/85 g)**
**Calories:** 138 (576 kJ)
**Protein:** 24.5 g
**Total fat:** 3.7 g
**Saturated fat:** 1.2 g
**Carbohydrates:** 0 g
**Fiber:** 0 g

The dark meat contains a similar range of nutrients, but has higher levels of all the minerals and a significant level of copper.

### THE HEALTHY EVIDENCE

A 2007 study published in the journal *Cancer Causes and Control* reported on the association between the intake of specific foods and pancreatic cancer. Researchers at the University of California San Francisco looked at the intake of various animal-protein foods, including eggs, dairy products, processed meats, specific meats, and poultry among people with and without pancreatic cancer. Consumption of turkey, as well as chicken, was associated with a lower risk of developing the cancer.

## In a Nutshell

**Origin:** North America

**Season:** Available year-round

**Why it's super:** High in vitamin B6, protein, niacin, phosphorus, selenium, and zinc; good source of vitamin B12, pantothenic acid, riboflavin, iron, potassium, and magnesium; dark meat higher in minerals and has significant level of copper

**Growing at home:** Not applicable

## Making the Most of Skinless Turkey

Consuming both light and dark turkey meat will provide the most diverse levels of nutrients. To make a nutrient-rich soup, combine leftover dark turkey meat with vegetables that are high in antioxidants, such as carrots, tomatoes, and peas, and add a high-fiber grain, such as barley. Use the light meat to add protein to fresh salads, such as romaine lettuce and tomatoes.

SEAFOOD

# Squid and Octopus

Squid and octopus are close relatives in the marine cephalopod family. Both release a dark inklike substance when threatened, and squid eaten as food is sometimes called calamari, an Italian word that derives from the Latin word *calamarium* for "ink pot."

Both creatures are an important food source in a number of cultures around the world. The body of both is the best source of the meat, which is white and firm, though the tentacles are also sliced into rings. The meat is prepared in a variety of ways, including frying and boiling, though small squid and octopus are also eaten raw and even alive in some Asian cultures.

Squid is an excellent source of vitamins B6 and B12, protein, pantothenic acid, niacin, riboflavin, selenium, and zinc, and a good source of vitamin E. Octopus has a similar nutritional profile but is also an excellent source of iron. Both contain omega-3 fatty acids, with squid supplying three times as much as octopus; however, in comparison, a high-fat finfish, such as salmon, contains more than four times as much as squid. Phosphatidylcholine, a beneficial phospholipids compound is also found in squid and octopus.

## THE HEALTHY EVIDENCE

A 2008 study published in the journal *Nutrition Research* reported on the effects of various marine extracts on colon cancer in rats, and a phospholipid compound, phosphatidylcholine (PC), contained in squid, was compared to other marine sources of the compound. The researchers found that squid PC slowed the growth of colon cancer and increased the rate of cancer cell apoptosis, or suicide.

## Making the Most of Squid and Octopus

The body meat of squid or octopus can be used whole, cut into flat pieces, or sliced crosswise into rings. The healthiest method of cooking is to boil the meat for one minute or less, and then place it on ice. To make a seafood salad, add fresh lemon juice, olive oil, seasonings, fresh chopped parsley, onion, tomato, and black olives.

## What's in a Serving?

**RAW SQUID**
**(3 ounces/85 g)**
**Calories:** 78 (327 kJ)
**Protein:** 13.2 g
**Total fat:** 1.2 g
**Saturated fat:** 0.3 g
**Carbohydrates:** 2.6 g
**Fiber:** 0 g

**RAW OCTOPUS**
**(3 ounces/85 g)**
**Calories:** 70 (292 kJ)
**Protein:** 12.7 g
**Total fat:** 0.9 g
**Saturated fat:** 0.2 g
**Carbohydrates:** 1.9 g
**Fiber:** 0 g

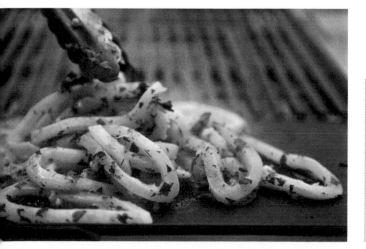

LEFT The meat of squid is firm, mild, and slightly sweet. It is suitable for eating raw or pickled, or after rapid frying or grilling.

## In a Nutshell

**Origin:** Oceans around the world
**Season:** Available year-round
**Why they're super:** High in vitamins B6 and B12, protein, pantothenic acid, niacin, riboflavin, selenium, and zinc (octopus is also high in iron); good source of vitamin E; contain omega-3 fatty acids and phosphatidylcholine
**Growing at home:** Not applicable

# Shellfish

The term "shellfish" can be used to refer generally to all water-dwelling invertebrates with a hard shell, but more specifically it denotes water-dwellers belonging to the group of invertebrates known as mollusks, or molluscs, all of which have a hinged, two-part shell. The most notable from a nutritional point of view are abalone, clams, mussels, oysters, scallops, and pipis.

A kind of sea snail with a broad flat shell, abalone is considered a delicacy in many cultures, notably China and Japan, and the shell, which is lined with mother of pearl, is used in jewelry. The word "clam" is used to refer to a wide range of mollusks (including mussels), but in a culinary context usually refers to the hard clam *Mercenaria mercenaria*, or, in Italy, the vongola *(Venerupis decussata)*. Popular uses include soups, or chowders, and pasta sauces. Likewise, "mussels" might refer to mollusks of a variety of families, but usually denotes those of the Mytilidae family, which have dark oval shells and are consumed around the world, on their own or in sauces or soups. Oysters are harvested from the seabed but also cultivated; they are often eaten raw. Consisting of a colorful fan-shaped shell containing two types of meat—the thick white muscle and the red roe—scallops are sought after by gourmets and shell-collectors alike. Another type of small mollusk, the pipi, is popular in Australia and New Zealand.

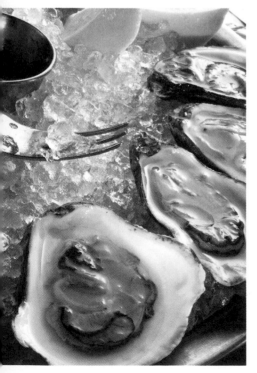

BELOW The oyster is not the only shellfish that can produce a pearl, but it does it far more often than others such as mussels and clams.

| What's in a Serving? | |
|---|---|
| **RAW ABALONE** | **RAW CLAMS** |
| **(3 ounces/85 g)** | **(3 ounces/85 g)** |
| **Calories:** 89 (373 kJ) | **Calories:** 63 (264 kJ) |
| **Protein:** 14.5 g | **Protein:** 10.9 g |
| **Total fat:** 0.7 g | **Total fat:** 0.8 g |
| **Saturated fat:** 0.1 g | **Saturated fat:** 0.1 g |
| **Carbohydrates:** 5.1 g | **Carbohydrates:** 2.2 g |
| **Fiber:** 0 g | **Fiber:** 0 g |

## EAT WITH CAUTION

Shellfish commonly induce food allergies, often severe ones resulting in anaphylactic shock, which can be fatal. Despite this, their nutrient-rich profile and flavor make them highly prized. Shellfish are excellent sources of protein and are low in calories and fat; they contain varying amounts of vitamins, minerals, and omega-3 fatty acids (generally, the higher the level of fat, the higher the level of omega-3 fatty acids).

## Making the Most of Shellfish

All of the key nutrients in shellfish will be retained regardless of the cooking method. Some shellfish can be eaten raw. Frying is best avoided because it will generally add calories; however, if you use olive or canola oil for frying or sautéeing, you can still make those recipes a reasonable choice, health-wise.

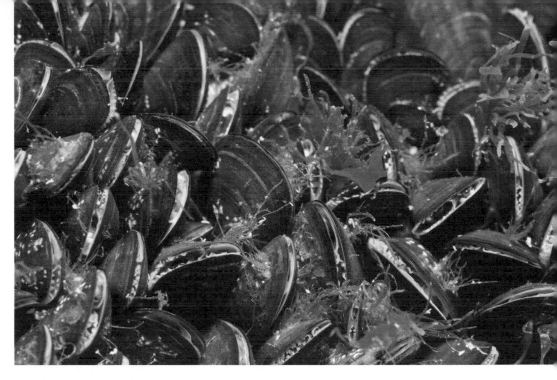

Abalone is high in vitamins B12, E, and K, pantothenic acid, thiamine, selenium, phosphorus, iron, and magnesium, and is a good source of vitamin B6, riboflavin, niacin, copper, potassium, and zinc. Clams are high in vitamins B12 and C, riboflavin, iron, selenium, manganese, phosphorus, and copper, and a good source of thiamine, niacin, potassium, and zinc. Mussels are an excellent source of vitamins B12 and C, riboflavin, manganese, selenium, iron, and phosphorus, and a good source of folate, thiamine, niacin, zinc, potassium, and magnesium. Oysters are high in vitamin B12, zinc, selenium, iron, manganese, and copper, and a good source of vitamin C, thiamine, niacin, magnesium, and phosphorus. Scallops are an excellent source of vitamin B12, selenium, phosphorus, and magnesium, and a good source of vitamin B6, niacin, potassium, and zinc.

*He was a bold man that first ate an oyster.*
Jonathan Swift, Anglo-Irish writer (1667–1745)

ABOVE Native to Ireland, the blue mussel has been an important food source for 20,000 years and has been cultivated for 800 years.

### In a Nutshell

**Origin:** Oceans around the world
**Season:** Available year-round
**Why they're super:** Excellent sources of protein, low in calories and fat, good-to-excellent sources of many vitamins and minerals
**Growing at home:** Not applicable

## THE HEALTHY EVIDENCE
In a 2009 review published in the *Asia Pacific Journal of Clinical Nutrition*, the authors cited numerous studies pointing to the anticlotting action and blood-pressure-lowering and anti-inflammatory effects of shellfish, all of which may help reduce the risk of cardio-vascular disease. In addition, the omega-3 fatty acids may promote improvements in visual function, attention-deficit conditions, depression, schizophrenia, and dementia.

### What's in a Serving?

| RAW MUSSELS (3 ounces/85 g) | RAW OYSTERS (3 ounces/85 g) | RAW SCALLOPS (3 ounces/85 g) |
|---|---|---|
| **Calories:** 73 (306 kJ) | **Calories:** 50 (210 kJ) | **Calories:** 75 (313 kJ) |
| **Protein:** 10.1 g | **Protein:** 4.4 g | **Protein:** 14.3 g |
| **Total fat:** 1.9 g | **Total fat:** 1.3 g | **Total fat:** 0.7 g |
| **Saturated fat:** 0.4 g | **Saturated fat:** 0.4 g | **Saturated fat:** 0.1 g |
| **Carbohydrates:** 3.1 g | **Carbohydrates:** 4.7 g | **Carbohydrates:** 2 g |
| **Fiber:** 0 g | **Fiber:** 0 g | **Fiber:** 0 g |

# Crustaceans

*A truly destitute man is not one
without riches, but the poor wretch who
has never partaken of lobster.*

Anonymous

Crustaceans are mainly aquatic creatures belonging to the large class of invertebrate creatures known as arthropods, which generally have a hard, segmented outer body and jointed appendages. Crustaceans have jointed legs, mandibles, and an exoskeleton all made of chitin, which they shed or molt to allow for growth. Chitin is a type of carbohydrate, which has industrial uses; research has shown that it may have several medical uses, as well.

## CLAWED CREATURES

The crustacean group includes crabs, lobster, prawns, shrimps, and crayfish. Crabs are among the most widely eaten crustaceans; some are eaten whole but more usually it is just the meat of the claws and, sometimes, legs that is consumed.

Sizable crustaceans with large claws, lobsters are considered a delicacy around the world and underpin lucrative fishing industries; they are usually boiled (often alive) and served either plain or in soups or rich dishes such as lobster thermidor. Prawns and shrimp are similar in appearance and the terms are often used interchangeably: however, prawns usually are larger and

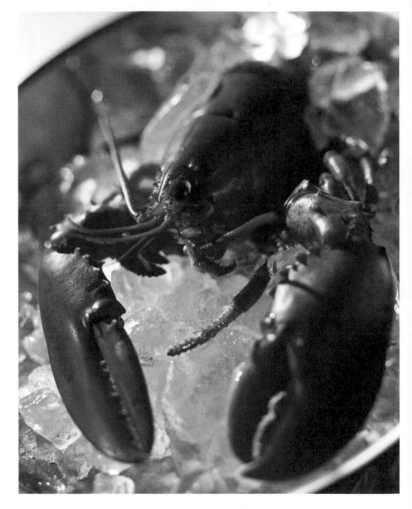

ABOVE In North America, lobster was considered a food of the poor until the mid-1800s, when improved transportation began to deliver fresh lobster to city areas and the food became fashionable.

have claws on three sets of legs, shrimps on just two. Both are cooked in a variety of ways—boiled, steamed, grilled, sautéed, or baked, with or without the shell—and served up in dishes ranging from salads to pasta sauces. Freshwater crustaceans that are related to and look like lobsters, crayfish are a popular food in China, Scandinavia, and the United States. In Australia, native freshwater crayfish are known as yabbies.

## Making the Most of Crustaceans

It is best to avoid frying crustaceans, as this will increase fat levels. Soups and stews are excellent methods of preparation, as the nutrients will be retained and consumed. Crustaceans make a good addition to fresh salads; boil them briskly (three minutes or so) and include colorful and antioxidant-containing vegetables to boost the nutrients further.

## What's in a Serving?

| RAW CRAB (3 ounces/85 g) | RAW CRAYFISH (3 ounces/85 g) | RAW LOBSTER (3 ounces/85 g) | RAW PRAWN (3 ounces/85 g) | RAW SHRIMP (3 ounces/85 g) |
|---|---|---|---|---|
| Calories: 74 (309 kJ) | Calories: 65 (271 kJ) | Calories: 76 (320 kJ) | Calories: 75 (315 kJ) | Calories: 90 (377 kJ) |
| Protein: 15.4 g | Protein: 14 g | Protein: 15.9 g | Protein: 17.4 g | Protein: 17.3 g |
| Total fat: 0.9 g | Total fat: 1 g | Total fat: 0.8 g | Total fat: 0.5 g | Total fat: 1.5 g |
| Saturated fat: 0.2 g | Saturated fat: 0 g | Saturated fat: 0.2 g | Saturated fat: 0.2 g | Saturated fat: 0.3 g |
| Carbohydrates: 0 g | Carbohydrates: 0 g | Carbohydrates: 0.4 g | Carbohydrates: 0 g | Carbohydrates: 0.8 g |
| Fiber: 0 g | Fiber: 0 g | Fiber: 0 g | Fiber: 0 g | Fiber: 0 g |

All the crustaceans are high in protein, low in fat and saturated fat, and contain varying amounts of omega-3 fatty acids, as well as vitamins and minerals. Crabs are high in vitamin B12, niacin, selenium, copper, zinc, and phosphorus, and a good source of vitamin B6, folate, thiamine, manganese, potassium, calcium, and magnesium. Lobster is an excellent source of vitamin B12, pantothenic acid, copper, selenium, phosphorus, and zinc, and a good source of vitamin E, niacin, potassium, and magnesium. Prawns are high in vitamins B6, B12, and E, niacin, selenium, and zinc, and a good source of manganese, potassium, and iron. Shrimps are generally high in vitamins B12 and D, niacin, selenium, phosphorus, iron, and copper, as well as a good source of vitamin E, zinc, and magnesium. Crayfish, yabbies, and bugs are high in vitamins B12 and E, selenium, phosphorus, copper, and manganese, and are a good source of vitamin B6, folate, pantothenic acid, niacin, potassium, zinc, and magnesium.

### THE HEALTHY EVIDENCE

Shellfish are known to be high in dietary cholesterol and for this reason many health agencies have recommended limiting intake of some of these foods to protect against cardiovascular disease. However, a 2010 study published in *Cellular and Molecular Biology* reported on the effects of prawns, which are high in dietary cholesterol, on blood cholesterol in men and found that the prawns produced no significant effects on levels of cholesterol or other lipids compared to a control diet of fish sticks. They concluded that "the consumption of cold water prawns, at least in healthy, male subjects, should not be restricted."

RIGHT The tiger prawn is named for the colorful stripes on its body. Much in demand as a food, it is the largest species of prawn, weighing up to 1½ pounds (0.7 kg) and reaching more than 12 inches (30 cm) in length.

## In a Nutshell

**Origin:** Worldwide
**Season:** Available year-round
**Why they're super:** High in protein; low in fat and saturated fat; contain omega-3 fatty acids, vitamins, and minerals
**Growing at home:** Not applicable

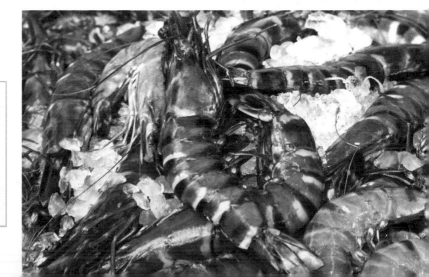

# Salmon

## What's in a Serving?

**RAW FARMED
ATLANTIC SALMON
(3 ounces/85 g)**
**Calories:** 177 (740 kJ)
**Protein:** 17.4 g
**Total fat:** 11.4 g
**Saturated fat:** 2.6 g
**Carbohydrates:** 0 g
**Fiber:** 0 g

**RAW WILD
ATLANTIC SALMON
(3 ounces/85 g)**
**Calories:** 121 (505 kJ)
**Protein:** 16.9 g
**Total fat:** 5.4 g
**Saturated fat:** 0.8 g
**Carbohydrates:** 0 g
**Fiber:** 0 g

**RAW SOCKEYE
SALMON
(3 ounces/85 g)**
**Calories:** 135 (545 kJ)
**Protein:** 18.7 g
**Total fat:** 6.2 g
**Saturated fat:** 0.9 g
**Carbohydrates:** 0 g
**Fiber:** 0 g

The term "salmon" is used to denote a number of different species in the Salmonidae family, which are found in the North Atlantic and Pacific oceans and adjacent rivers, and in the Great Lakes of North America. Among the best-known and most widespread species of salmon are Atlantic *(Salmo salar)*, chinook *(Oncorhynchus tshawytscha)*, chum *(Oncorhynchus keta)*, coho or silver *(Oncorhynchus kisutch)*, pink *(Oncorhynchus gorbuscha)*, and sockeye *(Oncorhynchus nerka)*.

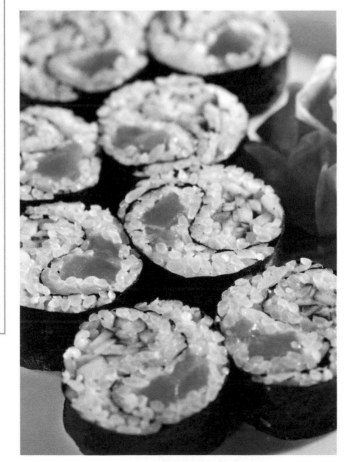

### Making the Most of Salmon

An excellent use for salmon is in a fresh green salad. Salmon's high protein, B vitamins, and omega-3 fatty acids complement the antioxidants and vitamin C in fresh greens. For a great flavor match-up, try an Asian dressing of soy sauce, honey, fresh diced ginger, and sesame oil.

Ever since the appearance, in the mid-1980s, of the first scientific studies showing that eating salmon could help counter heart disease, consumers around the world have embraced these fish. Salmon are an excellent source of vitamins B6, B12, and E, protein, pantothenic acid, niacin, thiamine, selenium, and phosphorus, and a good source of vitamin C, folate, riboflavin, potassium, and magnesium. Generally, salmon are also an excellent source of omega-3 fatty acids, though the amount varies according to the species: Atlantic has the highest levels, followed by chinook, pink, farmed coho and sockeye, wild coho, and chum.

**THE HEALTHY EVIDENCE**
Scientists have studied both the preventive and therapeutic effects of omega-3 fatty acids, in several diseases. For many of these

LEFT Salmon, both raw and smoked, is often used as an ingredient in sushi and sashimi, providing bright color as well as a host of beneficial nutrients.

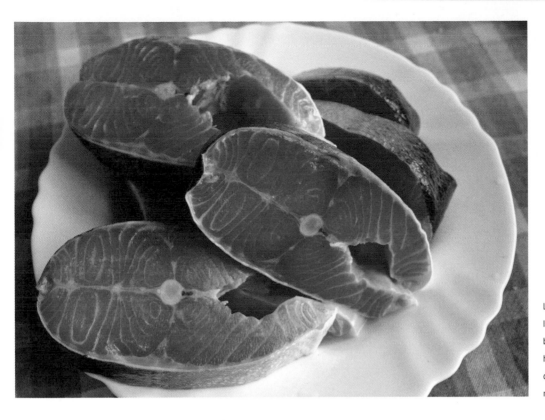

LEFT In North American Haida Indian folklore, salmon was first brought by a raven, which had heard that the chief's daughter had dreamed of a shiny fish and would not stop crying till she had one.

diseases, the protective mechanism is the inhibition of inflammation. In the case of cardiovascular disease, this is an important effect, but there are many other protective effects, as well. An important study published in the *Journal of the American Medical Association* and conducted by researchers at the University of Washington, in Seattle, reported that people consuming at least one 3-ounce (85-g) serving of fatty fish, such as salmon, a week had a 70 percent reduction in the risk for cardiac arrest. The researchers measured levels of omega-3 fatty acids in the subjects' red blood cells and noted that fatty acids "get incorporated into cell membranes and influence cell function in ways that reduce vulnerability."

*A hook's well lost to catch a salmon.*
Proverb

## In a Nutshell

**Origin:** North Atlantic and Pacific oceans and adjacent rivers
**Season:** Available year-round
**Why they're super:** High in vitamins B6, B12, and E, protein, pantothenic acid, niacin, thiamine, selenium, and phosphorus; good source of vitamin C, folate, riboflavin, potassium, and magnesium; contain omega-3 fatty acids
**Growing at home:** Not applicable

## Facts about Farmed Fish

Concerns have been raised about farmed salmon being high in toxins, especially polychlorinated biphenyls (PCBs) and methylmercury. However, a 2010 University of California review of all the studies of this issue found that PCB levels in both farmed and wild salmon are extremely low. The reviewers concluded that "the biggest risk is limiting or avoiding fish, which results in thousands of extra heart disease deaths per year." Farmed salmon has also been shown to be 40 percent higher in beneficial omega-3 fatty acids.

# Trout

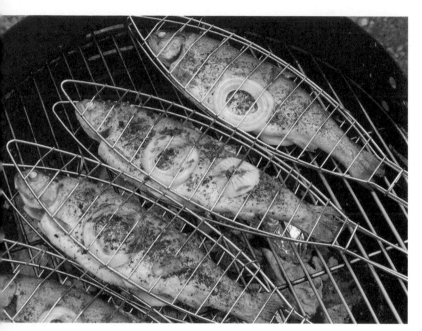

LEFT Trout are well suited to grilling, for two key reasons: their high-fat meat will hold together better than that of lower-fat fish, whose flesh tends to be more delicate, and the strong flavors of trout are seldom overpowered by the tastes imparted by the grill.

## In a Nutshell

**Origin:** North America, Europe, and Asia
**Season:** Available year-round
**Why they're super:** High in vitamins B6 and B12, protein, niacin, phosphorus, selenium, and potassium; good source of pantothenic acid, thiamine, riboflavin, manganese, magnesium, calcium, zinc, and copper; contain omega-3 fatty acids
**Growing at home:** Not applicable

## What's in a Serving?

**RAW RAINBOW TROUT**
**(3 ounces/85 g)**
**Calories:** 101 (423 kJ)
**Protein:** 17.4 g
**Total fat:** 2.9 g
**Saturated fat:** 0.6 g
**Carbohydrates:** 0 g
**Fiber:** 0 g

Trout are most familiar as freshwater fish, but they also live in the oceans. Various species are covered by the term "trout"; some are part of the Salmonidae family and thus related to salmon. Among the best-known species are brown trout *(Salmo trutta)* and rainbow trout *(Oncorhynchus mykiss)*. Like salmon, trout are high in fat, notably

## Making the Most of Trout

Here's an easy way to prepare fresh trout, which will also enhance absorption of some of the key nutrients. Combine the juice of three lemons with 3 tablespoons of olive oil, ¼ cup (15 g) chopped parsley, and coarse ground pepper. Dip eight trout fillets in the mixture, place them on a baking sheet, and top with slices of lemon, then place in a preheated 400°F (205°C) oven and bake for 15 minutes. Salt to taste.

omega-3 fatty acids, and this has made them increasingly popular with health-conscious consumers. As with salmon, trout can be purchased as farmed or wild. Trout are an excellent source of vitamins B6 and B12, protein, niacin, phosphorus, selenium, and potassium, and a good source of pantothenic acid, thiamine, riboflavin, manganese, magnesium, calcium, zinc, and copper. Trout also contain omega-3 fatty acids.

### THE HEALTHY EVIDENCE

A 2009 study published in the *Journal of Agricultural and Food Chemistry* reported on the effects of a peptide found in the skin of both trout and salmon on rats. The peptide, a protein strand, reduced levels of cholesterol and triglycerides. The authors concluded that such peptides "affect lipid absorption and metabolism and may be useful."

# Tuna

## What's in a Serving?

**RAW YELLOWFIN**
**(3 ounces/85 g)**
Calories: 92 (384 kJ)
Protein: 19.9 g
Total fat: 0.8 g
Saturated fat: 0.1 g
Carbohydrates: 0 g
Fiber: 0 g

**RAW BLUEFIN**
**(3 ounces/85 g)**
Calories: 122 (512 kJ)
Protein: 19.8 g
Total fat: 4.2 g
Saturated fat: 1.1 g
Carbohydrates: 0 g
Fiber: 0 g

**CANNED**
**ALBACORE/WHITE**
**(3 ounces/85 g)**
Calories: 109 (456 kJ)
Protein: 20.1 g
Total fat: 2.5 g
Saturated fat: 0.7 g
Carbohydrates: 0 g
Fiber: 0 g

**CANNED LIGHT TUNA**
**(3 ounces/85 g)**
Calories: 99 (414 kJ)
Protein: 21.7 g
Total fat: 0.7 g
Saturated fat: 0.2 g
Carbohydrates: 0 g
Fiber: 0 g

Tuna is perhaps the most familiar of fish, even to those who claim not to like eating fish. The more common types include albacore (also called white tuna), skipjack, bluefin, and yellowfin, the largest species, reaching up to 300 pounds (136 kg). So-called light tuna, often sold in cans, can be any tuna other than albacore; most often it is skipjack, but it can also be yellowfin, bigeye, and tongol.

All tunas are excellent sources of high-quality protein and low in fat. However, they vary in vitamin and mineral content, and in levels of omega-3 fatty acids. Bluefin tuna is high in vitamins A, B6, B12, niacin, thiamine, riboflavin, selenium, phosphorus, and magnesium, and a good source of pantothenic acid, potassium, and iron; a serving provides 1,104 milligrams of omega-3 fatty acids. Yellowfin is an excellent source of vitamin B6, niacin, thiamine, selenium, phosphorus, magnesium, and potassium, and a good source of vitamin B12 and pantothenic acid; a serving contains 196 milligrams of omega-3 fatty acids. Albacore (canned in water) is high in vitamin B12, niacin, selenium, and phosphorus, and a good source of vitamin B6, magnesium, potassium, and iron; a serving supplies 808 milligrams of omega-3 fatty acids. Light tuna (canned in water) is high in vitamins B12 and B6, niacin, selenium,

### In a Nutshell

**Origin:** Oceans worldwide
**Season:** Available year-round
**Why it's super:** High in protein, vitamins and minerals, and omega-3 fatty acids; low in fat
**Growing at home:** Not applicable

### Making the Most of Tuna

Select the varieties that are highest in omega-3 fatty acids, such as bluefin and canned albacore tuna. When purchasing packaged tuna, choose a product that is preserved in water instead of oil, to avoid the extra calories in the oil.

and phosphorus, and a good source of iron, magnesium, and potassium; a serving contains 238 milligrams of omega-3 fatty acids.

### THE HEALTHY EVIDENCE

Numerous studies have shown that omega-3 fatty acids are helpful in preventing several chronic diseases. A 2008 study published in the *Journal of Nutrition* reported that tuna oil significantly reduced damage to heart tissue in rats in which damage had been induced.

BELOW An important advantage of fresh tuna steaks over canned tuna is the significantly lower level of sodium in the fresh meat.

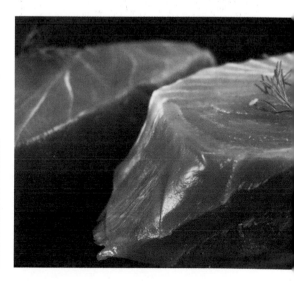

# Sardines and Pilchards

The terms "sardines" and "pilchards" are often used interchangeably but also mean slightly different things in different parts of the world. Usually, the word "sardine" refers to one of various types of small fish in the family Clupeidae, especially in the genuses *Sardina*, *Sardinops*, and *Sardinella*, and the word "pilchard" to one particular species, *Sardina pilchardus*. However, some authorities classify several species of fish as pilchards. UK fisheries, on the other hand, consider

## What's in a Serving?

| CANNED SARDINES (3.75 ounces/92 g) | CANNED PILCHARDS (3.75 ounces/92 g) |
|---|---|
| **Calories:** 191 (800 kJ) | **Calories:** 168 (702 kJ) |
| **Protein:** 22.7 g | **Protein:** 19.1 g |
| **Total fat:** 10.5 g | **Total fat:** 9.6 g |
| **Saturated fat:** 1.4 g | **Saturated fat:** 2.1 g |
| **Carbohydrates:** 0 g | **Carbohydrates:** 0 g |
| **Fiber:** 0 g | **Fiber:** 0 g |

## Making the Most of Sardines and Pilchards

The easiest way to include these nutrient-rich foods in your diet is by using canned sardines and pilchards. Add them to salads and sandwiches, use them as cracker toppers, or mix them with low-fat mayonnaise to make an excellent sauce for fish. Another option is to use them to make fish patties. Combine a can (200 g) of fish with 2 cups (420 g) of mashed potatoes, 1 cup (160 g) of finely chopped onion, an egg, and Italian herbs. Form into patties and bake at 400°F (200°C) for approximately 30 minutes, turning over after 15 minutes.

sardines to be young pilchards, and some other authorities suggest that length should be used as the criterion for classification, with fish over 6 inches (15 cm) in length qualifying as pilchards and smaller ones being termed sardines.

Both sardines and pilchards are available fresh in some areas, but are more commonly purchased in cans. During the canning process, the bones become soluble and edible, which makes the products high in calcium. Generally, sardines are an excellent source of vitamins B12 and D, niacin, riboflavin, protein, selenium, phosphorus, calcium, iron, and potassium, and a good source of vitamins B6 and E, thiamine, zinc, manganese, and magnesium. Pilchards are an excellent source of vitamins B6, B12, and D, niacin, riboflavin, protein, selenium, phosphorus, and potassium, and a good source of pantothenic acid, thiamine, magnesium, zinc, calcium, and iron. Both are, in addition, an excellent source of omega-3 fatty acids.

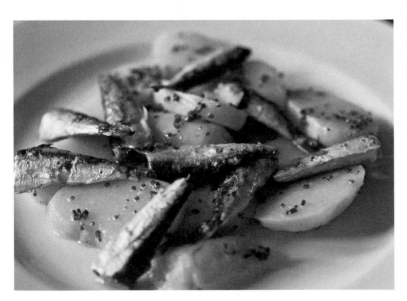

LEFT As with other oily fish, pilchards are well suited to grilling and baking, and their strong flavor is best accompanied by ingredients such as onion, garlic, oregano, basil, lemon, and tomato.

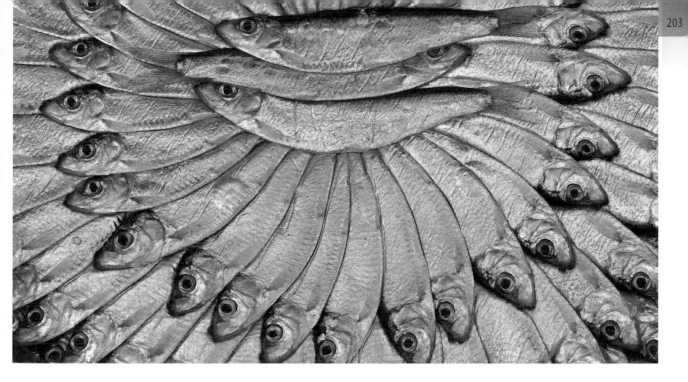

## THE HEALTHY EVIDENCE

Numerous studies have demonstrated the benefits of eating foods rich in omega-3 fatty acids, and sardines and pilchards both contain high levels. A 2009 study published in the *Journal of International Medical Research* reported on the effects of fish oil in elderly patients with heart failure. The fish oil significantly decreased blood levels of compounds that initiate inflammation. The authors concluded that fish oil "can reduce levels of plasma inflammatory markers in patients with heart failure and may offer a novel therapy for heart failure."

And as if the hefty supply of vitamins, minerals, and omega-3 fatty acids in sardines and pilchards were not enough, a 2009 study published in the journal *Bioscience, Biotechnology, and Biochemistry* highlighted another interesting compound in sardines. The Japanese researchers reported on the effects of sardine protein on hypertensive rats. The protein inhibited the action of an enzyme involved in raising blood pressure and, in combination with a common blood-pressure medication, the sardine protein improved glucose tolerance.

ABOVE Napoleon Bonaparte is credited with popularizing sardines in Europe by beginning the practice of canning the fish. His goal was to feed all the people of France with this nutritious food.

### In a Nutshell

**Origin:** Oceans worldwide

**Season:** Available year-round

**Why they're super:** Sardines: high in vitamins B12 and D, niacin, riboflavin, protein, selenium, phosphorus, calcium, iron, and potassium; good source of vitamin B6 and E, thiamine, zinc, manganese, and magnesium; contain omega-3 fatty acids.

Pilchards: high in vitamins B6, B12, and D, niacin, riboflavin, protein, selenium, phosphorus, and potassium; good source of pantothenic acid, thiamine, magnesium, zinc, calcium, and iron; contain omega-3 fatty acids.

**Growing at home:** Not applicable

*Life is rather like a tin of sardines; we're all of us looking for the key.*

Alan Bennett, English actor and writer (1934– )

# Mackerel

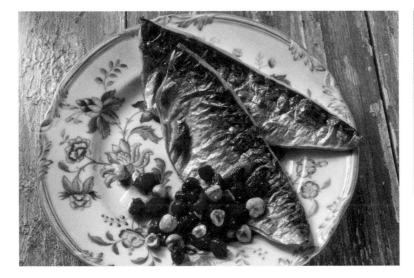

LEFT Mackerel is widely eaten in Europe, but although the fish is abundant in the North Atlantic and North Pacific oceans it is not much favored in North America and most of the harvest is frozen and exported.

## What's in a Serving?

RAW ATLANTIC
MACKEREL
(3 ounces/85 g)
**Calories:** 174 (729 kJ)
**Protein:** 15.8 g
**Total fat:** 11.8 g
**Saturated fat:** 2.8 g
**Carbohydrates:** 0 g
**Fiber:** 0 g

Mackerel includes many different species, most of which belong to the family Scombridae. They are all saltwater fish and are found in many areas of the world, notably in tropical seas, but they also inhabit bay areas. The largest species is the king mackerel *(Scomberomorus cavalla)*, which can reach lengths of up to 66 inches (1.68 m); other common varieties include Atlantic, Pacific jack, and Spanish mackerel.

## Making the Most of Mackerel

Here is a quick way to incorporate mackerel into your diet. In a food processor, chop finely a green pepper (capsicum), an onion, and a medium potato, and place the mixture in a bowl. Next, process for 30 seconds a 15-ounce (425-g) can of drained mackerel, an egg, and 2 teaspoons of any seasoning mix. Combine the result with the vegetable mixture and make into small patties. Coat with breadcrumbs, and sautée in canola oil for three minutes on each side before serving.

Mackerel is available fresh, as well as canned. Smoked mackerel is another popular product in some countries.

Mackerel is an excellent source of vitamins B6, B12, and D, protein, niacin, riboflavin, thiamine, selenium, magnesium, and phosphorus, and a good source of vitamins E and K, pantothenic acid, potassium, and iron. It is high in fat, which makes it an outstanding source of omega-3 fatty acids—indeed, Atlantic mackerel is higher in omega-3 fatty acids than most types of salmon, and Pacific jack is comparable to salmon in this regard.

### THE HEALTHY EVIDENCE

A 2005 study published in the *International Journal of Pharmaceutics* reported on the effects of three fish samples—two types of mackerel and one type of sardine—on inflammation, which plays an important role in promoting disease. In tests on laboratory samples and human volunteers, all three fish samples significantly reduced inflammation.

# Mullet

Mullet includes many species in the family Mugilidae, which occur throughout the world in tropical and temperate oceans; some also live in fresh water. In ancient times, notably in the Roman era, these fish were an important staple in the diets of many peoples of the Mediterranean region. In North America today, the word "mullet" usually refers to the striped mullet, *Mugil cephalus L*; in Europe, the term most often refers to various grey mullets in the family Mugilidae as well as some red mullets in the family Mullidae. Another name for mullet is goatfish.

Mullet is an excellent source of vitamin B6, protein, niacin, selenium, phosphorus, and potassium, as well as a good source of pantothenic acid, riboflavin, thiamine, magnesium, calcium, and iron. In addition, it contains omega-3 fatty acids.

### THE HEALTHY EVIDENCE

Mullet is not as widely appreciated as fish such as salmon or trout, yet it has an excellent nutritional profile, being low in calories and providing nutrients, high-quality protein, and a moderate amount of omega-3 fatty acids, which studies have shown to help combat heart disease. It is also generally cheaper than fish such as salmon and trout, and therefore represents an economical and convenient alternative that will still promote a healthy cardiovascular system.

## Making the Most of Mullet

A popular and nutritious recipe from Florida, which has an annual mullet festival, is a broiled mullet casserole. Place 2 pounds (0.9 kg) of mullet fillets in a glass dish. Combine 2 tablespoons each of orange juice and soy sauce with 1 teaspoon of black pepper, 2 teaspoons of oregano, and ¼ cup (40 g) grated onion. Pour over fillets and broil for five minutes, drain, and add this liquid to one 6-ounce (170-g) can of tomato paste and ½ cup (117 ml) of water. Top the fillets with one 16-ounce (450-g) package of frozen/thawed broccoli. Pour liquid over all and top with ⅓ cup (33 g) of grated Parmesan cheese. Bake at 350°F (180°C) for five minutes.

## What's in a Serving?

**RAW STRIPED MULLET**
**(3 ounces/85 g)**

**Calories:** 99 (416 kJ)
**Protein:** 16.5 g
**Total fat:** 3.2 g
**Saturated fat:** 1 g
**Carbohydrates:** 0 g
**Fiber:** 0 g

BELOW In the United States during the Depression, mullet became Florida's most valuable trading commodity.

## In a Nutshell

**Origin:** All tropical and temperate oceans
**Season:** Available year-round
**Why it's super:** High in vitamin B6, protein, niacin, selenium, phosphorus, and potassium; good source of pantothenic acid, riboflavin, thiamine, magnesium, calcium, and iron; contains omega-3 fatty acids
**Growing at home:** Not applicable

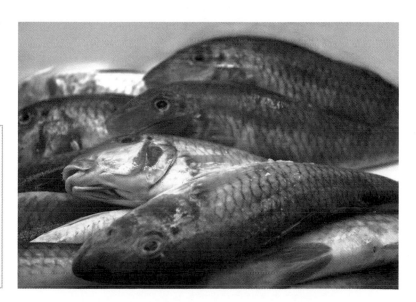

# Herring

✪ *Clupea* species

Herring include two species, *Clupea harengus*, which inhabits the North Atlantic Ocean and is particularly important to the commercial fishing industry, and *Clupea pallasii*, found in the North Pacific Ocean. Herring have been a valuable food source for thousands of years and have been preserved and prepared in countless ways—including raw, pickled, smoked, and cured—notably in the United Kingdom, where a whole smoked herring is known as a "bloater" and one that has been split and smoked is referred to as a "kipper." Despite the common idiomatic term "red herring," meaning a diversion from the truth, no species of herring is naturally red, though herring flesh that has been too heavily smoked may turn red.

Herring are an outstanding source of vitamin D, with one serving providing almost

## What's in a Serving?

**RAW HERRING**
**(3 ounces/85 g)**
**Calories:** 134 (562 kJ)
**Protein:** 15.3 g
**Total fat:** 7.7 g
**Saturated fat:** 1.7 g
**Carbohydrates:** 0 g
**Fiber:** 0 g

## In a Nutshell

**Origin:** All tropical and temperate oceans
**Season:** Available year-round
**Why they're super:** High in vitamins B6, B12, and D, protein, niacin, riboflavin, selenium, phosphorus, and potassium; good source of pantothenic acid, thiamine, magnesium, zinc, calcium, and iron; contains omega-3 fatty acids
**Growing at home:** Not applicable

three-and-a-half times the Daily Value. They are also an excellent source of vitamins B6 and B12, protein, niacin, riboflavin, selenium, phosphorus, and potassium, and a good source of pantothenic acid, thiamine, magnesium, zinc, calcium, and iron. They also contain a high level of omega-3 fatty acids.

### THE HEALTHY EVIDENCE

A 2009 study published in the *British Journal of Nutrition* reported on the effects of a diet containing herring on blood cholesterol levels in healthy men. Compared to a diet containing either lean pork or chicken, a diet containing 5 ounces (150 g) of herring five days a week significantly raised HDL cholesterol levels, which can protect against heart disease.

BELOW A northern European delicacy, rollmops are rolled herring fillets pickled in vinegar, onions, and chili.

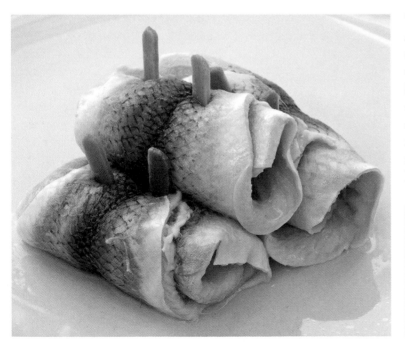

## Making the Most of Herring

To make a hearty salad loaded with nutrients, combine 9 ounces (255 g) of drained canned herring, two large potatoes, cooked and cubed, a diced cucumber, a large apple sliced, 2 tablespoons of light mayonnaise, and 6 tablespoons of low-fat yogurt.

# White Fish

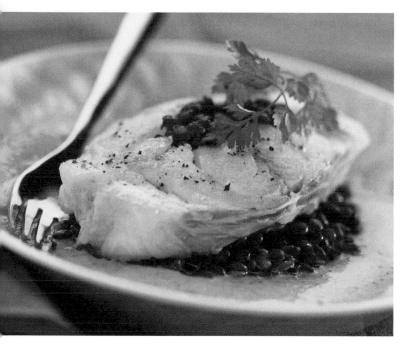

## Making the Most of White Fish

The delicate flavor of white fish can be enhanced by ingredients such as tomatoes, herbs, and garlic, which also add antioxidants and nutrients. In a roasting pan, combine 2 pints of cherry tomatoes, 1 tablespoon of olive oil, 12 garlic cloves, coarse salt, and cracked pepper, and ½ cup (12 g) of fresh basil leaves. Roast for 15 minutes at 425°F (220°C), then add 1 pound (0.45 kg) of white fish and cook for another seven to ten minutes till the fish is no longer translucent.

White fish is a collective and imprecise term used to refer to any species of fish that has white flesh, most usually cod, whiting, haddock, hake, Atlantic whitefish, or pollock, which are all common commercial fishes. These types of fish live on or near the bottom of the lake or seabed, in contrast with oily fish, such as salmon and trout, which live in the water column away from the bottom.

### In a Nutshell

**Origin:** Oceans, lakes, and rivers worldwide
**Season:** Available year-round
**Why it's super:** High in vitamin B12, protein, selenium, and phosphorus; good source of vitamin B6, niacin, potassium, and zinc; contains omega-3 fatty acids
**Growing at home:** Not applicable

### What's in a Serving?

**RAW WHITE FISH
(3 ounces/85 g)**
**Calories:** 114 (477 kJ)
**Protein:** 16.2 g
**Total fat:** 5 g
**Saturated fat:** 0.8 g
**Carbohydrates:** 0 g
**Fiber:** 0 g

White fish tends to be dry and delicate, even bland, with much less of a "fishy" taste than oily fish. It is lower in fat, and therefore lower in omega-3 fatty acids. Nevertheless, it makes an excellent substitute for meat, as it is high in quality protein and low in saturated fat. White fish is also an excellent source of vitamin B12, selenium, and phosphorus, and a good source of vitamin B6, niacin, potassium, and zinc.

### THE HEALTHY EVIDENCE

Many of the early studies that demonstrated the cardio-protective benefits of eating fish used white fish, which was then the most commonly eaten kind. So consuming white fish can be considered an effective way to protect your heart, though eating a variety of types of fish will provide the greatest benefit.

## DAIRY FOODS AND EGGS

# Skim Milk and Reduced-fat Milk

Commercially available milk comes in a wide variety of choices; whole milk, various kinds of reduced-fat milk, and fat-free milk, also called skim or skimmed milk. In addition, the milk may be fortified with vitamins A and D, as well as with calcium. Skim milk may contain a small amount of fat (usually less than 0.5 percent), but in many countries it can be labeled as "fat-free"; by comparison, whole milk has a fat content of 3.5 percent. Milk is also available in dried or powdered form, which can be used to boost the nutritive value of other foods.

Skim and reduced-fat milk are excellent sources of vitamins A, B12, and D, protein, riboflavin, calcium, phosphorus, potassium, and selenium. They are also good sources of vitamin B6, pantothenic acid, thiamine, magnesium, and zinc.

### What's in a Serving?

**FRESH SKIM MILK**
**(1 cup/235 ml)**
**Calories:** 83 (350 kJ)
**Protein:** 8.3 g
**Total fat:** 0.2 g
**Saturated fat:** 0.1 g
**Carbohydrates:** 12.2 g
**Fiber:** 0 g

### In a Nutshell

**Origin:** Europe and Asia
**Season:** Available year-round
**Why they're super:** High in vitamins A, B12, and D, protein, riboflavin, calcium, phosphorus, potassium, and selenium; good sources of vitamin B6, pantothenic acid, thiamine, magnesium, and zinc
**Growing at home:** Not applicable

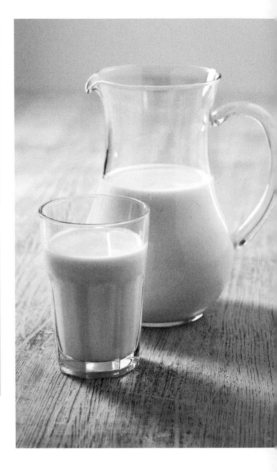

ABOVE For centuries, skim milk was considered a worthless byproduct and discarded. It was first promoted for its health benefits during World War II.

## THE HEALTHY EVIDENCE

One of the most important studies to emerge in the area of hypertension, or high blood pressure, was the Dietary Approaches to Stop Hypertension (DASH) study, which was reported in both the *New England Journal of Medicine* and the *Journal of the American Medical Association* in the late 1990s. The study demonstrated that, by adding low-fat dairy products (2.5 servings) as well as fruits and vegetables to a person's diet, blood pressure could be lowered in adults with hypertension. The resulting food plan became known as the DASH Diet.

### Making the Most of Milk

An economical and convenient way to store milk is in powdered form. Powdered skim milk can be added to most baking mixes to add protein and nutrients. For example, in a standard scone recipe, add ⅓ cup to ½ cup (22–34 g) of powdered milk. Other baking recipes to which powdered milk can be added include quick breads, such as banana bread, and fruit and oat bars.

# Cottage Cheese and Ricotta Cheese

Cottage cheese is a curd product. Curds are made by curdling milk with rennet, an enzyme obtained by soaking a calf's stomach in brine (vinegar, lemon juice, or another edible acid will have the same effect). Most of the liquid, known as whey, is then drained off, but some remains with the curd, giving it a loose, soft texture. Pressing rather than simply straining the curd produces a cheese called *queso blanco*, a Spanish phrase for "white cheese." Ricotta is made from the whey by using heat to precipitate out the remaining albumen protein, forming another, finer curd.

Cottage cheese is an excellent source of vitamin B12, protein, riboflavin, phosphorus, and selenium, and a good source of calcium. Ricotta is an excellent source of vitamin A, protein, riboflavin, calcium, phosphorus, zinc, and selenium, and a good source of vitamin B12 and magnesium.

## THE HEALTHY EVIDENCE

A 2004 review article published in the *European Journal of Nutrition* discussed the many benefits of ricotta. It noted, for example, that ricotta provides high-quality whey protein, which some studies suggest may be helpful in building muscle and in facilitating weight loss. It also cited ricotta's high content of essential amino acids. Cottage cheese has been shown to be similarly rich in protein, notably in the form of casein, also an especially high-quality protein.

---

### Making the Most of Cottage Cheese and Ricotta Cheese

Ricotta tends to be an ingredient in recipes, rather than being eaten on its own, and cottage cheese is often relegated to the low-calorie plate at a diner. For a healthy dessert, try mixing either of these nutrient-rich foods with an equal part of low-fat vanilla yogurt, cinnamon, and a touch of honey.

---

### What's in a Serving?

**FRESH COTTAGE CHEESE**
**(4 ounces/113 g)**
**Calories:** 81 (342 kJ)
**Protein:** 14 g
**Total fat:** 0.7 g
**Saturated fat:** 0.3 g
**Carbohydrates:** 3.1 g
**Fiber:** 0 g

**FRESH RICOTTA**
**(4 ounces/124 g)**
**Calories:** 171 (717 kJ)
**Protein:** 14.1 g
**Total fat:** 9.8 g
**Saturated fat:** 6.1 g
**Carbohydrates:** 6.4 g
**Fiber:** 0 g

---

### In a Nutshell

**Origin:** Europe
**Season:** Available year-round
**Why they're super:** Cottage cheese: high in vitamin B12, protein, riboflavin, phosphorus, and selenium; good source of calcium. Ricotta: high in vitamin A, protein, riboflavin, calcium, phosphorus, zinc, and selenium; good source of vitamin B12 and magnesium
**Growing at home:** Not applicable

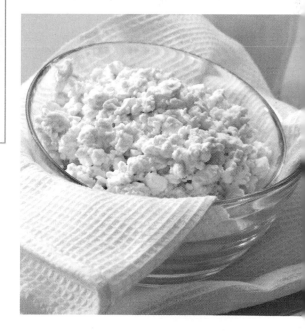

BELOW Cottage cheese has long been favored by people following diets, as it is high in protein and nutrients but low in fat and therefore makes an excellent substitute for full-fat cheeses and other calorie-rich foods.

# Yogurt

*Yogurt is very good for the stomach, the lumbar regions, appendicitis, and apotheosis.*

Eugene Ionesco, Romanian dramatist (1912–94)

The potential health benefits of yogurt were first highlighted for the modern consumer in the 1960s, through the work of a Nobel Prize winner, Russian microbiologist Dr. Ilya Metchnikoff. He postulated that ageing was caused by toxic bacteria in the colon and that lactic acid and friendly bacteria—so-called probiotics—commonly found in foods such as yogurt, could neutralize the bacteria and help prolong life. (He himself drank sour milk for most of his life.) While there is no evidence for yogurt prolonging lifespan, its active bacteria can almost certainly contribute to good health.

## Making the Most of Yogurt

Always choose yogurt that is made from low-fat or skim milk and declares it contains "live cultures." Yogurt can be added to almost any baked-goods recipe. When doing so, consider that it will replace up to half of the liquid; you can also typically omit at least half of the fat called for in the recipe. Another way to add more yogurt to your diet is to use it to make sauces and soups or stews.

## PROCESSES ANCIENT AND MODERN

Long before the Western world began its love affair with yogurt—5,000 years earlier in fact—yogurt was a staple food for peoples all over the world. In many ancient cultures, making fermented milk, which essentially describes yogurt, was the only way to preserve milk. Fermented cow's milk was, and still is, known as kefir, from the Persian *kef* (foam) and *shir* (milk).

When lactose is fermented, the bacteria produce lactic acid, which in turn acts upon the milk protein to change its texture. Current yogurt-making practices involve heating milk to 180°F (82°C) to eradicate unwanted bacteria and to prevent the development of curds. The milk is then quickly cooled to 110°F (43°C), and a culture of *Lactobacillus delbrueckii* subsp. *bulgaricus* and *Streptococcus salivarius* subsp. *thermophilus* bacteria is added. The yogurt is maintained at the same temperature for up to seven

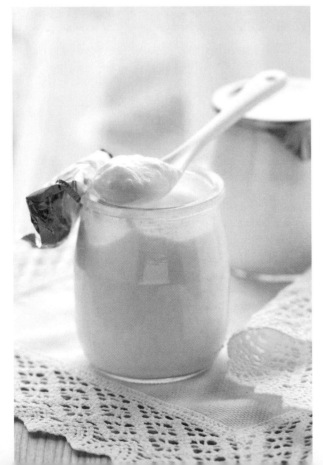

LEFT In the 1970s, yogurt gained widespread attention as a result of television adverts featuring a Turkish man said to be a daily yogurt eater and more than 100 years old.

## What's in a Serving?

**LOW-FAT YOGURT**
**(1 cup/245 g)**
**Calories:** 154 (649 kJ)
**Protein:** 12.9 g
**Total fat:** 3.8 g
**Saturated fat:** 2.5 g
**Carbohydrates:** 17.3 g
**Fiber:** 0 g

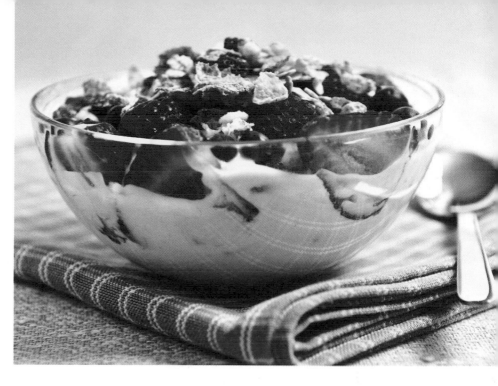

RIGHT Complementing yogurt with whole grains and berries makes for the perfect nutrient-rich meal: high protein, fiber, and antioxidants.

hours before it is ready to be packaged and refrigerated.

Yogurt is an excellent source of vitamin B12, protein, pantothenic acid, riboflavin, calcium, phosphorus, potassium, zinc, selenium, and magnesium, and a good source of vitamin B6, folate, and thiamine.

## THE HEALTHY EVIDENCE

Many of the potential health benefits of yogurt relate to the gastrointestinal tract (GIT), and specifically the colon. Some of the less glamorous, but certainly critical, benefits include promoting normal bowel movements and preventing constipation and other GIT problems, such as bloating and flatulence. However, another important benefit is reducing exposure of the GIT to pathogens, which can cause diseases such as cancer and inflammatory bowel disease.

Yogurt is also thought to help bolster the immune system. A review published in the

---

### Know Your Allies

A range of terms, potentially confusing, is used in relation to friendly bacteria in foods such as yogurts. Some standard definitions, based on the studies to date, include:

**Probiotics:** Live micro-organisms that, when consumed in adequate quantities, may confer health benefits

**Prebiotics:** Nondigestible food ingredients that stimulate the growth of one or more bacteria in the colon

**Synbiotics (or symbiotics):** A combination of prebiotics and probiotics

---

*American Journal of Clinical Nutrition* discussed possible mechanisms by which yogurt could enhance resistance to disease. According to a leading researcher in the area of immunology, Dr. S. Meydani, "yogurt may help make the immune system more resilient."

A study published in the journal *Cancer Causes and Control* reported on the link between colon cancer and yogurt. The study included more than 1,400 subjects with colon cancer from the Los Angeles area. Researchers assessed their previous food intake over the years leading up to their diagnoses. They found that yogurt intake was associated with a significantly decreased risk of developing colon cancer.

---

### In a Nutshell

**Origin:** Middle East

**Season:** Available year-round

**Why it's super:** High in vitamin B12, protein, pantothenic acid, riboflavin, calcium, phosphorus, potassium, zinc, selenium, and magnesium; good source of vitamin B6, folate, and thiamine

**Growing at home:** Not applicable

# Soy Milk

## What's in a Serving?

**LOW-FAT SOY MILK**
**(1 cup/227 g)**
**Calories:** 108 (451 kJ)
**Protein:** 5 g
**Total fat:** 3 g
**Saturated fat:** 0.5 g
**Carbohydrates:** 3.1 g
**Fiber:** 1 g

RIGHT A wide variety of soy-milk products is now available, including chocolate- and vanilla-flavored beverages.

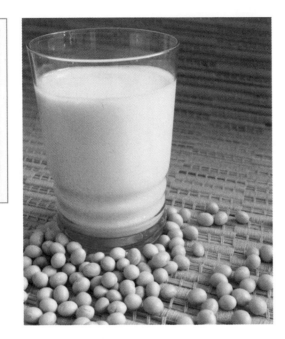

## In a Nutshell

**Origin:** Asia
**Season:** Available year-round
**Why it's super:** High in vitamins A, B12, and D, protein, riboflavin, and calcium; good source of iron; contains isoflavones and soy proteins
**Growing at home:** Not applicable

Soy milk is made by grinding presoaked soy beans in water; the milk can then be made into tofu (see p. 82) by adding a coagulating agent. Literary evidence for the production and use of soy milk dates back to the year CE 82 in China, the date of the earliest recorded use of the Mandarin Chinese word for soy milk, *doujiang*, with *dou* being the word for "bean" and *jiang* meaning "liquid." The Chinese name does not refer to milk, and that word may have become part of the name as a result of the earliest references in English to tofu-making, in which the water was called "the fresh milky liquid."

Many of the nutrients in soy milk vary by brand, as most are not naturally present and are added to the product. However, most brands of soy milk are an excellent source of vitamins A, B12, and D, protein, riboflavin, and calcium, and a good source of iron. Soy milk also contains isoflavones and soy proteins.

### THE HEALTHY EVIDENCE

Soy milk is useful as a substitute for cow's milk in people who are either allergic to the protein in milk or have lactose intolerance (lactose is the sugar in milk and is not contained in soy milk). Interest in other health benefits grew following a 1995 study published in the *New England Journal of Medicine*, which reported that soy lowered blood cholesterol levels. The beneficial compounds were assumed to be the phytosterols or phytoestrogens contained in soy, specifically the isoflavones genistein and daidzein. Since those early studies, however, researchers have suggested that the effect may also be related to the proteins in soy.

## Making the Most of Soy Milk

Choose low-fat soy milk. To add the milk to your diet, use it in place of cow's milk in recipes. Instant pudding mix works well with soy, although reducing the amount of liquid by about 25 percent will yield the best results. Soy milk can be substituted for most any liquid in baking to add nutrients and isoflavones.

# Eggs

Eggs are a versatile and nutritious food, though their precise nutritional content will vary according to what the chickens that produce them have been fed. Chicken eggs may come from factory-farmed chickens, which are generally kept in cages and not allowed to move freely, or free-range chickens, which are allowed to roam at will and placed in shelters only at night. In both cases, the chickens may be given antibiotics. Organic eggs come from free-range chickens that eat only organically grown feed that is free from animal byproducts and genetically modified organisms (GMOs), and are given antibiotics only in emergencies.

Eggs are an excellent source of protein, and the egg white or albumen is the highest-quality protein known. They are also an excellent source of vitamin B12, riboflavin, choline, phosphorus, and selenium, and a good source of vitamin B6, folate, pantothenic acid, and iron.

## THE HEALTHY EVIDENCE

A 2009 review article published in the journal *Nutrition Reviews* discussed the health benefits of choline, a compound that the Institute of Medicine added to the list of recommended nutrients in 1998. The authors noted that eggs are one of the best sources of choline, which has numerous roles in human metabolism. For example, choline may help prevent atherosclerosis, neurological disorders, and liver disease. The researchers suggested that, given the importance of choline in a wide range of critical functions, and the generally less-than-optimal intakes of the nutrient among the population, programs should be developed to encourage the intake of choline-rich foods such as eggs.

## Making the Most of Eggs

Although many health enthusiasts promote the eating of raw eggs, it's not recommended for at least two reasons. First, the high-quality protein in eggs is best absorbed by the body when they are cooked—protein absorption from raw eggs is almost half that of cooked eggs. Second, raw or undercooked eggs may contain the pathogenic bacteria salmonella.

## What's in a Serving?

**BOILED EGG**
**(1 large/50 g)**
**Calories:** 78 (324 kJ)
**Protein:** 6.3 g
**Total fat:** 5.3 g
**Saturated fat:** 1.6 g
**Carbohydrates:** 0.6 g
**Fiber:** 0 g

## In a Nutshell

**Origin:** Asia and Europe

**Season:** Available year-round

**Why they're super:** High in vitamin B12, protein, riboflavin, choline, phosphorus, and selenium; good source of vitamin B6, folate, pantothenic acid, and iron

**Growing at home:** Chickens are easy to rear at home

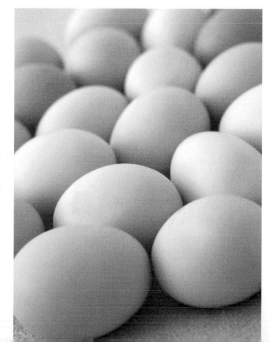

LEFT The belief that brown eggs are more nutritious than white is false: chickens with white earlobes lay white and those with red lobes lay brown; the nutrients are similar.

# Beverages and Treats

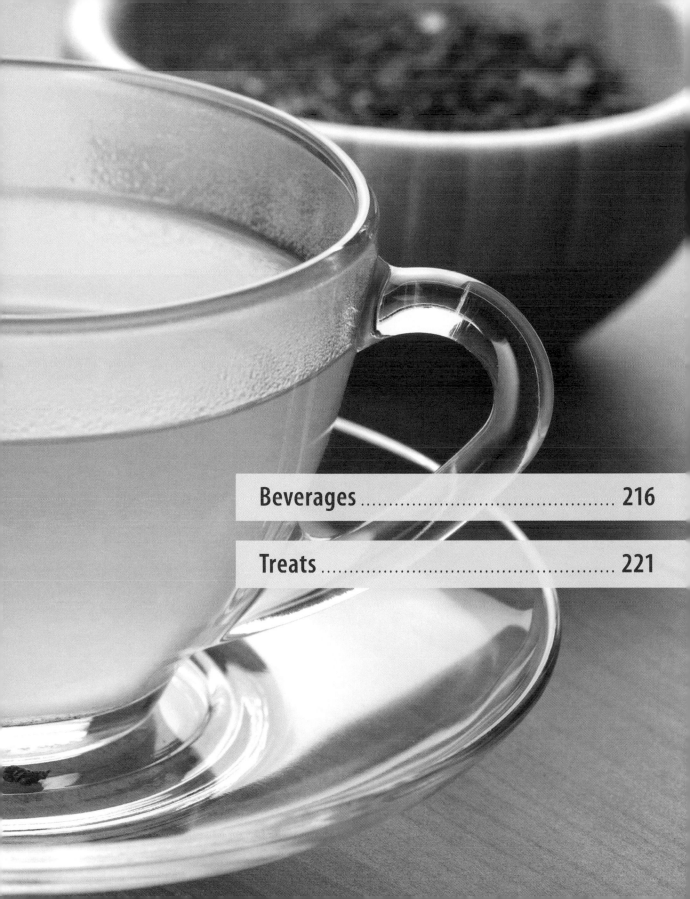

# BEVERAGES

# Tea

✿ *Camellia sinensis*

BELOW During the production of green tea, steaming or roasting is used to destroy oxidizing enzymes and thereby prevent oxidation and darkening of the leaves.

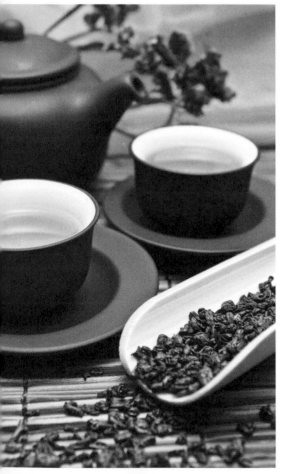

The word "tea" refers to the plant *Camellia sinensis*, or the leaves from this plant, or the beverage prepared from the leaves of this plant by adding it to boiling water. All of the various types of tea—black, white, yellow, green, and oolon—come from the *Camellia sinensis* plant (herbal teas, on the other hand, are created by an infusion of flowers, fruits, herbs, or other plants). Broadly, the differences have to do with how long the leaves are allowed to wilt and oxidize—the longer the oxidation, the darker the color.

The earliest written record of the use of tea is from China, in the first millennium BCE. Early Chinese texts cite the medical use of tea in the Han dynasty (206 BCE–CE 220), and literature from the Tang dynasty (CE 618–907) records the widespread use of tea as a beverage. Around CE 760–780, author Lu Yu compiled the first ever book on tea, *The Classic of Tea*, which described the cultivation of the tea plant and the brewing of the drink.

The Chinese saw drinking tea as an expression of harmony with people and nature, and various rituals developed around its consumption. In the fifteenth century, Buddhists introduced the Chinese tea ceremony to Japan, where it acquired immense significance through the medieval period and beyond. Variations on the Chinese tea ceremony also developed in Korea, Taiwan, Turkey, Thailand, and Vietnam.

## ABUNDANT ANTIOXIDANTS
Tea contains only a minimal amount of carbohydrate and very few calories; however, in addition it contains more than 700

### In a Nutshell

**Origin:** Southeast Asia
**Season:** Summer; products available year-round
**Why it's super:** High in antioxidant catechins
**Growing at home:** Tea can be grown in a garden or container in most climates; leaves can be harvested after three years

### Mythical Origins

Many myths surround the origins of tea. According to one, the Chinese emperor Shennong was drinking water that had just been boiled, when a gust of wind blew a few leaves from a nearby tree into the bowl. He was pleased with the flavor and its refreshing properties. A variation of this legend says that the emperor personally tested the medicinal properties of various herbs, and found that tea would act as an antidote if he ingested a poisonous herb.

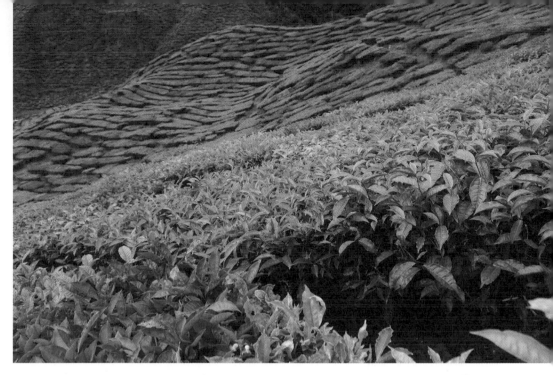

RIGHT Humans have been using the leaves of the *Camellia sinensis* plant for more than 5,000 years, and today it is second only to water as the most widely consumed beverage in the world.

other chemicals, among which are numerous antioxidant phyto-chemicals, which make teas of all kinds potentially highly beneficial in combating disease.

Tea also contains caffeine, and the amount varies among the types of tea and the length of time it is steeped. However, an average cup of black tea steeped for three minutes contains 47 milligrams, whereas an equivalent volume of brewed coffee contains 95 milligrams.

## THE HEALTHY EVIDENCE

A 2009 article published in the *American Journal of Obstetrics and Gynecology* analyzed a range of studies of the relationship between drinking tea and endometrial cancer. It found that an increase in tea intake of two cups daily was associated with a risk reduction of 25 percent for the cancer.

A 2009 review article published in the *Journal of Cardiovascular Pharmacology* discussed studies of the relationship between drinking tea and heart disease. The authors pointed out that tea contains a catechin, epigallocatechin-3-gallate (E3G), which appears to inhibit the production of molecules that promote cells called monocytes, which then stick to the lining of the blood vessels, a significant development in atherosclerosis.

### Making the Most of Tea

Most people enjoy drinking tea; however, even if you don't like the taste, there are still some simple ways to incorporate tea into your diet. The easiest method is to combine lightly brewed tea with a combination of juices. More highly flavored and citrus-based juices will mask the flavor best. Another option is to substitute tea for part of the normal liquid added to baked goods.

*If you are cold,*
*tea will warm you;*
*If you are too heated,*
*it will cool you;*
*If you are too depressed,*
*it will cheer you;*
*If you are excited,*
*it will calm you.*

William Gladstone, English statesman (1809–98)

### What's in a Serving?

**BREWED TEA**
**(1 cup/235 g)**
**Calories:** 2 (9 kJ)
**Protein:** 0 g
**Total fat:** 0 g
**Saturated fat:** 0 g
**Carbohydrates:** 0.7 g
**Fiber:** 0 g

# Coffee

- *Coffea arabica*
- *Coffea robusta*

First cultivated in Ethiopia in the sixth century CE, the coffee plant was most likely introduced to Europe by Muslims. French colonists established the first coffee plantations in the Americas in the 1700s. By the beginning of the next century, Brazil had become a major producer, and today it is the world's largest exporter. Other major producers include Colombia and Vietnam.

Coffee has long been one of the most popular beverages in the world, but also one of the most maligned, with regular reports of its detrimental effects. More recently, however, numerous studies have pointed to just the opposite: significant health benefits. Just 2 cups (470 ml) of coffee a day provide almost one-quarter of the Daily Value for riboflavin and are a good source of pantothenic acid, manganese, and potassium. Coffee also contains antioxidant polyphenols including caffeic acid, and a derivative of that compound known as chlorogenic acid. In addition, it contains caffeine, which has been shown to improve cognitive function and enhance physical performance.

## What's in a Serving?

**FRESH COFFEE**
**8 ounces (235 g)**
**Calories:** 2 (5 kJ)
**Protein:** 0.3 g
**Total fat:** 0.1 g
**Saturated fat:** 0 g
**Carbohydrates:** 0 g
**Fiber:** 0 g

BELOW Scientists have found that the aroma of coffee causes changes in the brains of rats, which result in both antioxidant activity and stress relaxation.

## Making the Most of Coffee

Adding sugar and cream can increase your calorie intake if you drink a lot of coffee. If a teaspoon of each is included in every cup, 4–8 cups of coffee a day will add 120–240 calories a day. To avoid this, try taking your coffee black, and use a low-calorie sweetener.

## THE HEALTHY EVIDENCE

A 2010 study published in the *American Journal of Clinical Nutrition* reported on the effects of coffee on blood markers of inflammation and oxidation, processes linked to cardiovascular disease and diabetes. When subjects began drinking coffee again after a one-month break, the markers declined and their HDL cholesterol, a helpful compound, increased. A 2009 study published in the *Archives of Internal Medicine* reported that, for every cup of coffee (including decaffeinated coffee) consumed daily, there was a 7 percent reduction in the risk of diabetes. And a 2010 study presented at the American Association for Cancer Research in Houston reported that men with the highest coffee intake were 60 percent less likely to develop advanced prostate cancer than non-coffee drinkers.

## In a Nutshell

**Origin:** Africa
**Season:** Available year-round
**Why it's super:** High in riboflavin; good source of pantothenic acid, manganese, and potassium; contains antioxidant polyphenols
**Growing at home:** Plant can be grown indoors; takes four to six years to bear fruit

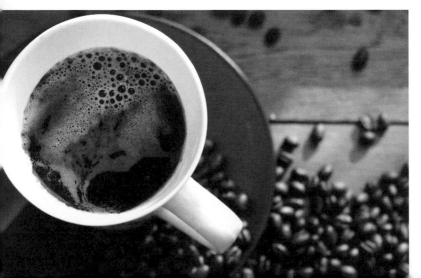

# Wheat and Barley Grass Juices

✪ *Hordeum vulgare* Barley Grass
✪ *Triticum* species Wheat Grass

## What's in a Serving?

**FRESH JUICE**

**(4 ounces/113 g)**

**Calories:** 24 (100 kJ)

**Protein:** 2.2 g

**Total fat:** 0 g

**Saturated fat:** 0 g

**Carbohydrates:** 2.3 g

**Fiber:** 1.5 g

**POWDER**

**(2 teaspoons/7 g)**

**Calories:** 30 (126 kJ)

**Protein:** 2 g

**Total fat:** 0 g

**Saturated fat:** 0 g

**Carbohydrates:** 4 g

**Fiber:** 2 g

The young grasses of both wheat and barley are used to make a range of health products including powders and tablets, but are most often consumed in the form of juices. The benefits of the grasses were first noted in 1930 by an agricultural chemist named Charles F. Schnabel. He made a powder from the grass juices and used it to treat his ailing hens; he found that it not only cured the birds but also caused them to produce more eggs than healthy hens. Given the dramatic results, he distributed his powder to family and friends as a supplement. Major companies soon invested in more research, and by 1940 the powder was in drug stores throughout North America.

Wheat grass and barley grass are excellent sources of vitamins A, C, and K, folate, biotin, riboflavin, selenium, manganese, and potassium. They are also good sources of vitamin E, fiber, iron, and calcium, and contain antioxidant carotenoids, mainly as beta-carotene.

### THE HEALTHY EVIDENCE

A 2007 review published in the journal *Nutrition and Cancer* reported on the effects of wheat grass juice on a side effect of chemotherapy, neutropenia, or low white blood cells. The study found that in 60 breast cancer patients on chemotherapy, wheat grass juice reduced the side effect.

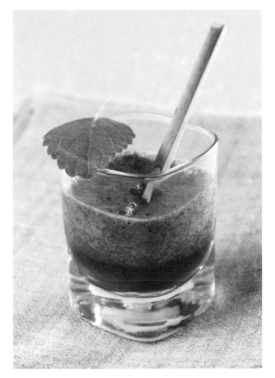

ABOVE Early researchers and promoters of grass juices claimed, without foundation, that the high content of chlorophyll in the juice, evident in its verdant color, could cure and prevent numerous diseases.

## In a Nutshell

**Origin:** Wheat grass: Fertile Crescent region of the Middle East; barley grass: Eurasia and northern Africa

**Season:** Summer; products available year-round

**Why they're super:** High in vitamins A, C, and K, folate, biotin, riboflavin, selenium, manganese, and potassium; good source of vitamin E, fiber, iron, and calcium; contain antioxidant carotenoids, primarily as beta-carotene

**Growing at home:** Both are easy to grow; kits and directions are available online

## Making the Most of Wheat and Barley Grass Juices

Both wheat and barley grasses can be purchased in juice or powder form, and both have similar nutritional values. The powders can be added to liquids, such as water or juice, and to a range of recipes. For example, they make an excellent addition to baked grains such as breads and muffins.

# Water

While many organisms can produce individual vitamins, no organism on earth can survive without water. Water is one of the six essential nutrients vital not only for life, but also for good health. At both ends of the life span, dehydration—a lack of adequate water in the body—is a critical and potentially life-threatening condition, with infants and the elderly at highest risk.

Water usually contains a host of naturally occurring compounds. Among the most desirable are essential minerals, such as calcium and iron. Unfortunately, however, we do not always know what is present in water, even bottled waters.

The US Institute of Medicine recommends a daily liquid intake of 4.7 pints (2.2 l) for women and 6.3 pints (3 l) for men, which includes water from foods, which usually averages about 20 percent of total water consumption. Drinking water as your main source of liquid will maintain hydration while avoiding the sugars, caffeine, and additives in so many other drinks, and is also thought to offer protection against kidney stones.

## THE HEALTHY EVIDENCE

A 2007 review published in the journal *Urologic Nursing* reported on the evidence

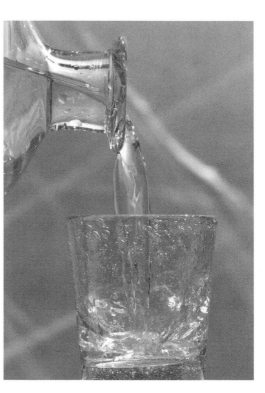

LEFT As well as environmental conditions, diet affects a person's water requirement. High intakes of salt and protein increase the amount needed by the body.

| What's in a Serving? |
| --- |
| **FRESH WATER** |
| **(1 cup/235 ml)** |
| **Calories:** 0 (0 kJ) |
| **Protein:** 0 g |
| **Total fat:** 0 g |
| **Saturated fat:** 0 g |
| **Carbohydrates:** 0 g |
| **Fiber:** 0 g |

## Making the Most of Water

Plan to drink plain water for at least part of your daily fluid intake. Bearing in mind that 20 percent will be supplied by food, aim to drink 4 pints (1.9 l) of water and other beverages a day if you are female and 5 pints (2.4 l) if you are male. If you have a history or family history of kidney stones, make sure at least half of your fluid is plain water.

## In a Nutshell

**Origin:** Ubiquitous

**Season:** Available year-round

**Why it's super:** Safest, most convenient form of hydration, may supply important minerals, protects against kidney stones; contains no carbohydrates or fat

**Growing at home:** Not applicable

for various dietary and nutritional factors on the development of kidney stones. Maintaining a high intake of fluids was a critical factor, and water was shown to have a protective effect. In contrast, some beverages were linked to an increased risk.

# TREATS

# Dark Chocolate

To the ancient Mayans, chocolate was more than a sweet indulgence, it played a pivotal role in their religious and social lives. More than 2,000 years ago, the Maya discovered the cacao tree, *Theobroma cacao*, in the rainforest, and made a spicy beverage from the ground seeds. The Maya traded with the Aztecs, and the cacao seeds soon became a form of currency among the Aztecs. The Spanish explorers brought the seeds back home in 1521 and added sugar and cinnamon to the beverage, but did not share the recipe with the rest of Europe for another 100 years. In the 1800s, technology made chocolate affordable to most people, and this resulted in the development of solid chocolate.

## What's in a Serving?

**DARK CHOCOLATE (1 ounce/28.4 g)**
**Calories:** 156 (653 kJ)
**Protein:** 1.5 g
**Total fat:** 9.1 g
**Saturated fat:** 5.4 g
**Carbohydrates:** 17 g
**Fiber:** 2 g

## In a Nutshell

**Origin:** Central America
**Season:** Available year-round
**Why it's super:** High in manganese, copper, iron, and magnesium; good source of fiber and phosphorus; contains antioxidant flavonols and theobromine
**Growing at home:** Not applicable

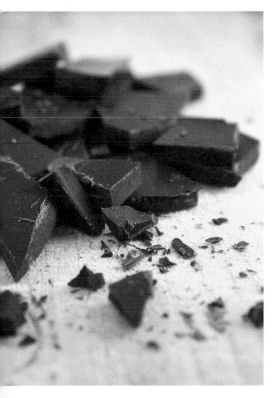

LEFT Some studies have noted that there is potential for people to become addicted to chocolate, partly as a result of an alkaloid compound, salsolinol, which binds to receptors in the brain.

Dark chocolate is an excellent source of manganese, copper, iron, and magnesium, and a good source of fiber and phosphorus. It contains antioxidant flavonols and theobromine, a relative of caffeine. Many dark chocolate products now label the content of cacao solids; choosing the highest percentage provides the greatest nutritional benefits.

### THE HEALTHY EVIDENCE

A 2009 review of the health effects of dark chocolate was published in the *Journal of Thrombosis and Thrombolysis*. The most important compounds in dark chocolate are flavonols, which, as antioxidants, have been shown to reduce the oxidation of LDL cholesterol, a contributing factor in heart disease. Studies have shown that flavonols can lower blood pressure, improve blood flow, and reduce blood clotting.

## Making the Most of Dark Chocolate

The enjoyment of simply eating a chunk of dark chocolate is hard to top. However, you can derive the same health benefits with less fat and fewer calories by using dark cocoa powder to make hot beverages or incorporating it in recipes—try using it to make a dark chocolate quick bread, and add a handful of dried cranberries to further increase the quota of antioxidants.

# Nutritional Supplements

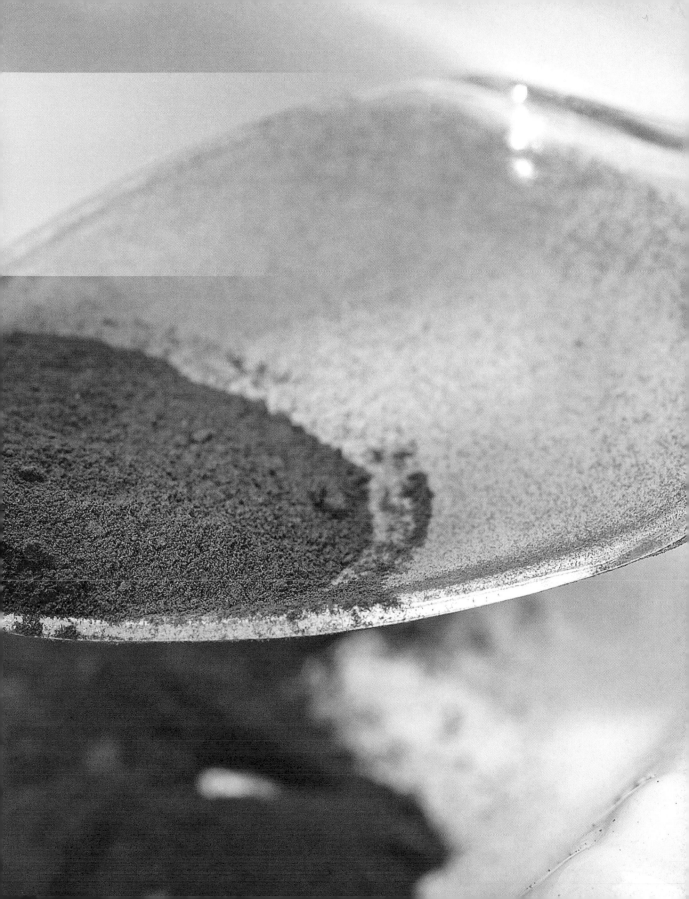

# Blue-green Algae

## What's in a Serving?

**POWDERED
BLUE-GREEN ALGAE**
(¼ teaspoon/1 g)
**Calories:** 4 (17 kJ)
**Protein:** 0.7 g
**Total fat:** 0 g
**Saturated fat:** 0 g
**Carbohydrates:** 0.2 g
**Fiber:** 0 g

Blue-green algae form a large group of organisms, also known as cyanobacteria (a reference to their blue, or cyan, color), found in the ocean, fresh water, and soil crusts of arid areas. Fossilized remains of blue-green algae suggest that they have existed for as long as 3.5 billion years. Recently, these algae have been found in the most barren areas of Antarctica and the Arctic, where little other life exists, surviving only on rocks just below the surface of the ocean and lakes. They even appear to inhabit underground layers of rocks such as limestone.

Interest in the use of algae as a low-cost and nutritious food source grew through the 1950s and 1960s, and they were first made into a nutritional supplement in the 1970s. Today blue-green algae can be purchased in powder or tablet form. They are an excellent source of protein, vitamins A, B12 (a mere ¼ teaspoon of the powder contains an entire day's supply), and C, and manganese, and also contain carotenoids as beta-carotene and other antioxidants.

### THE HEALTHY EVIDENCE

In a 2010 study published in the journal *Trials*, researchers at the Western Australian Centre for Health and Ageing reported on the effects of supplementation with specific

## Making the Most of Blue-green Algae

Powdered blue-green algae can be combined with dry ingredients in recipes for baked goods, and not much is needed to derive the nutritional benefits. You can also boost the antioxidant content of almost any food by adding just ¼ teaspoon of powdered blue-green algae per serving.

B vitamins, including B12, on 300 older adults who reported significant depression. They found that the supplementation was associated with a statistically significant improvement in their subjects' condition and concluded, "we anticipate that our findings will have implications for clinical practice and health policy development."

BELOW Blue-green algae are cultivated commercially to produce a range of supplements. The largest US source is Upper Klamath Lake in Oregon.

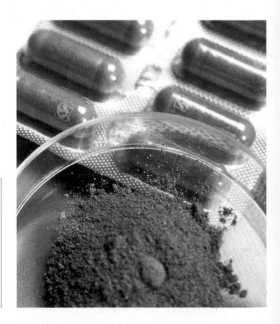

## In a Nutshell

**Origin:** Oceans, freshwater lakes, and soil crusts worldwide

**Season:** Available year-round

**Why they're super:** High in vitamins A, B12, C, protein, and manganese; contain beta-carotene and other antioxidants

**Growing at home:** Not applicable

# Spirulina

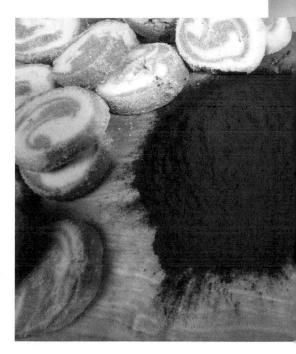

ABOVE Powdered spirulina can be used to add nutrients to sweet snacks such as cookies and cakes, and is sometimes included in energy bars.

## What's in a Serving?

**POWDERED SPIRULINA**
(¼ cup/28 g)
**Calories:** 81 (340 kJ)
**Protein:** 16 g
**Total fat:** 2.2 g
**Saturated fat:** 0.7 g
**Carbohydrates:** 6.7 g
**Fiber:** 1 g

Spirulina is a specific type of blue-green algae, or rather two types, as it is derived from two species, *Arthrospira platensis* and *Arthrospira maxima*. It was harvested from the surfaces of lakes by the Aztecs, who made it into cakes that were an important part of their diet. More recently, it has been cultivated in artificial ponds so that it can be collected and used as a nutritional supplement. Its benefits have been recognized among health-food enthusiasts since the 1970s, but it is still unfamiliar among the wider population.

Spirulina can be purchased whole and dried, as flakes, powder, and tablets. It is an excellent source of protein, pantothenic acid, thiamine, riboflavin, niacin, copper, iron, manganese, magnesium, and potassium, and a good source of vitamins B6, C, E, and K and folate. It also contains numerous phytochemicals, including antioxidants.

### THE HEALTHY EVIDENCE

A 2009 review published in the *Journal of Medicinal Food* discussed studies of the health effects of spirulina. The authors noted that studies carried out using both animal and human subjects pointed to a beneficial effect on blood cholesterol, triglyceride levels, and blood pressure, which in turn suggests

## In a Nutshell

**Origin:** Oceans and lakes worldwide
**Season:** Available year-round
**Why it's super:** High in protein, pantothenic acid, thiamine, riboflavin, niacin, copper, iron, manganese, magnesium, and potassium; good source of vitamins B6, C, E, and K and folate; contains antioxidants
**Growing at home:** Not applicable

a potentially significant role for spirulina in the prevention of cardiovascular disease.

Another 2009 study, published in the *International Journal of Biological Sciences*, reported on spirulina's effects on liver cancer in rats. The authors discussed other studies demonstrating the algae's antioxidant, anti-inflammatory, and anticancer properties, and reported that the rats that received spirulina were protected against induced liver cancer. This led them to propose that spirulina may have a use in preventing this cancer.

## Making the Most of Spirulina

Dried spirulina is more readily available than fresh spirulina, and it can be used in many recipes, thereby adding abundant antioxidants and nutrients. Try it in soups, stews, and dips, and include it in smoothie beverages. For a healthy guacamole dip, combine the following ingredients in a blender until smooth: 2 avocados, juice from 1 lemon, 2 teaspoons of minced garlic, ¼ cup (28 g) of spirulina, 1 tomato, 1 onion, and salt and pepper to taste.

# Chlorella

Chlorella is a species of one-celled green algae in the phylum *Chlorophyta*. Its name is a combination of the Greek word for green, *chloros*, and the Latin suffix indicating small size, *ella*. The Greek word also indicates that the organism contains chlorophyll and uses the process of photosynthesis to generate energy.

Concerns in the 1950s and 1960s about an impending population explosion and subsequent food shortages led many researchers to propose widespread use of chlorella as a nutrient-rich and low-cost food source. Many prestigious scientific research institutions, notably the Stanford Research Institute, undertook serious studies of the algae that received extensive media coverage and led to wider use of the algae as a nutritional supplement.

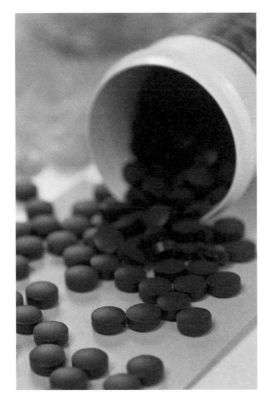

## Making the Most of Chlorella

Dried chlorella can be added to most foods to boost nutrients and antioxidants. Try adding a few tablespoons to your favorite stew recipe, especially a highly flavored stew with a thick consistency, or mix it in sauces, such as pasta sauces.

### In a Nutshell

**Origin:** Oceans and lakes worldwide
**Season:** Available year-round
**Why it's super:** High in vitamins A and B6, protein, riboflavin, thiamine, niacin, iron, zinc, magnesium, and phosphorus; contains beta-carotene and other antioxidants
**Growing at home:** Not applicable

LEFT In their natural state, chlorella algae cannot be digested by the human intestine. Chemical treatment is therefore required to break down the algae's strong cell walls before they can be used in supplements.

Chlorella can now be purchased as dried granules and in tablet form. It is an excellent source of vitamins A and B6, protein, riboflavin, thiamine, niacin, iron, zinc, magnesium, and phosphorus. It also contains antioxidant carotenoids, including beta-carotene, and other antioxidants.

### What's in a Serving?

**DRIED CHLORELLA**
**(2 tablespoons/15 g)**
**Calories:** 63 (264 kJ)
**Protein:** 9.3 g
**Total fat:** 1.8 g
**Saturated fat:** 0.3 g
**Carbohydrates:** 2.4 g
**Fiber:** 1.8 g

## THE HEALTHY EVIDENCE

A 2009 study published in the *Annals of the New York Academy of Sciences* reported on the health benefits of chlorella. The authors noted that it has "many biological merits for promoting health," including enhancing the immune system and helping to prevent cancer. They found that chlorella extract reduced the accumulation of fat in human fat cells and theorized that it may be useful as an anti-obesity agent. Another study published in the *Journal of Agricultural and Food Chemistry* reported that chlorella reduced the growth of human colon cancer cells, concluding that it might be a "useful functional ingredient in the prevention of human cancers."

# Whey Protein

Whey is the liquid byproduct of cheese production, and whey protein is a mixture of globular proteins that is isolated from the whey by filtering and drying. Three forms of whey protein are produced: isolate, hydrolysate, and concentrate. The isolate contains no fat, while the concentrate contains a small amount. The hydrolysate is treated (hydrolyzed) to degrade the proteins and make them easier for the body to absorb, but it is more expensive for this reason and therefore less widely used.

Whey protein is of particular interest for its bioactive compounds, which may possess anti-inflammatory and anticancer properties. These tend to be found at a higher level, not surprisingly, in the concentrate. Most commercial whey products contain a combination of the isolate and the concentrate. Whey

BELOW Whey protein enhances the synthesis of glutathione, an important antioxidant that has been shown to bolster the immune system.

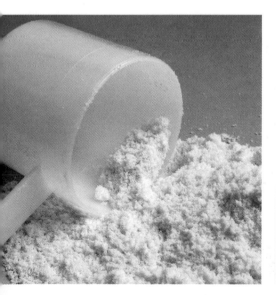

## Making the Most of Whey Protein

Powdered whey protein makes an excellent addition to baked grains, such as banana or other fruited quick breads. It can also be used to add high-quality protein to cookies, milkshakes, and smoothies.

protein is most commonly available in powdered form, but is also incorporated in snack bars and shakes.

An excellent source of protein, calcium, and phosphorus, whey protein is also a good source of potassium. Its bioactive compounds may enhance immune function and have antioxidant action.

### THE HEALTHY EVIDENCE

Dietary protein plays a role in weight regulation through its impact on hormones that affect appetite. A 2009 study published in the journal *Physiology and Behavior* reported on the effects of whey protein on appetite. It compared the effects of three different proteins in breakfasts—casein, soy, and whey—at varying levels of intake. The results showed that even at the lowest level of intake whey protein decreased hunger more than either casein or soy; and at the highest level, whey protein elicited stronger responses in hormone levels than the other proteins.

## What's in a Serving?

**WHEY PROTEIN POWDER**
(⅓ cup/33 g)
**Calories:** 135 (17 kJ)
**Protein:** 26 g
**Total fat:** 1 g
**Saturated fat:** 0.5 g
**Carbohydrates:** 3 g
**Fiber:** 0 g

## In a Nutshell

**Origin:** Europe and Asia; derived from cow's milk
**Season:** Available year-round
**Why it's super:** High in protein, calcium, and phosphorus; good source of potassium
**Growing at home:** Not applicable

# Yeast

Although many species of yeast are pathogens that cause sicknesses in humans, the yeast species *Saccharomyces cerevisiae* has been used for baking and the fermentation or brewing of drinks, notably wine and beer, for centuries. Indeed, it was probably one of the first organisms to be used domestically—baking stoves and grinding stones for making yeast bread have been discovered by archaeologists in Egyptian ruins dating back more than 4,000 years.

For most of history, people made use of this microorganism without understanding its nature. Only in 1860 did Louis Pasteur show that it was yeast organisms that caused the fermentation of wine and beer. In 1876, at the Centennial Exposition in Philadelphia, Charles L. Fleischmann introduced a

### In a Nutshell

**Origin:** Worldwide

**Season:** Available year-round

**Why it's super:** High in vitamins B6 and B12, folate, fiber, protein, riboflavin, thiamine, niacin, selenium, and zinc

**Growing at home:** Not applicable

commercial yeast product and a baked bread made with a yeast he had isolated and preserved in the form of a small cake. His product revolutionized baking and made the mass production and consumption of bread possible. The company he founded, the Fleischmann Yeast Company, went on to become the world's leading yeast producer.

RIGHT The yeast in brewer's yeast and other dietary yeasts has to be deactivated. Otherwise it would continue to grow in the body and deprive it of important nutrients.

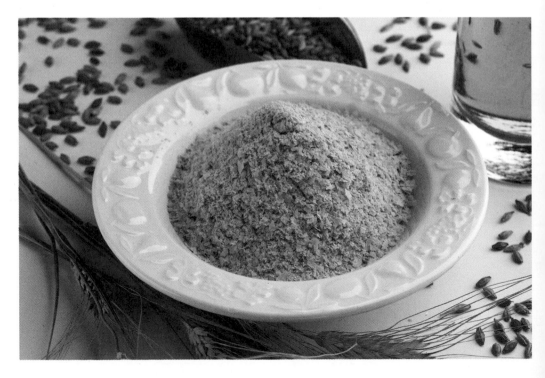

*Three things are good
in little measure and evil in large:
yeast, salt, and hesitation.*

The Talmud

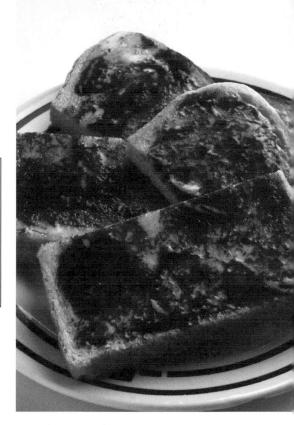

---

### Yeast Spreads

An extract of brewer's yeast is used to make Marmite, a food spread that is especially popular in the United Kingdom. A dark brown paste, with a potent, salty flavor, Marmite is an excellent source of several vitamins and minerals including vitamin B12, folate, thiamine, niacin, and iron. Another version of Marmite is made in New Zealand, and yeast extract is also used to make a similar product in Australia, called Vegemite, and another in Switzerland, called Cenovis.

---

## NUTRITIONAL PRODUCTS

Further scientific research established many of the health benefits of yeast, and led to its use as a nutritional supplement. Initially, it was the yeast byproduct of the beer-brewing process, so-called brewer's yeast, that became a popular supplement, particularly among vegetarians, who favored it for its high vitamin B content. This kind of yeast has a characteristic bitter hops flavor. A newer product is nutritional yeast, which is also derived from the beer-making process but subsequently treated in a different way. It is grown in a medium of enriched molasses, then pasteurized to kill off the yeast. This gives the product a different texture and flavor, akin to cheese, which leads many people, especially vegans, to use it as a substitute for Parmesan.

Now widely available as flakes or powders, brewer's and nutritional yeast are excellent sources of vitamins B6 and B12, folate, fiber, protein, riboflavin, thiamine, niacin, selenium, and zinc.

## THE HEALTHY EVIDENCE

Phytate is a compound found in many nutritious plant foods, which prevents absorption of nutrients, such as zinc and iron.

RIGHT Spreads such as Marmite are a convenient way to incorporate yeast in your diet, and are often especially popular with children.

A 2009 study published in *Animal Science Journal* reported that brewer's yeast produces an enzyme, known as phytase, which can degrade phytate and thereby prevent it from interfering with nutrient absorption.

A 2008 review published in *Urologic Nursing* discussed the benefits of yeast. The author, a researcher at the University of Michigan in Ann Arbor, noted that several studies have pointed to a potential immune-enhancing effect—most notably a randomized trial among adults, which showed that yeast significantly reduced both the incidence and duration of seasonal influenza.

---

### Making the Most of Brewer's Yeast

Yeast is a concentrated source of numerous nutrients, so a single tablespoon can significantly increase the nutritive value of almost any food. Try it in cold or hot cereal, or yogurt, or add it to sauces, soups, and casseroles, and to bread and muffins. Kept in a cool, dry place, yeast will keep for up to six to eight months; stored in the refrigerator, it will stay fresh for up to three years.

# REFERENCE

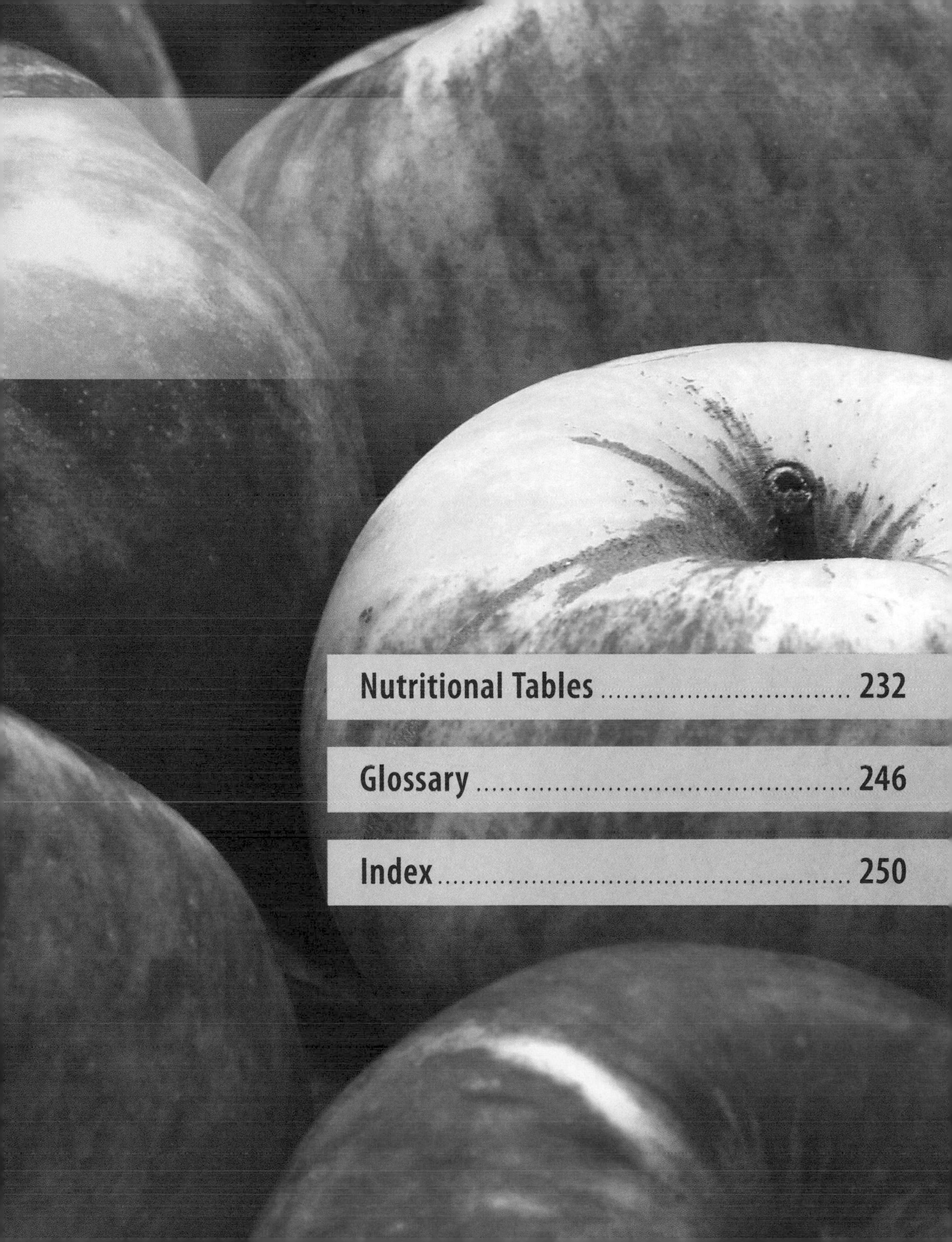

# Nutritional Tables

The tables below are intended as a quick-reference guide to the nutritional content of the "superfoods" in this book. The foods are listed under their chapter headings, and then in the order in which they appear within their chapter. Alongside the common name (or names) for the food are listed the botanical or scientific name (where relevant), and a typical serving size. For further details on the specific content of each serving, turn to the relevant page in the book and look under the heading "What's in a Serving?"

As noted in the Introduction (see p. 11), the best yardstick of the level of a nutrient in a food is the

## Vegetables

| Common Name | Scientific Name | SERVING SIZE | VITAMIN A | THIAMINE (B1) |
|---|---|---|---|---|
| Asparagus | *Asparagus officinalis* | 1 cup/180 g | ★★ | ★★ |
| Chard and Leaf Beets | *Beta vulgaris* var. *flavescens, Beta vulgaris* var. *flavescens* subsp. *cicla* | 1 cup/175 g | ★★ | |
| Chinese Mustard | *Brassica juncea* var. *rugosa* | 1 cup/140 g | ★★ | |
| Kale | *Brassica oleracea,* Acephala group | 1 cup/130 g | ★★ | |
| Collard | *Brassica oleracea,* Acephala group | 1 cup/190 g | ★★ | |
| Chinese Broccoli | *Brassica oleracea,* Alboglabra group | 1 cup/88 g | ★★ | ★ |
| Cauliflower | *Brassica oleracea,* Botrytis group | 1 cup/124 g | | |
| Cabbage | *Brassica oleracea,* Capitata group | 1 cup/150 g | | |
| Broccoli | *Brassica oleracea,* Cymosa group | 1 cup/156 g | ★★ | |
| Brussels Sprouts | *Brassica oleracea,* Gemmifera group | 1 cup/156 g | ★★ | |
| Asian Greens | *Brassica rapa* var. *chinensis, Brassica rapa* var. *nipposinica, Brassica rapa* var. *pekinensis, Brassica rapa* var. *rosularis* | 1 cup/170 g | ★★ | |
| Endive | *Cichorium endivia* | 2 cups/100 g | ★★ | |
| Globe Artichoke | *Cynara scolymus* | 1 cup/168 g | | |
| Arugula or Rocket | *Eruca sativa* | 2 cups/40 g | ★★ | |
| Fennel | *Foeniculum vulgare* | 1 tbsp/5.8 g | | |
| Romaine or Cos Lettuce | *Lactuca sativa* | 2 cups/94 g | ★★ | ★ |
| Alfalfa Sprouts | *Medicago sativa* | 2 cups/66 g | | |
| Watercress | *Nasturtium officinale* | 2 cups/68 g | ★★ | |
| Purslane | *Portulaca oleracea* | 1 cup/115 g | ★★ | |
| Spinach | *Spinacia oleracea* | 1 cup/180 g | ★★ | ★ |
| Okra | *Abelmoschus esculentus* | 1 cup/160 g | ★ | |
| Bell Pepper or Capsicum | *Capsicum annuum* | 1 cup/149 g | ★★ | ★ |
| Chili Pepper | *Capsicum annuum* | 3 tbsp/28g | ★ | |
| Summer Squash | *Cucurbita pepo* | 1 cup/180 g | ★★ | ★ |
| Winter Squash or Pumpkin | *Cucurbita maxima, Cucurbita moschata, Cucurbita pepo* | ½ cup/102–123 g | ★★ | |

percentage of the Daily Value of the nutrient a standard serving provides. Throughout this book, if a food provides 5–9 percent of the Daily Value of a nutrient, it is said to be a good source of that nutrient; and if it supplies 10 percent or more, it is considered an excellent source. In the tables below, these levels are indicated with one and two stars, respectively. Note that the absence of a star does not necessarily indicate that the food does not contain the nutrient at all. The level may be very low, or, in some cases, the food may not have been analyzed for that particular nutrient. This is especially true of nonnutrient constituents, such as antioxidants.

| PANTOTHENIC ACID (B5) | VITAMIN B6 | FOLATE (B9) | VITAMIN B12 | VITAMIN C | VITAMIN D | VITAMIN E | VITAMIN K | FIBER | PROTEIN | CALCIUM | IRON | MAGNESIUM | PHOSPHORUS | POTASSIUM | SODIUM | ZINC | COPPER | MANGANESE | SELENIUM | ANTIOXIDANTS |
|---|---|---|---|---|---|---|---|---|---|---|---|---|---|---|---|---|---|---|---|---|
|  |  | ★★ |  | ★★ |  |  | ★★ | ★★ |  |  |  |  |  | ★★ |  |  | ★★ | ★★ |  | ★★ |
|  |  | ★★ |  | ★★ | ★★ | ★★ | ★★ |  |  | ★ | ★★ | ★★ |  | ★★ |  |  | ★ | ★★ |  | ★★ |
|  |  | ★★ |  | ★★ |  |  | ★★ | ★★ |  | ★★ |  |  |  | ★★ |  |  | ★★ | ★★ |  | ★★ |
|  |  | ★★ |  | ★ |  |  | ★★ | ★ |  | ★ |  |  |  | ★ |  |  | ★ | ★ |  | ★★ |
|  |  | ★★ |  | ★★ |  |  | ★★ | ★★ |  | ★★ |  |  |  | ★★ |  |  |  | ★★ |  | ★★ |
|  |  | ★★ |  | ★★ |  |  | ★★ | ★ |  | ★ |  |  |  | ★ |  |  |  | ★ |  | ★ |
|  | ★ | ★ |  | ★★ |  |  | ★★ | ★ |  |  |  |  |  |  |  |  |  | ★ |  |  |
|  | ★ | ★ |  | ★★ |  |  | ★★ | ★ |  |  |  |  |  | ★ |  |  |  | ★ |  |  |
|  |  | ★★ |  | ★★ |  |  | ★★ | ★★ |  |  |  |  | ★ |  | ★ |  |  |  | ★ |  | ★ |
|  |  | ★★ |  | ★★ |  |  | ★★ | ★ |  |  |  |  | ★ |  | ★ |  |  |  | ★ |  | ★ |
| ★★ | ★★ | ★★ |  | ★★ |  |  | ★★ |  |  | ★★ | ★★ |  |  | ★★ |  |  |  | ★★ |  | ★★ |
| ★ |  | ★★ |  | ★ |  |  | ★★ | ★★ |  |  |  |  |  | ★ |  |  |  | ★★ |  | ★ |
|  |  | ★★ |  | ★ |  |  | ★★ | ★★ |  |  | ★ |  |  | ★★ |  |  |  |  |  | ★ |
|  |  | ★★ |  | ★★ |  |  | ★★ |  |  | ★ |  | ★ |  |  |  |  |  |  |  | ★★ |
|  |  |  |  |  |  |  |  | ★★ | ★★ | ★ | ★ |  |  |  |  |  |  | ★ |  | ★★ |
|  |  | ★★ |  | ★★ |  |  | ★★ | ★ |  |  | ★ |  | ★ | ★ |  |  |  | ★★ |  | ★★ |
|  |  | ★ |  | ★ |  |  |  | ★ |  |  |  |  |  |  |  |  | ★ | ★ |  |  |
|  |  |  |  | ★★ |  |  | ★★ |  |  | ★ |  |  |  | ★ |  |  |  | ★ |  | ★★ |
|  |  |  |  | ★★ |  |  |  |  |  | ★ |  | ★ |  | ★ |  |  | ★ | ★ |  | ★★ |
|  | ★★ | ★★ |  | ★★ | ★★ | ★★ | ★★ |  |  | ★★ | ★★ | ★★ |  | ★★ |  | ★ | ★★ | ★★ |  | ★★ |
|  | ★ | ★ |  | ★★ |  | ★★ | ★★ |  |  | ★ |  | ★ |  | ★ |  |  | ★ | ★ |  | ★ |
| ★ | ★★ | ★★ |  | ★★ |  | ★ | ★★ |  |  |  |  |  |  | ★ |  |  |  | ★ |  | ★★ |
|  | ★ |  |  | ★★ |  |  | ★ |  |  |  |  |  |  |  |  |  |  |  |  |  |
|  | ★ | ★ |  | ★ |  |  | ★ |  |  |  |  | ★ |  | ★ |  |  | ★ | ★ |  | ★★ |
|  |  | ★★ |  |  |  |  | ★★ |  |  |  |  |  |  | ★★ |  |  |  | ★★ |  | ★★ |

# Vegetables

| Common Name | Scientific Name | Serving Size | Vitamin A | Thiamine (B1) |
|---|---|---|---|---|
| Tomato | *Lycopersicon esculentum* | 1 cup/180 g | ★★ | |
| Bitter Melon or Goya | *Momordica charantia* | 1 cup/180 g | | ★ |
| Mung Sprouts | *Phaseolus aureus* | 2 cups/208 g | | |
| Pea Sprouts | *Pisum sativum* var. *macrocarpon* | 2 cups/208 g | ★★ | |
| Green Beans | *Phaseolus coccineus, Phaseolus vulgaris, Vigna unguiculata* | 1 cup/125 g | ★★ | |
| Peas | *Pisum sativum, Pisum sativum* var. *macrocarpon* | 1 cup/160 g | ★★ | ★★ |
| Eggplant or Aubergine | *Solanum melongena* | 1 cup/99 g | | ★ |
| Broad or Fava Bean | *Vicia faba* | 1 cup/126 g | ★ | ★ |
| Onion | *Allium cepa* | ½ cup/105 g | | |
| Leek | *Allium porrum* | ½ cup/52 g | | |
| Beetroot or Beet | *Beta vulgaris* | 1 cup/170 g | | |
| Turnips | *Brassica napus* var. *napobrassica, Brassica napus* var. *rapifera* | 1 cup/156 g | | |
| Turnip Greens | *Brassica napus* var. *napobrassica, Brassica napus* var. *rapifera* | 1 cup/156 g | ★★ | |
| Carrot | *Daucus carota* | 1 cup/156 g | ★★ | ★ |
| Sweet Potato or Kumara | *Ipomoea batatas* | 1 cup/200 g | ★★ | ★★ |
| Jicama | *Pachyrhizus erosus* | 1 cup/120 g | | |
| Dulse | *Palmaria palmata* | ⅓ cup/7 g | | ★ |
| Nori | *Porphyra* species | 4 sheets/10 g | ★★ | |
| Kombu | *Saccharina japonica* | ½ cup/40 g | | |
| Wakame | *Undaria pinnatifida* | ½ cup/40 g | | |

# Mushrooms

| Common Name | Scientific Name | Serving Size | Vitamin A | Thiamine (B1) |
|---|---|---|---|---|
| White, Brown, and Field Mushrooms | *Agaricus bisporus, Agaricus campestris* | 1 cup/72 g | | ★ |
| Porcini or Cep | *Boletus edulis* | 1 cup/75 g | | ★ |
| Chanterelle or Girole | *Cantharellus cibarius* | 1 cup/54 g | | |
| Enoki | *Flammulina velutipes* | 1 cup/65 g | | |
| Maitake | *Grifola frondosa* | 1 cup/70 g | | ★ |
| Shimeji | *Hypsizygus marmoreus* | 1 cup/114 g | | ★ |
| Shiitake | *Lentinula edodes* | 1 piece/76 g | | |
| Morel | *Morchella esculenta* | 1 cup/66 g | | |
| Oyster Mushroom | *Pleurotus ostreatus* | 1 cup/86 g | | |
| Straw Mushroom | *Volvariella volvacea* | 1 cup/114 g | | |

| PANTOTHENIC ACID (B5) | VITAMIN B6 | FOLATE (B9) | VITAMIN B12 | VITAMIN C | VITAMIN D | VITAMIN E | VITAMIN K | FIBER | PROTEIN | CALCIUM | IRON | MAGNESIUM | PHOSPHORUS | POTASSIUM | SODIUM | ZINC | COPPER | MANGANESE | SELENIUM | ANTIOXIDANTS |
|---|---|---|---|---|---|---|---|---|---|---|---|---|---|---|---|---|---|---|---|---|
|  | ★ | ★ |  | ★★ |  |  | ★★ | ★ |  |  |  |  |  | ★ |  |  |  | ★ |  | ★ |
|  |  | ★★ |  | ★★ |  |  | ★ | ★★ |  |  |  |  |  | ★★ |  | ★ |  |  |  |  |
| ★ | ★ | ★★ |  | ★★ |  |  | ★★ | ★ |  |  | ★ | ★ |  | ★ |  |  | ★ | ★ |  |  |
| ★ | ★ | ★★ |  | ★★ |  | ★★ | ★★ | ★ |  |  | ★ | ★ |  | ★ |  |  | ★ | ★ |  | ★★ |
|  |  | ★ |  | ★★ |  |  | ★★ | ★★ |  | ★ | ★ | ★ |  | ★ |  |  | ★ | ★★ |  | ★ |
|  | ★★ | ★★ |  | ★★ |  |  | ★★ | ★★ | ★★ |  | ★ | ★ |  | ★ |  | ★ | ★ |  |  | ★ |
|  | ★ |  |  |  |  |  |  | ★ |  |  |  |  |  | ★ |  |  |  | ★ | ★ |  |
|  |  | ★★ |  | ★ |  |  |  | ★ | ★★ |  | ★ | ★ |  | ★ |  |  |  | ★ | ★★ |  |
|  | ★ |  |  | ★ |  |  |  | ★ |  |  |  |  |  | ★ |  |  |  | ★ |  | ★★ |
|  |  |  |  | ★ |  |  | ★ |  |  |  |  |  |  |  |  |  |  | ★ |  |  |
|  | ★ | ★★ |  | ★ |  |  | ★★ | ★★ |  |  | ★ | ★ |  | ★ |  |  |  | ★★ |  | ★★ |
|  | ★ |  |  | ★★ |  |  | ★★ | ★★ |  | ★ |  |  |  | ★ |  |  |  | ★ |  | ★★ |
| ★★ | ★★ | ★★ |  | ★★ |  | ★★ | ★★ | ★★ | ★★ |  |  |  |  | ★★ |  |  | ★★ | ★★ |  | ★★ |
|  | ★ | ★ |  | ★ |  | ★ | ★★ | ★★ |  |  |  |  |  | ★ |  |  |  | ★ |  | ★★ |
| ★★ | ★★ |  |  | ★★ |  | ★ |  | ★★ | ★ | ★ | ★ | ★★ |  | ★★ |  |  | ★★ | ★★ |  | ★★ |
|  |  | ★★ |  |  |  |  |  | ★★ |  |  |  |  |  | ★ |  |  |  |  |  | ★★ |
|  | ★★ |  | ★★ |  |  |  |  | ★ |  |  |  | ★★ |  | ★★ |  |  |  |  |  | ★★ |
|  |  | ★★ |  | ★★ |  |  | ★★ |  | ★ |  |  | ★ |  | ★★ |  |  |  |  |  | ★★ |
|  |  | ★★ |  |  |  |  | ★★ |  |  | ★ | ★ | ★★ |  |  |  |  |  |  |  | ★★ |
|  |  | ★★ |  |  |  |  |  | ★ |  |  |  | ★ |  |  |  |  |  | ★★ |  | ★★ |

| PANTOTHENIC ACID (B5) | VITAMIN B6 | FOLATE (B9) | VITAMIN B12 | VITAMIN C | VITAMIN D | VITAMIN E | VITAMIN K | FIBER | PROTEIN | CALCIUM | IRON | MAGNESIUM | PHOSPHORUS | POTASSIUM | SODIUM | ZINC | COPPER | MANGANESE | SELENIUM | ANTIOXIDANTS |
|---|---|---|---|---|---|---|---|---|---|---|---|---|---|---|---|---|---|---|---|---|
| ★★ |  |  |  |  |  |  |  |  |  |  |  |  |  | ★★ |  | ★ | ★★ | ★ | ★★ |  |
| ★★ |  | ★★ |  |  |  |  |  | ★★ |  |  |  |  |  |  |  | ★★ |  |  |  | ★ |
| ★ |  |  |  |  |  | ★★ |  |  |  |  | ★★ |  |  | ★★ |  |  | ★★ |  |  |  |
| ★★ |  |  |  |  |  |  |  |  |  |  |  |  |  | ★ |  |  |  |  |  | ★ |
|  |  | ★ |  |  |  |  |  |  |  |  |  |  |  |  |  |  | ★★ |  |  |  |
|  |  |  |  |  |  |  | ★ |  |  |  |  |  |  | ★★ |  |  |  |  |  |  |
| ★★ | ★ |  |  |  |  |  |  |  |  |  |  |  |  |  |  | ★ | ★★ | ★ | ★★ |  |
|  |  |  |  |  |  |  |  | ★★ |  |  |  |  |  | ★ |  | ★ | ★★ | ★★ |  |  |
| ★★ | ★ |  |  |  |  | ★ |  | ★★ |  |  |  |  |  | ★★ |  | ★ | ★★ |  |  |  |
| ★ |  | ★★ |  |  |  |  |  | ★★ |  |  |  |  |  | ★ |  | ★★ | ★★ | ★★ | ★★ | ★ |

# Legumes

| Common Name | Scientific Name | SERVING SIZE | VITAMIN A | THIAMINE (B1) |
|---|---|---|---|---|
| Pigeon Pea | *Cajanus cajan* | 1 cup/168 g | | ★★ |
| Chickpea or Garbanzo | *Cicer arietinum* | 1 cup/164 g | | ★★ |
| Soybean | *Glycine max* | 1 cup/180 g | | ★★ |
| Lentil | *Lens culinaris* | 1 cup/198 g | | ★★ |
| Beans | *Lupinus* species, *Phaseolus* species | 1 cup/172 g | | ★★ |
| Split Pea | *Pisum sativum* | 1 cup/196 g | | ★★ |
| Black-eyed Pea | *Vigna unguiculata* | 1 cup/172 g | | ★★ |

# Fruits

| Common Name | Scientific Name | SERVING SIZE | VITAMIN A | THIAMINE (B1) |
|---|---|---|---|---|
| Limes | *Citrus aurantifolia, Citrus hystrix, Citrus latifolia* | 2.4 ounces/67 g | | |
| Kumquat | *Citrus japonica* | 1.3 ounces/38 g | | |
| Oranges | *Citrus aurantium, Citrus aurantium* subsp. *bergamia, Citrus reticulata* x *Citrus sinensis, Citrus sinensis* | 5 ounces/141 g | ★ | ★★ |
| Lemons | *Citrus ichangensis, Citrus limetta, Citrus limon, Citrus* x *meyeri* | 3 ounces/84 g | | |
| Grapefruit | *Citrus* x *paradisi* | 1 cup/230 g | ★ | ★ |
| Tangerine, Mandarin, or Clementine | *Citrus reticulata* | 1 cup/195 g | ★★ | ★ |
| Tangelo | *Citrus* x *tangelo* | 1 cup/99 g | | |
| Avocado | *Persea americana* | 1 cup/150 g | | ★ |
| Date | *Phoenix dactylifera* | 2.6 ounces/72 g | | |
| Apricot | *Prunus armeniaca* | 1 cup/165 g | ★★ | |
| Sweet Cherries | *Prunus avium* | 1 cup/154 g | | |
| Sour Cherries | *Prunus cerasus* | 1 cup/155 g | ★★ | |
| Plums | *Prunus* x *domestica, Prunus institia, Prunus nigra, Prunus salicina, Prunus spinosa* | 1 cup/165 g | ★★ | |
| Nectarine | *Prunus persica* | 5.5 ounces/156 g | ★★ | |
| Peach | *Prunus persica* | 6.2 ounces/175 g | ★★ | |
| Japanese Persimmon | *Diospyros kaki* | 5.9 ounces/168 g | ★★ | |
| Apple | *Malus* x *domestica* | 6.4 ounces/182 g | | |
| Pears | *Pyrus communis, Pyrus pyrifolia* | 6.3 ounces/178 g | | |
| Pineapple | *Ananas comosus* | 1 cup/165 g | | ★ |
| Papaya | *Carica papaya* | 10.7 ounces/304 g | ★★ | ★ |
| Acai Berry (juice) | *Euterpe oleracea* | 1 cup/235 ml | | |

| PANTOTHENIC ACID (B5) | VITAMIN B6 | FOLATE (B9) | VITAMIN B12 | VITAMIN C | VITAMIN D | VITAMIN E | VITAMIN K | FIBER | PROTEIN | CALCIUM | IRON | MAGNESIUM | PHOSPHORUS | POTASSIUM | SODIUM | ZINC | COPPER | MANGANESE | SELENIUM | ANTIOXIDANTS |
|---|---|---|---|---|---|---|---|---|---|---|---|---|---|---|---|---|---|---|---|---|
| ★ |  | ★★ |  |  |  |  |  | ★★ | ★★ | ★ | ★★ | ★★ |  | ★★ |  | ★★ | ★★ | ★★ | ★ | ★ |
| ★ | ★★ | ★★ |  |  |  |  | ★ | ★★ | ★★ | ★ | ★★ | ★★ |  | ★★ |  | ★★ | ★★ | ★★ | ★ | ★ |
| ★ |  | ★★ |  | ★ |  |  | ★★ | ★★ | ★★ | ★★ | ★★ | ★★ |  | ★★ |  | ★★ | ★★ | ★★ | ★★ |  |
| ★★ | ★★ | ★★ |  | ★ |  |  |  | ★★ | ★★ |  | ★★ |  |  | ★★ |  | ★★ | ★★ | ★★ |  | ★ |
|  |  | ★★ |  |  |  |  |  | ★★ | ★★ | ★ | ★★ | ★★ |  | ★★ |  | ★★ | ★★ | ★★ |  |  |
| ★★ | ★ | ★★ |  |  |  |  | ★★ | ★★ | ★★ |  | ★★ | ★★ |  | ★★ |  | ★★ | ★★ | ★★ |  |  |
| ★ | ★ | ★★ |  |  |  |  |  | ★★ | ★★ |  | ★★ | ★★ |  | ★★ |  | ★★ | ★★ | ★★ | ★ |  |

| PANTOTHENIC ACID (B5) | VITAMIN B6 | FOLATE (B9) | VITAMIN B12 | VITAMIN C | VITAMIN D | VITAMIN E | VITAMIN K | FIBER | PROTEIN | CALCIUM | IRON | MAGNESIUM | PHOSPHORUS | POTASSIUM | SODIUM | ZINC | COPPER | MANGANESE | SELENIUM | ANTIOXIDANTS |
|---|---|---|---|---|---|---|---|---|---|---|---|---|---|---|---|---|---|---|---|---|
|  |  |  |  | ★★ |  |  |  | ★ |  |  |  |  |  |  |  |  |  |  |  |  |
|  |  |  |  | ★★ |  |  |  | ★ |  |  |  |  |  |  |  |  |  |  |  | ★ |
| ★ | ★ | ★ |  | ★★ |  |  |  | ★★ |  | ★ |  | ★ |  | ★ |  |  |  |  |  | ★ |
|  |  |  |  | ★★ |  |  |  | ★★ |  |  |  |  |  |  |  |  |  |  |  | ★ |
| ★ | ★ |  |  | ★★ |  |  |  | ★★ |  |  |  | ★ |  | ★★ |  |  | ★ |  | ★ | ★ |
|  | ★ | ★ |  | ★★ |  |  |  | ★★ |  | ★ |  | ★ |  | ★★ |  |  |  |  |  | ★ |
|  |  | ★ |  | ★★ |  |  |  | ★★ |  |  |  |  |  | ★ |  |  |  |  |  | ★ |
| ★★ | ★★ | ★★ |  | ★★ |  | ★★ | ★★ | ★★ |  |  | ★ | ★★ | ★ | ★★ |  | ★ | ★★ | ★★ |  | ★ |
| ★ | ★ |  |  | ★★ |  |  |  | ★★ |  | ★ |  |  |  | ★★ |  |  | ★★ | ★★ |  |  |
|  |  |  |  | ★★ |  | ★ | ★ | ★★ | ★ |  |  |  |  | ★★ |  |  | ★ | ★ |  | ★ |
|  |  |  |  | ★★ |  |  |  | ★★ |  |  |  |  |  | ★★ |  |  | ★ | ★ |  |  |
|  |  |  |  | ★★ |  |  |  | ★★ |  |  |  |  |  | ★ |  |  | ★ | ★ |  | ★ |
|  |  |  |  | ★★ |  |  | ★★ | ★★ |  |  |  |  |  | ★ |  |  | ★ |  |  | ★ |
|  |  |  |  | ★★ |  | ★ |  | ★★ |  |  |  |  |  | ★ |  |  | ★ |  |  | ★ |
|  |  |  |  | ★★ |  | ★ | ★ | ★★ |  |  |  |  |  | ★★ |  |  | ★ | ★ |  | ★ |
|  | ★ |  |  | ★★ |  | ★ | ★ | ★★ |  |  |  |  |  | ★ |  |  | ★ | ★★ |  | ★ |
|  |  |  |  | ★ |  |  | ★ | ★★ |  |  |  |  |  | ★ |  |  |  |  |  | ★ |
|  |  |  |  | ★ |  |  | ★ | ★★ |  |  |  |  |  | ★ |  |  | ★ |  |  | ★ |
|  | ★ | ★ |  | ★★ |  |  |  |  |  |  |  |  |  | ★ |  | ★ |  | ★ | ★★ |  | ★ |
| ★ |  | ★★ |  | ★★ |  | ★★ | ★★ | ★★ |  | ★ | ★ |  |  | ★★ |  |  | ★ |  |  | ★ |
|  |  |  |  | ★★ |  | ★★ |  |  |  |  |  | ★★ |  | ★ |  |  |  |  |  | ★ |

# Fruits

| Common Name | Scientific Name | SERVING SIZE | VITAMIN A | THIAMINE (B1) | |
|---|---|---|---|---|---|
| Mango | *Mangifera indica* | 7.3 ounces/207 g | ★★ | ★ | |
| Noni (juice) | *Morinda citrifolia* | 2 ounces/60 ml | | | |
| Banana | *Musa acuminata* | 4.2 ounces/118 g | | | |
| Guavas | *Psidium guajava, Psidium littorale* | 1 cup/165 g | ★★ | ★ | |
| Kiwi Fruits | *Actinidia arguta, Actinidia chinensis, Actinidia deliciosa* | 1 cup/180 g | | | |
| Watermelon | *Citrullus lanatus* | 10 ounces/286 g | ★★ | ★ | |
| Cantaloupe or Rockmelon | *Cucumism melo var. cantalupensis* | 1 cup/177 g | ★★ | ★ | |
| Passionfruit | *Passiflora edulis* | 1 cup/236 g | ★★ | | |
| Grape | *Vitis vinifera* | 1 cup/92 g | | ★ | |
| Fig | *Ficus carica* | ½ cup/75 g | | ★ | |
| Strawberry | *Fragaria* x *ananassa* | 1 cup/166 g | | | |
| Goji Berry or Wolfberry | *Lycium barbarum, Lycium chinense* | ¼ cup/28 g | ★★ | | |
| Pomegranate (juice) | *Punica granatum* | 1 cup/235 ml | | | |
| Blackberry | *Rubus fruticosus* | 1 cup/144 g | ★ | | |
| Raspberry | *Rubus idaeus* | 1 cup/123 g | | | |
| Loganberry | *Rubus* x *loganbaccus* | 1 cup/147 g | | ★ | |
| Elderberry | *Sambucus nigra* | 1 cup/145 g | ★★ | ★ | |
| Blueberries | *Vaccinium ashei, Vaccinium corymbosum, Vaccinium lamarckii* | 1 cup/148 g | | | |
| Cranberries | *Vaccinium macrocarpon, Vaccinium oxycoccus* | ½ cup/50 g | | | |
| Bilberry (juice) | *Vaccinium myrtillus* | ½ cup/120 ml | | | |

# Nuts and Oils

| Common Name | Scientific Name | SERVING SIZE | VITAMIN A | THIAMINE (B1) | |
|---|---|---|---|---|---|
| Cashew | *Anacardium occidentale* | 1 ounce/28.4 g | | | |
| Brazil Nut | *Bertholletia excelsa* | 1 ounce/28.4 g | | | |
| Pecan | *Carya illinoinensis* | 1 ounce/28.4 g | | ★ | |
| Hazelnuts | *Corylus avellana, Corylus maxima* | 1 ounce/28.4 g | | | |
| Pumpkin Seed | *Cucurbita maxima* | 1 ounce/28.4 g | | | |
| Sunflower Seed | *Helianthus annuus* | 1 ounce/28.4 g | | | |
| Walnuts | *Juglans cinerea, Juglans nigra, Juglans regia* | 1 ounce/28.4 g | | ★ | |
| Flax Seed or Linseed | *Linum usitatissimum* | ¼ cup/28 g | | ★★ | |
| Macadamia | *Macadamia integrifolia* | 1 ounce/28.4 g | | ★★ | |
| Pistachio | *Pistachia vera* | 1 ounce/28.4 g | | ★★ | |

| PANTOTHENIC ACID (B5) | VITAMIN B6 | FOLATE (B9) | VITAMIN B12 | VITAMIN C | VITAMIN D | VITAMIN E | VITAMIN K | FIBER | PROTEIN | CALCIUM | IRON | MAGNESIUM | PHOSPHORUS | POTASSIUM | SODIUM | ZINC | COPPER | MANGANESE | SELENIUM | ANTIOXIDANTS |
|---|---|---|---|---|---|---|---|---|---|---|---|---|---|---|---|---|---|---|---|---|
|  | ★★ | ★ |  | ★★ |  | ★★ | ★★ | ★★ |  |  |  | ★ |  | ★ |  |  | ★★ |  |  | ★ |
|  |  |  |  | ★ |  |  |  |  |  |  |  |  |  |  |  | ★ |  |  |  | ★ |
|  | ★★ | ★ |  | ★★ |  |  |  | ★★ |  |  |  | ★ |  | ★★ |  |  | ★ | ★★ |  | ★ |
| ★ | ★ | ★★ |  | ★★ |  | ★ | ★ | ★★ | ★ |  |  | ★ | ★ | ★★ |  |  | ★★ | ★★ |  | ★ |
|  | ★ | ★★ |  | ★★ |  | ★★ | ★★ | ★★ |  | ★ |  | ★ | ★ | ★★ |  |  | ★★ | ★ |  | ★ |
|  | ★ |  |  | ★★ |  | ★ |  |  |  |  |  | ★ |  | ★ |  |  | ★ |  |  | ★ |
|  | ★ | ★ |  | ★★ |  |  | ★ |  |  |  |  | ★ |  | ★ |  |  |  |  |  | ★ |
|  | ★★ | ★ |  | ★★ |  |  |  | ★★ | ★★ |  | ★★ | ★★ | ★★ | ★★ |  |  | ★★ |  |  | ★ |
|  | ★ |  |  | ★ |  | ★★ |  |  |  |  |  |  |  | ★ |  |  |  | ★★ |  | ★ |
|  | ★ |  |  |  |  |  | ★★ | ★★ | ★ | ★★ | ★ | ★★ | ★ | ★★ |  |  | ★★ | ★★ |  | ★ |
|  |  | ★★ |  | ★★ |  |  | ★ | ★★ |  | ★ |  |  | ★ |  | ★ |  |  |  | ★★ |  | ★ |
|  |  |  |  | ★★ |  |  |  | ★★ |  | ★ |  |  |  |  |  |  |  |  |  |  | ★ |
| ★ | ★ | ★★ |  |  |  | ★ | ★★ |  |  |  |  |  |  | ★★ |  |  |  | ★★ |  | ★ |
|  |  | ★★ |  | ★★ |  | ★ | ★★ | ★★ |  |  | ★ | ★ |  | ★ |  | ★ | ★★ | ★★ |  | ★ |
|  |  | ★ |  | ★★ |  | ★ | ★★ | ★★ |  |  | ★ | ★ |  | ★ |  |  | ★ | ★★ |  | ★ |
|  | ★ | ★★ |  | ★★ |  | ★ | ★★ | ★★ |  |  | ★ | ★ |  | ★ |  |  | ★ | ★★ |  | ★ |
|  | ★★ |  |  | ★★ |  |  |  | ★★ |  | ★ | ★★ |  | ★ | ★★ |  |  |  |  |  | ★ |
|  |  |  |  | ★★ |  |  | ★★ | ★★ |  |  |  |  |  |  |  |  |  | ★★ |  | ★ |
|  |  |  |  | ★★ |  |  |  | ★ |  |  |  |  |  |  |  |  |  | ★ |  | ★ |
|  |  |  |  | ★★ |  |  |  |  |  |  |  |  |  |  |  |  |  |  |  | ★ |

| PANTOTHENIC ACID (B5) | VITAMIN B6 | FOLATE (B9) | VITAMIN B12 | VITAMIN C | VITAMIN D | VITAMIN E | VITAMIN K | FIBER | PROTEIN | CALCIUM | IRON | MAGNESIUM | PHOSPHORUS | POTASSIUM | SODIUM | ZINC | COPPER | MANGANESE | SELENIUM | ANTIOXIDANTS |
|---|---|---|---|---|---|---|---|---|---|---|---|---|---|---|---|---|---|---|---|---|
|  |  | ★ |  |  |  |  | ★★ |  | ★ |  | ★ | ★★ | ★★ | ★ |  | ★ | ★★ | ★ | ★ |  |
|  |  |  |  |  |  | ★★ |  | ★★ | ★ |  |  | ★★ | ★★ |  |  | ★★ | ★★ | ★★ | ★★ |  |
|  |  |  |  |  |  |  |  | ★★ | ★ |  |  | ★ | ★ |  |  | ★ | ★★ | ★★ |  |  |
|  |  |  |  |  |  | ★★ |  | ★★ |  | ★ |  | ★★ | ★ | ★ |  | ★ | ★★ | ★★ |  |  |
|  |  |  |  |  |  |  |  | ★★ | ★ |  | ★ | ★★ |  | ★ |  | ★★ | ★ | ★ |  |  |
| ★★ | ★★ | ★★ |  |  |  | ★★ |  | ★★ | ★★ | ★ |  | ★ | ★★ | ★ |  | ★ | ★★ | ★★ | ★★ |  |
|  | ★ | ★ |  |  |  |  |  | ★ | ★ |  | ★ | ★★ | ★ |  |  | ★ | ★★ | ★★ |  | ★ |
|  | ★ | ★ |  |  |  |  |  | ★★ | ★★ | ★ | ★ | ★★ | ★★ | ★ |  | ★ | ★★ |  | ★ |  |
|  |  |  |  |  |  |  |  | ★ |  |  |  | ★ | ★ |  |  |  | ★ | ★★ | ★★ |  |
|  | ★★ |  |  |  |  |  | ★ | ★★ | ★★ |  | ★ | ★ | ★★ | ★ |  |  | ★★ | ★★ |  | ★ |

# Nuts and Oils

| Common Name | Scientific Name | SERVING SIZE | VITAMIN A | THIAMINE (B1) |
|---|---|---|---|---|
| Olive Oil | *Olea europaea* | 1 tbsp/13.5 g | | |
| Almond | *Prunus dulcis* | 1 ounce/28.4 g | | |
| Sesame Seed | *Sesamum orientale* | 2 tbsp/18 g | | ★ |

# Herbs and Spices

| Common Name | Scientific Name | SERVING SIZE | VITAMIN A | THIAMINE (B1) |
|---|---|---|---|---|
| Garlic | *Allium sativum, Allium scordoprasum, Allium ursinum* | 4 cloves/12 g | | |
| Cinnamon Cassia | *Cinnamomum aromaticum* | 1 tbsp/7.8 g | | |
| Turmeric | *Curcuma longa* | 1 tbsp/6.8 g | | |
| Basil | *Ocimum basilicum* | 1 cup/24 g | ★★ | |
| Marjoram and Oregano | *Origanum majorana, Origanum onites, Origanum vulgare* | 2 tsp/3.6 g | | |
| Rosemary | *Rosmarinus officinalis* | 2 tsp/2.4 g | | |
| Parsley | *Petroselinum crispum* | 1 cup/60 g | ★★ | |
| Sage | *Salvia officinalis* | 2 tsp/1.4 g | | |
| Thyme | *Thymus x citriodora, Thymus serpyllum, Thymus vulgaris* | 2 tsp/2.8 g | | |
| Ginger | *Zingiber officinale* | ¼ cup/24 g | | |

# Grains

| Common Name | Scientific Name | SERVING SIZE | VITAMIN A | THIAMINE (B1) |
|---|---|---|---|---|
| Oats | *Avena sativa* | ½ cup/41 g | | ★★ |
| Bran | *Avena sativa, Hordeum vulgare* | ½ cup/47 g | | ★★ |
| Quinoa | *Chenopodium quinoa* | 1 cup/185 g | | ★★ |
| Millet | *Eleusine coracana, Panicum miliaceum, Pennisetum glaucum, Setaria italica* | 1 cup/174 g | | ★★ |
| Buckwheat | *Fagopyrum esculentum* | ¼ cup/41 g | | ★ |
| Barley | *Hordeum vulgare* | 1 cup/157 g | | ★ |
| Brown Rice | *Oryza sativa* | 1 cup/195 g | | ★★ |
| Whole Wheat Berries | *Triticum* species | 1 cup/195 g | | ★★ |
| Bulgur | *Triticum* species | 1 cup/182 g | | ★ |
| Wheat Germ | *Triticum* species | ½ cup/57 g | | ★★ |
| Whole-wheat Pasta | *Triticum* species | 1 cup/57 g | | ★★ |

| PANTOTHENIC ACID (B5) | VITAMIN B6 | FOLATE (B9) | VITAMIN B12 | VITAMIN C | VITAMIN D | VITAMIN E | VITAMIN K | FIBER | PROTEIN | CALCIUM | IRON | MAGNESIUM | PHOSPHORUS | POTASSIUM | SODIUM | ZINC | COPPER | MANGANESE | SELENIUM | ANTIOXIDANTS |
|---|---|---|---|---|---|---|---|---|---|---|---|---|---|---|---|---|---|---|---|---|
|  |  |  |  |  |  | ★ | ★ |  |  |  |  |  |  |  |  |  |  |  |  | ★ |
|  |  |  |  |  |  | ★★ |  | ★★ | ★★ | ★ | ★ | ★★ | ★★ | ★ |  | ★ | ★★ | ★★ |  | ★ |
|  | ★ |  |  |  |  |  |  | ★★ | ★ | ★★ | ★★ | ★★ |  |  |  | ★★ | ★★ | ★★ |  | ★ |

| PANTOTHENIC ACID (B5) | VITAMIN B6 | FOLATE (B9) | VITAMIN B12 | VITAMIN C | VITAMIN D | VITAMIN E | VITAMIN K | FIBER | PROTEIN | CALCIUM | IRON | MAGNESIUM | PHOSPHORUS | POTASSIUM | SODIUM | ZINC | COPPER | MANGANESE | SELENIUM | ANTIOXIDANTS |
|---|---|---|---|---|---|---|---|---|---|---|---|---|---|---|---|---|---|---|---|---|
|  | ★ |  |  | ★ |  |  |  |  |  |  |  |  |  |  |  |  |  | ★★ |  | ★ |
|  |  |  |  |  |  |  |  | ★★ |  | ★ |  |  |  |  |  |  |  | ★★ |  | ★ |
|  | ★ |  |  |  |  |  |  | ★ |  |  | ★★ |  |  | ★ |  |  |  | ★★ |  | ★ |
|  |  | ★ |  |  |  |  | ★★ |  |  |  |  |  |  |  |  |  |  | ★ |  | ★ |
|  |  |  |  |  |  |  | ★★ | ★ |  | ★ | ★ |  |  |  |  |  |  | ★ |  | ★ |
|  |  |  |  |  |  | ★ |  |  |  |  | ★ |  |  |  |  |  |  |  |  | ★ |
|  |  | ★★ |  | ★★ |  |  | ★★ | ★★ |  | ★ | ★★ | ★ |  | ★ |  |  |  | ★ |  | ★ |
|  |  |  |  |  |  |  | ★ |  |  |  |  |  |  |  |  |  |  |  |  | ★ |
|  |  |  |  |  |  |  | ★★ |  |  |  | ★★ |  |  |  |  |  |  | ★ |  | ★ |
|  |  |  |  |  |  |  |  |  |  |  |  |  |  |  |  |  |  |  |  | ★★ |

| PANTOTHENIC ACID (B5) | VITAMIN B6 | FOLATE (B9) | VITAMIN B12 | VITAMIN C | VITAMIN D | VITAMIN E | VITAMIN K | FIBER | PROTEIN | CALCIUM | IRON | MAGNESIUM | PHOSPHORUS | POTASSIUM | SODIUM | ZINC | COPPER | MANGANESE | SELENIUM | ANTIOXIDANTS |
|---|---|---|---|---|---|---|---|---|---|---|---|---|---|---|---|---|---|---|---|---|
| ★ |  |  |  |  |  |  |  | ★★ | ★★ |  | ★★ | ★★ | ★★ | ★ |  | ★★ | ★★ | ★★ | ★★ | ★ |
| ★ |  | ★ |  |  |  |  |  | ★★ | ★★ |  | ★★ | ★★ | ★★ | ★ |  | ★ | ★ | ★★ | ★★ | ★ |
|  | ★★ | ★★ |  |  |  | ★ |  | ★★ | ★★ |  | ★★ | ★★ | ★★ | ★ |  | ★★ | ★★ | ★★ | ★ | ★ |
|  | ★ | ★ |  |  |  |  |  | ★ | ★★ |  | ★ | ★★ | ★★ |  |  | ★★ | ★★ | ★★ |  | ★ |
| ★ | ★ |  |  |  |  |  |  | ★★ |  |  | ★ | ★★ | ★★ |  |  | ★ | ★★ | ★★ | ★ | ★ |
|  | ★ | ★ |  |  |  |  |  | ★★ |  |  | ★★ | ★ | ★ |  |  | ★ | ★ | ★★ | ★★ | ★ |
|  | ★★ |  |  |  |  |  |  | ★★ | ★ |  | ★ | ★★ | ★★ |  |  | ★ | ★ | ★★ | ★★ | ★ |
|  | ★ | ★ |  |  |  |  |  | ★★ | ★ |  | ★ | ★★ | ★★ | ★ |  | ★ | ★ | ★★ |  |  |
| ★ | ★ | ★ |  |  |  |  |  | ★★ | ★★ |  | ★★ | ★★ | ★ |  |  | ★ | ★ | ★★ |  | ★ |
| ★★ | ★★ | ★★ |  | ★ |  | ★★ | ★ | ★★ | ★★ | ★ | ★★ | ★★ | ★★ | ★★ |  | ★★ | ★★ | ★★ | ★★ | ★ |
|  | ★ | ★ |  |  |  |  |  | ★★ | ★★ |  | ★ |  |  |  |  |  | ★★ | ★★ |  | ★ |

# Grains

| Common Name | Scientific Name | SERVING SIZE | VITAMIN A | THIAMINE (B1) |
|---|---|---|---|---|
| Whole-wheat Bread | *Triticum* species | 2 slices/52 g | | ★★ |
| Spelt | *Triticum spelta* | 1 cup/194 g | | ★★ |
| Wild Rice | *Zizania aquatica, Zizania latifolia, Zizania palustris, Zizania texana* | 1 cup/164 g | | |
| Corn or Maize | *Zea mays* | 1 cup/149 g | ★ | ★★ |

# Meat, Seafood, and Dairy Foods

| Common Name | Scientific Name | SERVING SIZE | VITAMIN A | THIAMINE (B1) |
|---|---|---|---|---|
| Lean Red Meats (beef and lamb) | | 3 ounces/85 g | | ★ |
| Game (venison and kangaroo) | | 3 ounces/85 g | | ★★ |
| Liver | | 3 ounces/85 g | ★★ | ★★ |
| Pork | | 3 ounces/85 g | | ★★ |
| Veal | | 3 ounces/85 g | | |
| Skinless Chicken | | 3 ounces/85 g | | |
| Skinless Turkey | | 3 ounces/85 g | | |
| Squid | | 3 ounces/85 g | | |
| Octopus | | 3 ounces/85 g | | |
| Abalone | | 3 ounces/85 g | | ★★ |
| Clams | | 3 ounces/85 g | | ★ |
| Mussels | | 3 ounces/85 g | | ★ |
| Oysters | | 3 ounces/85 g | | ★ |
| Scallops | | 3 ounces/85 g | | |
| Crab | | 3 ounces/85 g | | ★ |
| Crayfish | | 3 ounces/85 g | | |
| Lobster | | 3 ounces/85 g | | |
| Prawn | | 3 ounces/85 g | | |
| Shrimp | | 3 ounces/85 g | | |
| Salmon | | 3 ounces/85 g | | ★★ |
| Trout | | 3 ounces/85 g | | ★ |
| Albacore Tuna | | 3 ounces/85 g | | |
| Bluefin Tuna | | 3 ounces/85 g | ★★ | ★★ |
| Light Tuna (canned) | | 3 ounces/85 g | | |
| Yellowfin Tuna | | 3 ounces/85 g | | ★★ |
| Sardines | | 3.75 ounces/92 g | | ★ |

| PANTOTHENIC ACID (B5) | VITAMIN B6 | FOLATE (B9) | VITAMIN B12 | VITAMIN C | VITAMIN D | VITAMIN E | VITAMIN K | FIBER | PROTEIN | CALCIUM | IRON | MAGNESIUM | PHOSPHORUS | POTASSIUM | SODIUM | ZINC | COPPER | MANGANESE | SELENIUM | ANTIOXIDANTS |
|---|---|---|---|---|---|---|---|---|---|---|---|---|---|---|---|---|---|---|---|---|
|  | ★ | ★★ |  |  |  |  |  | ★★ | ★★ |  | ★ | ★★ | ★★ |  |  | ★ | ★ | ★★ | ★★ | ★ |
|  | ★ | ★ |  |  |  |  |  | ★★ | ★★ |  | ★★ | ★★ | ★★ | ★ |  | ★★ | ★★ | ★★ | ★ | ★ |
|  | ★★ | ★★ |  |  |  |  |  | ★★ | ★★ |  | ★ | ★★ | ★★ | ★ |  | ★★ | ★★ | ★★ |  |  |
| ★★ | ★ | ★★ |  | ★★ |  |  |  | ★★ | ★★ |  |  | ★★ | ★★ | ★★ |  | ★ |  | ★★ |  | ★ |

| PANTOTHENIC ACID (B5) | VITAMIN B6 | FOLATE (B9) | VITAMIN B12 | VITAMIN C | VITAMIN D | VITAMIN E | VITAMIN K | FIBER | PROTEIN | CALCIUM | IRON | MAGNESIUM | PHOSPHORUS | POTASSIUM | SODIUM | ZINC | COPPER | MANGANESE | SELENIUM | ANTIOXIDANTS |
|---|---|---|---|---|---|---|---|---|---|---|---|---|---|---|---|---|---|---|---|---|
| ★ | ★★ |  | ★★ |  |  |  |  |  | ★★ |  | ★ | ★ | ★★ | ★ |  | ★★ |  |  | ★★ |  |
| ★ | ★★ |  | ★★ |  |  |  |  |  | ★★ |  | ★★ | ★ | ★★ | ★★ |  | ★★ | ★★ |  | ★★ |  |
| ★★ |  | ★★ | ★★ |  |  |  |  |  | ★★ |  | ★★ |  | ★★ | ★ |  | ★★ | ★★ | ★★ | ★★ |  |
| ★ | ★★ |  | ★★ |  |  |  |  |  | ★★ |  | ★ | ★ | ★★ | ★★ |  | ★★ |  |  | ★★ |  |
| ★ | ★★ |  | ★★ |  |  |  |  |  | ★★ |  |  | ★ | ★★ | ★★ |  | ★★ | ★ |  | ★★ |  |
| ★ | ★★ |  | ★ |  |  |  |  |  | ★★ |  | ★ | ★ | ★★ | ★ |  | ★ |  |  | ★★ |  |
| ★ | ★★ |  | ★ |  |  |  |  |  | ★★ |  | ★ | ★ | ★★ | ★ |  | ★★ |  |  | ★★ |  |
| ★★ | ★★ |  | ★★ |  |  | ★ |  |  | ★★ |  |  |  |  |  |  | ★★ |  |  | ★★ |  |
| ★★ | ★★ |  | ★★ |  |  | ★ |  |  | ★★ |  | ★★ |  |  |  |  | ★★ |  |  | ★★ |  |
| ★★ | ★ |  | ★★ |  |  | ★★ | ★★ |  |  |  | ★★ | ★★ | ★★ | ★ |  | ★ | ★ |  | ★★ |  |
|  |  |  | ★★ | ★★ |  |  |  |  |  |  | ★★ |  | ★★ | ★ |  | ★ | ★★ | ★★ | ★★ |  |
|  |  | ★ | ★★ | ★★ |  |  |  |  |  |  | ★★ | ★ | ★★ | ★ |  | ★ |  | ★★ | ★★ |  |
|  |  |  | ★★ | ★ |  |  |  |  |  |  | ★★ | ★ | ★ |  |  | ★★ | ★★ | ★★ | ★★ |  |
|  | ★ |  | ★★ |  |  |  |  |  |  |  |  | ★★ | ★★ | ★ |  | ★ |  |  | ★★ |  |
|  | ★ | ★ | ★★ |  |  |  |  |  |  | ★ |  | ★ | ★★ | ★ |  | ★★ | ★★ | ★ | ★★ |  |
| ★ | ★ | ★ | ★★ |  |  | ★★ |  |  |  |  |  | ★ | ★★ | ★ |  | ★ | ★★ | ★★ | ★★ |  |
| ★★ |  |  | ★★ |  |  | ★ |  |  |  |  |  | ★ | ★★ | ★ |  | ★★ | ★★ |  | ★★ |  |
|  | ★★ |  | ★★ |  |  | ★★ |  |  |  |  | ★ |  |  | ★ |  | ★★ |  | ★ | ★★ |  |
|  |  |  | ★★ |  | ★★ | ★ |  |  |  |  | ★★ | ★ | ★★ |  |  | ★ | ★★ |  | ★★ |  |
| ★★ | ★★ | ★ | ★★ | ★ |  | ★★ |  |  | ★★ |  |  | ★ | ★★ | ★ |  |  |  |  | ★★ |  |
| ★ | ★★ |  | ★★ |  |  |  |  |  | ★★ | ★ |  | ★ | ★★ | ★★ |  | ★ | ★ | ★ | ★★ |  |
|  | ★ |  | ★★ |  |  |  |  |  |  |  | ★ | ★ | ★★ | ★ |  |  |  |  | ★★ |  |
| ★ | ★★ |  | ★★ |  |  |  |  |  |  |  | ★ | ★★ | ★★ | ★ |  |  |  |  | ★★ |  |
|  | ★★ |  | ★★ |  |  |  |  |  |  |  | ★ | ★ | ★★ | ★ |  |  |  |  | ★★ |  |
| ★ | ★★ |  | ★ |  |  |  |  |  |  |  |  | ★★ | ★★ | ★★ |  |  |  |  | ★★ |  |
|  | ★ |  | ★★ |  | ★★ | ★ |  | ★★ | ★★ | ★★ | ★ | ★★ | ★★ |  |  | ★ |  |  | ★ | ★★ |

# Meat, Seafood, and Dairy Foods

| Common Name | Scientific Name | SERVING SIZE | VITAMIN A | THIAMINE (B1) |
|---|---|---|---|---|
| Pilchards | | 3.75 ounces/92 g | | ★ |
| Mackerel | | 3 ounces/85 g | | ★★ |
| Mullet | | 3 ounces/85 g | | ★ |
| Herring | | 3 ounces/85 g | | ★ |
| White Fish | | 3 ounces/85 g | | |
| Skim Milk and Reduced-fat Milk | | 1 cup/235 ml | ★★ | ★ |
| Cottage Cheese | | 4 ounces/113 g | | |
| Ricotta Cheese | | 4 ounces/124 g | ★★ | |
| Yogurt | | 1 cup/245 g | | ★ |
| Soy Milk | | 1 cup/227 g | ★★ | |
| Eggs | | 1 large/50 g | | |

# Beverages and Treats

| Common Name | Scientific Name | SERVING SIZE | VITAMIN A | THIAMINE (B1) |
|---|---|---|---|---|
| Tea | *Camellia sinensis* | 1 cup/235 g | | |
| Coffee | *Coffea arabica, Coffea robusta* | 8 ounces/235 g | | |
| Wheat and Barley Grass Juice | *Hordeum vulgare, Triticum* species | 4 ounces/113 g | ★★ | |
| Water | | 1 cup/235 ml | | |
| Dark Chocolate | | 1 ounce/28.4 g | | |

# Nutritional Supplements

| Common Name | Scientific Name | SERVING SIZE | VITAMIN A | THIAMINE (B1) |
|---|---|---|---|---|
| Blue-green Algae | | ¼ tsp/1 g | ★★ | |
| Spirulina | | ¼ cup/28 g | | ★★ |
| Chlorella | | 2 tbsp/15 g | ★★ | ★★ |
| Whey Protein | | ⅓ cup/33 g | | |
| Yeast | | 1 tbsp/15 g | | ★★ |

| PANTOTHENIC ACID (B5) | VITAMIN B6 | FOLATE (B9) | VITAMIN B12 | VITAMIN C | VITAMIN D | VITAMIN E | VITAMIN K | FIBER | PROTEIN | CALCIUM | IRON | MAGNESIUM | PHOSPHORUS | POTASSIUM | SODIUM | ZINC | COPPER | MANGANESE | SELENIUM | ANTIOXIDANTS |
|---|---|---|---|---|---|---|---|---|---|---|---|---|---|---|---|---|---|---|---|---|
| ★ | ★★ |  | ★★ |  | ★★ |  |  |  | ★★ | ★ | ★ | ★ | ★★ | ★★ |  | ★ |  |  | ★★ |  |
| ★ | ★★ |  | ★★ |  | ★★ | ★ | ★ |  | ★★ |  |  | ★ | ★★ | ★★ | ★ |  |  |  | ★★ |  |
| ★ | ★★ |  |  |  |  |  |  |  | ★★ | ★ | ★ | ★ | ★★ | ★★ |  |  |  |  | ★★ |  |
| ★ | ★★ |  | ★★ |  | ★★ |  |  |  | ★★ | ★ | ★ | ★ | ★★ | ★★ |  | ★ |  |  | ★★ |  |
|  | ★ |  | ★★ |  |  |  |  |  | ★★ |  |  |  | ★★ | ★ |  | ★ |  |  | ★★ |  |
| ★ | ★ |  | ★★ |  | ★★ |  |  |  | ★★ | ★★ |  | ★ | ★★ | ★★ |  | ★ |  |  | ★★ |  |
|  |  |  | ★★ |  |  |  |  |  | ★★ | ★ |  |  | ★★ |  |  |  |  |  | ★★ |  |
|  |  | ★ |  |  |  |  |  |  | ★★ | ★★ |  | ★ | ★★ |  |  |  | ★★ |  | ★★ |  |
| ★★ | ★ | ★ | ★★ |  |  |  |  |  | ★★ | ★★ |  | ★★ | ★★ | ★★ |  |  | ★★ |  | ★★ |  |
|  |  |  | ★★ |  | ★★ |  |  |  | ★★ | ★★ | ★ |  |  |  |  |  |  |  |  |  |
| ★ | ★ | ★ | ★★ |  |  |  |  |  | ★★ |  | ★ |  | ★★ |  |  |  |  |  | ★★ |  |

| PANTOTHENIC ACID (B5) | VITAMIN B6 | FOLATE (B9) | VITAMIN B12 | VITAMIN C | VITAMIN D | VITAMIN E | VITAMIN K | FIBER | PROTEIN | CALCIUM | IRON | MAGNESIUM | PHOSPHORUS | POTASSIUM | SODIUM | ZINC | COPPER | MANGANESE | SELENIUM | ANTIOXIDANTS |
|---|---|---|---|---|---|---|---|---|---|---|---|---|---|---|---|---|---|---|---|---|
|  |  |  |  |  |  |  |  |  |  |  |  |  |  |  |  |  |  |  |  | ★★ |
| ★ |  |  |  |  |  |  |  |  |  |  |  |  |  | ★ |  |  |  | ★ |  | ★ |
|  |  | ★★ |  | ★★ |  | ★ | ★★ | ★ |  |  | ★ | ★ |  | ★★ |  |  |  | ★★ | ★★ | ★ |
|  |  |  |  |  |  |  |  | ★ |  |  | ★★ | ★★ | ★ |  |  |  | ★★ | ★★ |  | ★ |

| PANTOTHENIC ACID (B5) | VITAMIN B6 | FOLATE (B9) | VITAMIN B12 | VITAMIN C | VITAMIN D | VITAMIN E | VITAMIN K | FIBER | PROTEIN | CALCIUM | IRON | MAGNESIUM | PHOSPHORUS | POTASSIUM | SODIUM | ZINC | COPPER | MANGANESE | SELENIUM | ANTIOXIDANTS |
|---|---|---|---|---|---|---|---|---|---|---|---|---|---|---|---|---|---|---|---|---|
|  |  |  | ★★ | ★★ |  |  |  |  | ★★ |  |  |  |  |  |  |  |  | ★★ |  | ★ |
| ★★ | ★ | ★ |  | ★ |  | ★ | ★ |  | ★★ |  | ★★ | ★★ |  | ★★ |  |  |  | ★★ | ★★ | ★ |
|  | ★★ |  |  |  |  |  |  |  | ★★ |  | ★★ | ★★ | ★★ |  |  | ★★ |  |  |  | ★ |
|  |  |  |  |  |  |  |  |  | ★★ | ★★ |  |  | ★★ | ★ |  |  |  |  |  |  |
|  | ★★ | ★★ | ★★ |  |  |  | ★★ |  | ★★ |  |  |  |  |  |  | ★★ |  |  | ★★ |  |

# Glossary

**Alpha-linolenic acid (ALA)** An omega-3 fatty acid that is an essential nutrient. It is found in some plants, notably walnuts, canola, soybean, flaxseed/linseed, and olive. The body can convert a small amount, which varies from 8 to 15 percent, to two other omega-3 fatty acids, docosahexaenoic acid (DHA) and eicosapentaenoic acid (EPA), the oils also found in fish, which may reduce the risk of cardiovascular disease and some inflammatory conditions. It is not clear if ALA has health benefits independent of its conversion to EPA and DHA, although some studies suggest it may.

**Annual** A plant that completes its life cycle within the span of one growing season. It is planted and germinates in the spring, then grows, flowers, sets seed, and finally dies after the frosts in autumn.

**Anthocyanins** A group of compounds of the flavonoid family of polyphenols, which produce purple and red pigments in fruits and vegetables. They are potent antioxidants and may protect against cardiovascular disease, cancer, and other diseases and conditions in which oxidative damage is important. Foods high in anthocyanins include blueberries, cranberries, blackberries, blackcurrants, redcurrants, cherries, and purple grapes.

**Antioxidants** Compounds that help prevent oxidative damage in the body by becoming oxidized themselves. Oxidative damage may be the underlying cause of cardiovascular disease, cancer, diabetes, and other diseases and conditions. Vitamins C and E, selenium, and phytochemicals such as carotenoids and polyphenols all have antioxidant properties.

**Atherosclerosis** The development within the blood vessels of plaque, consisting of cholesterol, other lipids, calcium, and cellular debris. It is the underlying process of cardiovascular disease, which can in turn lead to heart attacks and strokes. As atherosclerosis progresses, the growing plaques narrow the blood vessels and reduce blood flow. The trigger for a cardiovascular event is the rupture of plaques resulting in the formation of a blood clot, which can block the flow of blood to the heart, brain, or extremities.

**Beta-carotene** A carotenoid compound, a yellow-orange pigment, found in many fruits and vegetables. It functions as an antioxidant, and is a precursor to retinol, the active form of vitamin A in the body. Good sources include carrots, apricots, cantaloupes or rockmelons, and dark leafy greens.

**Beta-glucans** A group of compounds found in the cell walls of plants, fungi, bacteria, and yeast. Research shows that they may enhance the immune system, lower levels of LDL cholesterol, and help in the treatment of cancer. Good sources include some types of mushrooms, bran from some grains, and particular types of seaweed.

**Beta-sitosterol** One of numerous plant sterols, which have a chemical structure similar to cholesterol. Studies indicate that it may lower levels of cholesterol in the blood. Dietary sources include nuts, seeds, berries, wheat germ, bran from various grains, soybeans, and some vegetable oils.

**Calorie** A unit of measure of energy obtained from food, being the heat required to raise the temperature of 1 kilogram of water by 1°C. It is also expressed as kilojoules, with 1 calorie equalling 4.184 kilojoules. In general, the average adult requires 1500 to 2800 calories per day, depending on age, gender, and activity level. Also known as kilocalorie.

**Carbohydrates** A group of essential nutrients that serve as the major energy source for the body, providing 4 calories (16.7 kJ) per gram. Carbohydrates include starches, sugars, and fiber. Simple carbohydrates, or sugars, include those naturally occurring in fruit (fructose) and milk (lactose). So-called added sugars are those used as ingredients in commercial products such as soft drinks, candy, and desserts. In addition to causing dental caries, sugar contributes no nutrients but significant calories, which can lead to a low nutrient-dense diet, and consequent weight gain.

**Carotenoids** A group of more than 600 compounds that provide red and yellow pigments in plants. About 50 of them can be converted to active vitamin A, or retinol, by the liver. These include the five principal carotenoids found in human plasma: alpha-carotene, beta-carotene, lutein, crypto-xanthin, and lycopene. Many carotenoids function as antioxidants; in addition, they inhibit cell proliferation, a key step in cancer development, and they may enhance immune function.

**Cholesterol** A waxy compound made by the liver and contained in animal products. It is an important constituent of cell membranes and a precursor for some hormones. Cholesterol is carried in the blood by lipoproteins, notably high-density lipoprotein (HDL) and low-density lipo-protein (LDL). HDL carries cholesterol away from arteries and to the liver for removal; high HDL levels protect against heart attacks. Conversely, high levels of LDL promote atherosclerosis and increase the risk of heart attack and stroke. Dietary sources of cholesterol include organ meats, dairy products, higher-fat meats, and eggs.

**Cruciferous** Sulfur-containing vegetables of the family Cruciferae, such as broccoli, cauliflower, kale, and brussels sprouts. They contain compounds known as indoles and dithiolthiones, which have piqued the interest of cancer researchers in recent years because of their ability to inhibit the growth of cancer cells.

**Cryptoxanthin** A carotenoid that occurs naturally in fruits and vegetables and can be converted by the human body to active vitamin A. It functions as an antioxidant, and may therefore help prevent chronic diseases. Good sources include corn, oranges, and paprika.

**Cultivar** An agricultural or horticultural variety originating and constant under cultivation—the word is a contraction of "cultivated variety." Cultivar names, which must conform to an international code, must not use Latin, must be enclosed in single quotes, and are capitalized, such as 'Golden Delicious'.

**Daily Value** A reference standard used on food labels, which expresses the content of nutrients and other constituents in a typical serving of the food as a percentage of the amount you need each day. In some countries, this is called the Daily Intake (DI).

**Endosperm** The nutritive and reproductive tissue within a seed plant, which forms inside the embryo sac as a result of the division of the endosperm nucleus. In grain products, it contains the starch and some protein.

**Fat** An essential nutrient that is a lipid and organic in nature. The fat in foods and the fat stored in the human body are both in the form of triglyceride, which consists of a glycerol backbone connected to three fatty acids. The fatty acid chains may have double bonds between carbon atoms, in which case the fat is unsaturated, or no double bonds, in which case it is saturated. A high intake of saturated fat is associated with high blood cholesterol, while some types of unsaturated fat may improve blood cholesterol levels. Both types of dietary fat provide 9 calories (37.7 kJ) per gram, which is more than twice that provided by carbohydrate and protein.

**Fiber** Indigestible materials in plants, of two types: insoluble fiber and soluble fiber. Insoluble fiber aids in waste elimination, which may help prevent constipation and diverticulosis; sources include wheat bran, whole-grain breads and cereals, and vegetables. Soluble fiber reduces blood glucose and lowers blood cholesterol; good sources include fruits (especially apples and citrus fruits), legumes, oats, and barley.

**Fish oil** See Omega-3 fatty acids

**Flavonoids** A group of polyphenol compounds abundant in fruits, vegetables, nuts, tea, and coffee. They include flavanols (which include catechins), flavones, flavonols, flavanones, isoflavones, and anthocyanins. Studies show that many

function as antioxidants and possess other biological activities that may be beneficial to health. The strongest evidence is the link between a higher intake of flavonoids and a lower risk of atherosclerosis, which leads to heart attack and stroke.

**Flavonols** A group of flavonoid compounds with biological activities that may be beneficial to health. Some important flavonols include kaempferol, myricetin, and quercetin. In addition to acting as antioxidants, flavonols are important for blood flow and blood pressure, which in turn are important for cardiovascular health, and also in the prevention of DNA damage and cancer. Good, readily available sources include apples, apricots, beans, broccoli, cherries, cranberries, kale, pears, onions, and grapes.

**Free radicals** See Oxidative damage

**Germ** The nutrient-rich innermost part of the whole-grain kernel, which is part of the reproductive seed of a cereal grain. It contains fiber, B vitamins, vitamin E, minerals, and essential fatty acids. The milling process removes the germ and the bran (the fiber-rich outer layer), which improves the shelf life but also eliminates key nutrients. Whole-grain products include the germ.

**Gluten** A protein in wheat and other grains, which is responsible for the elastic quality of breads and other baked goods. Gluten contains another protein fraction, gliadin, which causes damage to the small intestine of people with celiac disease. Such people must avoid wheat, oats, rye, and barley. Products labeled as "gluten-free" cannot contain any form of gluten as an ingredient.

**Glycemic Index (GI)** A measure of the extent to which a food containing carbohydrate affects blood glucose and insulin as compared to a reference food (usually glucose or white bread). Examples of foods with a low GI include legumes, most vegetables, most fruits, and whole-grain breads and cereals. In general, the higher the content of fiber and fat, the lower the GI of a specific food. In particular, people with diabetes may benefit from a diet that focuses on foods with low GIs, because this will provide more controlled levels of blood glucose.

**Glycemic Load (GL)** A system for ranking foods based on the Glycemic Index (GI), which represents the effect on blood glucose and insulin levels, and takes into account the amount of carbohydrate consumed in a specific serving. It uses the following formula: (GI x the amount of carbohydrate in grams in a serving)/100. In general, GI and GL are likely to be similar, though the GL may be lower if a typical serving is small.

**Hybrid** In horticulture, the offspring of two plants of different varieties, species, or genera. In a scientific name, a hybrid is indicated by the use of "x," as in *Citrus reticulata x Citrus sinensis.*

**Isothiocyanates** A group of sulfur-containing compounds that possess biological activities that may be beneficial to health. Some isothiocyanates, such as sulforaphane, may be powerful cancer-preventive agents. Others, such as those contained in garlic (thiosulfinate allicin and S-allylcysteine), may also lower LDL cholesterol and inhibit platelet aggregation, which can help prevent cardiovascular disease.

**Lipids** A group of non-water-soluble compounds that includes triglyceride, phospholipids, and sterols. Triglyceride is the form of fat found in foods and stored in the body; phospholipids are important in the formation of the cell membrane; sterols include cholesterol, steroid hormones, and phytosterols in plants.

**Lutein** A carotenoid compound which also occurs as zeaxanthin. Both are powerful antioxidants. Lutein is found in the peripheral retina of the eye, and zeaxanthin is contained in the central macula. Studies have shown that higher intakes of lutein and zeaxanthin inhibit the formation of cataracts and reduce macular degeneration. Dark, leafy green vegetables are the best source.

**Monounsaturated fats** Unsaturated fats (see **Fat**) that have one double bond between adjacent carbon atoms on a fatty-acid chain. They may have beneficial effects on cardiovascular disease, such as reducing LDL cholesterol, and some contain anti-oxidant phytochemicals that may help prevent cancer. Examples of these fats as foods include olive oil, canola oil, peanut oil, and sesame oil, avocados, and many nuts and seeds.

**Nutrient** A substance necessary for body function and vital to life. The essential nutrients are those that cannot be made by the body and must be obtained from food. The six classes are carbohydrates, protein, fats, vitamins, minerals, and water.

**Omega-3 fatty acids (OFAs)** Unsaturated fats found primarily in fish, but also in some plants. Three important OFA groups include alpha-linolenic acid, eicosapentaenoic acid (EPA), and docosahexaenoic acid (DHA). EPA and DHA are found only in fish oils. These oils may lower blood pressure, improve cardiovascular function, alleviate arthritic symptoms, and strengthen immune function.

**Oxidative damage** Damage caused by a range of compounds known as reactive oxygen species (ROS), most notably those referred to as free radicals. ROSs are produced in the body in response to environmental pollutants, cigarette smoke, sunlight, and oxidized compounds in foods. In addition, the body produces ROSs during the immune response, intense exercise, and normal metabolism. ROSs are thought to be involved in cardiovascular disease, cancer, and other diseases and conditions. Compounds that combat oxidative damage are called antioxidants.

**Perennial** A plant that does not keep a woody skeleton above ground all year, but instead dies below the ground and re-emerges in spring.

**Phenols** A large group of polyphenol compounds found in many plants. Studies have shown that they demonstrate important biological activity, in particular potent antioxidant capability. Good sources include rosemary, raspberries, and pomegranates. Also referred to as phenolics and phenolic acids.

**Phytochemicals** Chemicals that occur naturally in plants, also called phytonutrients. More than 4,000 have been identified and many may possess beneficial health effects.

**Phytoestrogens** Compounds found in some plants, which have chemical structures similar to that of the female hormone estrogen. Important phytoestrogens include two flavonoids, the isoflavones and flavones. Studies have shown that an intake of phytoestrogens can result in a reduction in breast and prostate cancers and cardiovascular disease. Food sources include nuts, seeds, and soy products.

**Phytosterols** A group of compounds that are similar to cholesterol in humans and animals. Along with a similar related group, phytostanols, they have been shown to lower blood cholesterol by blocking absorption of cholesterol from the diet. Important phytosterols include sitosterol, beta-sitosterol, and campesterol. Several health agencies have endorsed these compounds as effective cholesterol-lowering agents, and they are currently being added to margarine products.

**Polyphenols** A large group of compounds found in almost all plants, consisting of three subgroups: tannins, lignins, and flavonoids. Many function as antioxidants and some display other biological activities that may be beneficial for human health.

**Precursor or Provitamin** A compound that the body can convert to the active form of a vitamin. An example is beta-carotene, which does not possess vitamin A activity until the body converts it to retinol, the active form of vitamin A.

**Protein** Broadly, a type of essential nutrient that contains nitrogen and provides the body with energy (at a rate of 4 calories/ 16.7 kJ per gram). It is a key structural component of many body tissues. There are different forms of protein, and they can also function as enzymes, antibodies, and hormones, but all consist of chains of amino acids, nine of which must be obtained through diet.

**Quercetin** A flavonol compound noted for its antioxidant activity. Studies have shown it can help protect against ulcers and stomach cancers. Good sources include onions, tea, asparagus, and grapefruit and other citrus fruits.

**Reactive oxygen species (ROSs)** See Oxidative damage

**Saponins** Compounds found in some grains, grapes, legumes, and soy beans, which often confer a bitter taste, as in quinoa. Some studies indicate that they may inhibit the proliferation of cancer cells and interfere with cholesterol absorption, helping to lower blood cholesterol levels. However, saponins may also interfere with the absorption of fat-soluble vitamins.

**Species** A genetically distinct group sharing a common gene pool and reproductive isolation from all other groups.

**Sulforaphane** A compound belonging to the family of isothiocyanates found in cruciferous vegetables. It is an antioxidant and also stimulates the liver's production of enzymes to neutralize toxins that can cause damage to cell membranes and DNA, which may in turn lead to cancer. Epidemiological studies have linked sulforaphane intake with lower rates of breast and prostate cancer, and lower blood pressure. Rich sources include broccoli, broccoli sprouts, cauliflower, cabbage, and kale.

**Tannins** Polyphenol compounds present in plants, which confer bitterness or astringency in foods. They have been shown to be powerful antioxidants and may therefore protect against diseases such as cancer and heart disease, though they can also interfere with the absorption of essential trace minerals, such as iron. Good sources include tea, coffee, nuts, and pomegranate.

**Triglyceride** See Fat

**Variety** A subcategory of a species, which has an appearance distinct from other varieties of the species but can still hybridize with them.

**Vitamins** Essential nutrients that promote and regulate chemical processes in the body. An inadequate intake of a particular vitamin results in a deficiency, which can manifest itself in different ways (including rashes, nerve damage, anemia, and osteoporosis); providing the vitamin reverses the deficiency. Vitamins cannot be produced by the body, are needed in only small amounts, and have no calorie value.

**Zeaxanthin** See Lutein

# Index

Page numbers in *italics* indicate an illustration and its caption.

# Acknowledgments

The publishers would like to thank David Kidd, Philippa Sandall, and Belinda Vance for their help during the conceptualization process prior to production, John Reinhard for his contributions to writing and research, and Mary Etta Moorachian for her assistance with the nutritional tables.

# Picture Credits